Handbook of Evidence-based Radiation Oncology

Eric K. Hansen, MD
Resident Physician
Department of Radiation Oncology
University of California San Francisco
San Francisco, California

Mack Roach, III, MD
Interim Chair of Radiation Oncology,
Professor of Radiation Oncology & Urology, &
Director of Clinical Research
University of California San Francisco
San Francisco, California

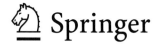 Springer

Eric K. Hansen
Resident Physician
Department of Radiation Oncology
University of California San Francisco
San Francisco, California

Mack Roach, III
Interim Chair of Radiation Oncology,
Professor of Radiation Oncology & Urology, &
Director of Clinical Research
University of California San Francisco
San Francisco, California

Library of Congress Control Number: 2005938664

ISBN-10: 0-387-30647-1   Printed on acid-free paper.
ISBN-13: 978-0387-30647-6

9 8 7 6 5 4 3 2 1

springer.com

Preface

Management of patients in radiation oncology is constantly evolving as the medical literature continues to grow exponentially. Our practices have become increasingly evidence-based. In this setting, it is critical to have a practical and rapid reference. The *Handbook of Evidence-based Radiation Oncology* is designed with this purpose in mind.

Each clinical chapter is organized in a concise manner. First, important "pearls" of epidemiology, anatomy, pathology, and presentation are highlighted. The key facets of the workup are then listed followed by staging and/or risk classification systems. Treatment recommendations are provided based on stage, histology, and/or risk classification. Brief summaries of key trials and studies provide the rationale for the treatment recommendations. Practical guidelines for radiation techniques are described. Finally, complications of treatment and follow-up guidelines are listed.

This handbook grew out of a practical need for a rapid reference for students, resident physicians, fellows, and other practitioners of radiation oncology. In order to be concise and portable, we limited the number of pages and references provided so that our Handbook did not become a textbook. Numerous sources were used to compile the information in each chapter, including the primary literature, each of the outstanding radiation oncology reference books (*Textbook of Radiation Oncology*; *Principles and Practice of Radiation Oncology*; *Radiation Oncology Rationale Technique Results*; *Clinical Radiation Oncology*; and *Pediatric Radiation Oncology*), the National Comprehensive Cancer Network Guidelines (at www.nccn.org), the National Cancer Institute's Physician Data Query Cancer Information Summaries (at www.cancer.gov), the American Society for Therapeutic Radiology & Oncology Annual Meeting Educational Sessions, and the notes of the radiation oncology residents at UCSF. Because a lengthy book could easily be written for many of the individual chapters, readers are encouraged to refer to the primary literature and the sources listed above for further details and references not listed in this handbook.

The handbook provides guidelines and suggestions, but it cannot replace the experience of clinicians skilled in the art of radiation oncology. The recommended doses and tolerances in this Handbook are suggestions only. It is the professional responsibility of the practitioner, relying on experience and knowledge of the patient, to determine the best treatment for each individual. Moreover, changes in care may become necessary and appropriate as new research is published, clinical experience is expanded, and/or changes occur in government regulations.

We thank all of the contributors for their hours of hard work. We owe them a debt of gratitude for their excellent chapters and their promptness, which made the task of editing this handbook much easier.

Eric K. Hansen
Mack Roach, III

Contents

Handbook of
Evidence-based
Radiation Oncology

Contributors

All contributors are members of the Department of Radiation Oncology, University of California San Francisco, San Francisco, California

Jeff Bellerose, BS
Physics staff, Illustrator

Alison Bevan, MD, PhD
Assistant Adjunct Professor

M. Kara Bucci, MD
Assistant Professor of Clinical Radiation Oncology

Allen Chen, MD
Resident Physician

Hans T. Chung, MD, FRCPC
GU Radiation Oncology Fellow

Joy L. Coleman, MD
Resident Physician

Charlotte Y. Dai, MD, PhD
Resident Physician

Amy M. Gillis, MD
Resident Physician

Alexander R. Gottschalk, MD, PhD
Assistant Professor in Residence

Daphne A. Haas-Kogan, MD
Associate Professor of Radiation Oncology & Neurosurgery, & Vice-Chair of Radiation Oncology, Director of Basic Science Research

Eric K. Hansen, MD
Resident Physician

I-Chow Joe Hsu, MD
Associate Professor of Clinical Radiation Oncology

Kim Huang, MD
Clinical Instructor

David A. Larson, MD, PhD
Professor of Radiation Oncology & Neurosurgery, & Vice-Chair
of Radiation Oncology

Brian Lee, MD, PhD
Resident Physician

Lawrence W. Margolis, MD
Professor Emeritus

Laura E. Millender, MD
Resident Physician

Kavita K. Mishra, MD, MPH
Resident Physician

Brian Missett, MD
Resident Physician

Jean L. Nakamura, MD
Assistant Adjunct Professor

Catherine Park, MD
Assistant Professor in Residence

Jeanne Marie Quivey, MD, FACR
Professor of Clinical Radiation Oncology

James L. Rembert, MD
Resident Physician

Mack Roach, III, MD
Interim Chair of Radiation Oncology, Professor of Radiation
Oncology & Urology, & Director of Clinical Research

Naomi R. Schechter, MD
Assistant Professor of Clinical Radiation Oncology

Joycelyn L. Speight, MD, PhD
Assistant Clinical Professor

Alice Wang-Chesebro, MD
Resident Physician

William M. Wara, MD, FACR
Professor & Chairman of Radiation Oncology

Handbook of
Evidence-based
Radiation Oncology

Chapter 1
Skin Cancer

James Rembert and Lawrence W. Margolis

PEARLS

- Most common malignancy in U.S.
- Main histologic types: BCC (65%), SCC (35%), adnexal (5%), melanoma (1.5%)
- More common in men (4:1)
- Median age: 68 (SCC and BCC)
- Most common predisposing factor: UV exposure
- Other predisposing factors: chronic irritation, trauma, occupational exposure, genetic disorders (phenylketonuria, basal cell nevus syndrome [Gorlin's], xeroderma pigmentosum, giant congenital nevi), immunosuppression (drug-induced, leukemia/lymphoma, HIV)
- Common routes of spread: lateral & deep along path of least resistance, perineural invasion (60–70% are asymptomatic), & regional LN
- <u>Basal cell carcinoma</u>:
  - Pathologic subtypes: nodulo-ulcerative (50%), superficial (33%), morphea-form (sclerosing), infiltrative, pigmented, fibroepithelial tumor of Pinkus, & basosquamous (rare, almost always on face, metastatic rate same as SCC)
  - Only ~1% perineural spread (mostly with recurrent or locally advanced), & "skip areas" common
  - Grow very slowly & <0.1% metastasize (regional LN > lung, liver, bones)
- <u>Squamous cell carcinoma</u>:
  - Pathologic subtypes: *Bowen's disease (CIS)* grows slowly as a sharply demarcated plaque, & is treated with surgery, cryotherapy, topical 5-FU, or RT (40 Gy/10 fx). *Erythroplasia of Queyrat* is Bowen's of the penis. *Marjolin's ulcer* is SCC within a burn scar. *Verrucous* carcinoma is low grade, exophytic, & often anogenital, oral, or on the plantar surface foot. *Spindle cell* presents most commonly on sun-exposed areas of Caucasians >40 yo

- 2–15% PNI (associated with nodal involvement & base of skull invasion)
- Nodal involvement:
  - Well differentiated: 1%
  - Poorly differentiated, recurrent, >3 cm greatest dimension, >4 mm depth, or located on lips: 10%
  - Located on burn scars/osteomyelitic site: 10–30%
- Distant Mets: 2% to lung, liver, bones
- <u>Adnexal and eccrine carcinomas</u> of the skin are more aggressive than SCC with propensity for nodal and hematogenous spread
- <u>Melanoma and Merkel cell carcinomas</u> will be briefly discussed after the following discussion of SCC/BCC

WORKUP

- H&P. Palpate for non-superficial extent of tumor. For head/face lesions do a detailed CN exam. Evaluate regional LN
- Biopsy
- CT/MRI if PNI or LN involvement suspected, & for lesions of medial/lateral canthi to rule out orbit involvement. CT is useful to rule out suspected bone invasion

STAGING: NON-MELANOMA SKIN CANCER

Primary tumor
TX: Primary tumor cannot be assessed
T0: No evidence of primary tumor
Tis: Carcinoma *in situ*
T1: Tumor 2 cm or less in greatest dimension
T2: Tumor more than 2 cm, but not more than 5 cm, in greatest dimension
T3: Tumor more than 5 cm in greatest dimension
T4: Tumor invades deep extradermal structures (i.e. cartilage, skeletal muscle, or bone)

Note: In case of multiple simultaneous tumors, the tumor with the highest T category will be classified and the number of separate tumors will be indicated in parentheses, e.g., T2 (5).

Regional lymph nodes
NX: No regional lymph node metastasis cannot be assessed
N0: No regional lymph node metastasis
N1: Regional lymph node metastasis

Distant metastasis
MX: Distant metastasis cannot be assessed
M0: No distant metastasis
M1: Distant metastasis

Stage Grouping	~5 yr Local Control:	
0: TisN0M0	All comers:	Moh's 99%, other tx ~90%
I : T1N0M0	RT for SCC:	T1 98%, T2 80%, T3 50%
II: T2-3N0M0	RT for BCC:	up to 5–10% better than SCC
III: T4N0M0, AnyTN1M0		
IV: M1		

Used with the permission of the American Joint Committee on Cancer (AJCC), Chicago, Illinois. The original source for this material is the AJCC Cancer Staging Manual, Sixth Edition (2002) published by Springer-Verlag New York, www.springeronline.com.

TREATMENT RECOMMENDATIONS

- Six major therapies: cryotherapy, curretage/electrodesiccation, chemotherapy, surgical excision, Moh's microsurgery, & RT
- Treatment indications:
  - *Cryotherapy*: small, superficial BCC & well-differentiated SCC with distinct margins
  - *Curretage & electrodesiccation*: same indications as cryotherapy but typically not used for recurrences or cancers overlying scar tissue, cartilage, or bone
  - *Chemotherapy*:
    - *Topical 5-FU*: only for tumors confined to epidermis
    - *Systemic*: not typically used but PR 60–70%, CR 30%
  - *Surgical excision*: reconstructive advances have made more patients surgical candidates
  - *Moh's micrographic surgery*: maximal skin sparing through concomitant pathologic examination of each horizontal and deep margin; if perineural invasion present should be followed by post-op RT
  - *RT*: typically recommended for primary and recurrent lesions of the central face >5 mm (especially for the eyelids, tip/ala of the nose, & lips) and large lesions (>2 cm) on the ears, forehead, & scalp that would potentially have poor functional and cosmetic outcomes after Moh's
- Positive margins after excision:

- 1/3 BCC recur if lateral margin + and >50% if deep margin +
- Most SCC recur at + margin and can recur loco-regionally with <50% salvage rate if LN+
- Both types should be retreated with re-excision or radiotherapy if +margin. For SCC, retreatment should be done immediately
- *Post-op RT indications*: + margins, PNI of named nerve, >3 cm primary, extensive skeletal muscle invasion, bone/cartilage invasion, & SCC of the parotid
- *Relative RT contraindications*: age <50 (cosmetic results worsen over time), postradiation recurrences (suboptimal salvage rates with re-irradiation – use Moh's), area prone to repeated trauma (dorsum of hand, bony prominence, belt line), poor blood supply (below knees/elbows), high occupational sun exposure, impaired lymphatics, exposed cartilage/bone, Gorlin's syndrome, CD4 count <200

RADIATION TECHNIQUES
Simulation and field design
- Superficial/orthovoltage X-rays and megavoltage electrons are most commonly used to cure skin cancers
- Orthovoltage advantages: less margin on skin surface, less expensive than electrons, Dmax at skin surface, skin collimation with lead cutout (0.95 mm Pb for <150 kV beam; 1.9 mm Pb for >150 kV beam)
- Most common orthovoltage energies: 50, 100, 150, 200, 250, 300 kV; must specify filter/HVL
- Select an energy so that the 90% depth dose encompasses tumor (90% IDL: 50 kV [0.7 mm Al] ~1 mm; 100 kV [4–7 mm Al] ~5 mm; 150 kV [0.52 mm Cu] 1.0 cm)
- Orthovoltage is not appropriate for >1 cm deep lesions
- f factor (roentgen-rad conversion): increases dramatically below 300 kV, which can lead to much higher dose to tissue with high atomic number (e.g., bone). Thus if carcinomas invade bone, megavoltage beams give a more homogeneous distribution. There is little variation in dose delivered to cartilage regardless of orthovoltage energy
- Must specify filtration (HVLs) in orthovoltage beams; generally choose thickest filter providing a dose rate >50 cGy/min (Al typically for 50/100 kV and Cu for higher energy; now most machines provide only one filter per energy)
- RBE of orthovoltage X-rays is 10–15% higher than RBE of megavoltage electrons/photons, so must raise daily &

total doses by 10–15% with megavoltage electrons/photons compared to suggested orthovoltage doses

- Lead shields should be used to block the lens, cornea, nasal septum, teeth, etc. as appropriate
- Backscattered electrons/photons can lead to conjunctival/mucosal irritation. For eyelids, thin coating of dental acrylic/wax should be used, for other areas a thicker coating should be applied
- General orthovoltage margins
    - Tumor size <2 cm = 0.5–1.0 cm horizontal margin; tumor size >2 cm = 1.5–2 cm horizontal margin. Deep margin should be at least 0.5 cm deeper than the suspected depth of tumor
    - Additional margin is needed in these circumstances:
        - <u>Electrons</u>: lateral constriction of isodose curves in deep portion of tumor volume increases with decreasing field sizes, so add 0.5 cm additional margin at skin surface
        - <u>Recurrent and morphea-form BCC</u>: infiltrate more widely, so add extra 0.5–1.0 cm margin at skin surface
        - <u>High-risk SCC</u>: 2 cm margin around tumor should be used if possible AND consider including regional LN
        - <u>PNI</u>: if present, include named nerve retrograde to the skull base. Consider IMRT and coverage of regional LN
- Nodal treatment should be considered for recurrences after surgery and is indicated for poorly differentiated, >3 cm tumors, and/or large infiltrative-ulcerative SCC
- Irradiation of a <u>graft</u> should not begin until after it is well-healed and healthy (usually 6–8 weeks) and the entire graft should be included in the target volume

Dose prescriptions (orthovoltage)

- <2 cm: 3 Gy/fx to 45–51 Gy
- >2 cm (no cartilage involvement): 2.5 Gy/fx to 50–55 Gy
- >2 cm (cartilage involved): 2 Gy/fx to 60–66 Gy
- For electrons, add 10–15% to the daily & total dose to account for lower RBE. When treating cartilage always keep daily dose <3 Gy/fx
- Prescription points: orthovoltage = Dmax, electrons = Dmax or 95%

Special recommendations by anatomic site

- Dorsum of hand and feet
  - Generally avoid RT at these locations due to high risk of necrosis due to repeated trauma to the region. If ≤4 mm in thickness, radioactive surface molds can be used
  - As a rule, lesions beyond elbow and knees are at risk of poor healing and ulceration after RT due to poor vascular supply, especially for elderly
- Eyelid
  - Surgery preferred for lesions 5 mm or less
  - Radiation is very effective for lesions 0.5–2 cm. With lead shielding, the lens dose is negligible as is the risk of RT-induced cataracts. Ophthalmic anesthetic drops are applied prior to insertion of shield.
  - Ectropion/epiphora can occur regardless of treatment modality. 50% are improved with corrective surgery
  - Mild conjunctivitis can occur due to use of eye-shields and from RT
  - Lacri-lube ophthalmic ointment can improve burning/pruritis
  - For tumors 0.5–2 cm recommended dose is 48 Gy/16 fx over 3.5 wks with 100 kV/0.19 mmCu or equivalent
- Lip
  - RT/Moh's/surgery are all good options
  - Place lead shield behind lip to shield teeth/mandible
  - For tumors <2.0 cm, recommended dose is 48 Gy/16 fx using 150 kV x-rays with 0.52 mm Cu HVL or 6 to 9 MeV electrons with appropriate bolus. Energy selection may vary depending on the depth of the lesion being treated, see above
  - Include neck nodes if SCC recurrent, grade 3, >3 cm greatest dimension or >4 mm thickness
- Nose and ear
  - Place wax covered lead strip in nose to prevent irritation
  - Include nasolabial fold for nasal ala lesions
  - Use wax bolus on irregular surfaces for homogeneity
  - For tumors 0.5–2.0 cm, recommended dose is 52.8 Gy/16 fx over 3.5 wks with electrons or 45–51 Gy/15–17 fx using orthovoltage
  - Selection of electron and orthovoltage energy will depend on depth of the lesion, see above

Dose limitations
- Cartilage: chondritis rare if <3 Gy/d given
- Skin: larger volumes of tissue do not tolerate radiation as well and thus require smaller daily fxs; moist desquamation is expected
- Bone: see f factor discussion above

COMPLICATIONS
- Telangectasias, skin atrophy, hypopigmentation, skin necrosis (~3%), osteoradionecrosis (~1%), chondritis/cartilage necrosis (rare if fx <300 cGy/d), hair loss/loss of sweat glands

FOLLOW-UP (Adapted From NCCN 2005 RECOMMENDATIONS)
- BCC: H&P, complete skin exam q 6–12 mo for life
- SCC localized: H&P q 3–6 mo for 2 yrs, then q 6–12 mo for 3 yrs, then q 1 yr for life
- SCC regional: H&P q 3 mo for 2 yrs, then q 4 mo for 1 yr, then q 6 mo for 2 yr, then q 1 yr for life

MERKEL CELL CARCINOMA (MCC)

- Rare, deadly (mortality rate > melanoma), neuroendocrine malignancy of the skin
- No consensus on management due to lack of randomized data to compare treatment modalities
- included in AJCC non-melanoma skin staging, many institutions (including UCSF) use a simpler system: stage I = localized (IA ≤2 cm; IB >2 cm); II = LN+; III = DM
- Local recurrences common (post surgery alone ~75%, with adjuvant RT ~15%)
- ~20% have +LN at diagnosis, & sentinel LN biopsy is rapidly becoming the standard means of assessing nodal status and should be performed before resection of the primary site
- Distant metastases develop in 50–60% of cases usually within 10 mo of diagnosis
- Role of chemotherapy is unclear, but with the high rate of DM it is often given either concurrently or after RT. Platinum-based regimens similar to those for SCLC are commonly used (cisplatin or carboplatin with etoposide or irinotecan)

- The UCSF approach to radiotherapy for MCC is as follows:
  - Clinically N0 nodes: 45–50 Gy/1.8–2.0 Gy fx
  - Microscopic disease/– margins: 45–50 Gy/1.8–2.0 Gy fx
  - Microscopic disease/+ margins: 55–60 Gy/1.8–2.0 Gy fx
  - Macroscopic disease: 55–60 Gy/1.8–2.0 Gy fx
  - Cover primary site, in-transit lymphatics, regional LN with wide margins
  - Consider eliminating RT to regional LN if SLN negative, or if regional LND performed for positive SLN, but patient cN0
  - Margins on primary site = 5 cm
- 3 yr DSS for stage I–II ~75%
- 3 yr OS by stage: I ~70–80%, II ~50–60%, III ~30%
- Data suggest almost no MCC-related deaths occur after 3 yrs from diagnosis

MELANOMA

PEARLS

- Incidence increasing rapidly
- 15% derive from preexisting melanocytic nevi
- <10% develop in noncutaneous sites
- Gender difference in predominant locations: M = trunk, F = extremities
- ~15% have +LN at diagnosis (~5% for T1, ~25% for >T1)
- ~5% have DM at diagnosis (1/3 with no evidence of primary)
- Subtypes: superficial spreading (~65%), nodular (~25%), lentigo maligna (least common – 7%), acral lentiginous (5% in whites, but most common form in dark-skinned populations)
- Lentigo maligna has the best prognosis with LN mets in only 10% cases, and 10 yr OS 85% after WLE alone. Hutchinson's freckle = lentigo maligna involving epidermis only
- Acral lentiginous generally presents on palms, soles, or sub-ungual
- Most powerful prognostic factor for recurrence and survival: Sentinel LN status
- Other prognostic factors: ulceration, thickness (Breslow measured depth, Clark related to histologic level of dermis), anatomic site (trunk worse), gender (male worse), age (young better), number of nodes

WORKUP

- <1 mm thick lesions – same as for SCC/BCC
- >1 mm thick lesions – need CXR, LFTs, CBC, evaluation of suspicious nodes, pelvic CT if inguino-femoral adenopathy

STAGING

- Clark levels: I = epidermis only, II = invasion of papillary dermis (localized), III = filling papillary dermis compressing reticular dermis, IV = invading reticular dermis, V = invades subcutaneous tissues

---

Primary tumor

TX: Primary tumor cannot be assessed
T0:   No evidence of primary tumor
Tis: Melanoma *in situ*
T1:   Melanoma ≤1.0 mm with or without ulceration
    T1a: Melanoma ≤1.0 mm in thickness and level II or III, no ulceration
    T1b: Melanoma ≤1.0 mm in thickness and level IV or V, or with ulceration
T2:   Melanoma 1.01–2.0 mm in thickness with or without ulceration
    T2a: Melanoma 1.01–2.0 mm in thickness, no ulceration
    T2b: Melanoma 1.01–2.0 mm in thickness, with ulceration
T3:   Melanoma 2.01–4.0 mm in thickness with or without ulceration
    T3a: Melanoma 2.01–4.0 mm in thickness, no ulceration
    T3b: Melanoma 2.01–4.0 mm in thickness, with ulceration
T4:   Melanoma greater than 4.0 mm in thickness with or without ulceration
    T4a: Melanoma >4.0 mm in thickness, no ulceration
    T4b: Melanoma >4.0 mm in thickness, with ulceration

Regional lymph nodes

NX: No regional lymph node metastasis cannot be assessed
N0:   No regional lymph node metastasis
N1:   Metastasis in one lymph node
    N1a: Clinically occult (microscopic) metastasis
    N1b: Clinically apparent (macroscopic) metastasis
N2:   Metastasis in 2 to 3 regional nodes or intralymphatic regional metastasis
    N2a: Clinically occult (microscopic) metastasis
    N2b: Clinically apparent (macroscopic) metastasis
    N2c: Satellite or in-transit metastasis without nodal metastasis

---

N3: Metastasis in 4 or more regional nodes, or matted metastatic nodes, or in-transit metastasis or satellite(s) with metastasis in regional node(s)

Distant metastasis
MX: Distant metastasis cannot be assessed
M0: No distant metastasis
M1: Distant metastasis
   M1a: Metastasis to skin, subcutaneous tissues, or distant lymph nodes
   M1b: Metastasis to lung
   M1c: Metastasis to all other visceral sites or distant metastasis at any site associated with an elevated LDH

Clinical Stage Grouping[1]		Pathologic Stage Grouping[2]		5 yr survival	
0:	TisN0M0	0:	TisN0M0	IA:	>95%
IA:	T1aN0M0	IA:	T1aN0M0	IB:	~90%
IB:	T1b-2aN0M0	IB:	T1b-2aN0M0	IIA:	~80%
IIA:	T2b-3aN0M0	IIA:	T2b-3aN0M0	IIB:	~65%
IIB:	T3b-4aN0M0	IIB:	T3b-4aN0M0	IIC:	~45%
IIC:	T4bN0M0	IIC:	T4bN0M0	IIIA:	~65%
III:	AnyT N1-3M0	IIIA:	T1-4aN1a/2aM0	IIIB:	~50%
IV:	M1	IIIB:	T1-4bN1a/2aM0		(30–50%
			T1-4aN1b/2bM0		if N2c)
			T1-4a/bN2cM0	IV:	~7-20%
		IIIC:	T1-4bN1b/2bM0		
			AnyTN3M1		
		IV:	M1		

Notes: [1]Clinical staging includes microstaging of the primary melanoma and clinical/radiological evaluation for metastases. By convention, it should be used after complete excision of the primary melanoma with clinical assessment for regional and distant mets. [2]Pathologic staging includes microstaging of the primary melanoma and pathologic information about the regional lymph nodes after partial or complete lymphadenectomy. Pathologic Stage 0 or Stage IA patients are the exception; they do not require pathologic evaluation of their lymph nodes.

Staging portions of the above table used with the permission of the American Joint Committee on Cancer (AJCC), Chicago, Illinois. The original source for this material is the AJCC Cancer Staging Manual, Sixth Edition (2002) published by Springer-Verlag New York, www.springeronline.com.

TREATMENT RECOMMENDATIONS
Primary
- Surgery: SLN biopsy followed by WLE and completion regional LN dissection if SLN+
- Minimum surgical margins: Tis = 5 mm, T1 = 1 cm, T2-T4 = 2 cm; retrospective studies suggest no benefit in LC, DFS, OS with >2 cm margins
- Primary RT rarely indicated with the exception of lentigo maligna melanomas on the face that would cause severe cosmetic/functional deficits with surgery. These can be treated with a 1.5 cm margin with 50 Gy/20 fx with 100–250 kV photons. For medically inoperable patients, hyperthermia can improve response and local control, especially for tumors >4 cm [Overgaard]

Adjuvant
- N–, 1–4 mm without ulceration, ≤1 mm with ulceration = None standard
- <4 mm with ulceration/Clark IV–V = clinical trial, if available, or observation
- >4 mm or N+ = high-dose interferon alpha, clinical trial, or observation
- RT indicated for multiple or matted LN, ECE

STUDIES
- Interferon alpha: [ECOG 1684/1690/1694]. 3 randomized trials established a role for high-dose IFN∝ in T4/N+ patients. IFN∝ provides ~10% absolute improvement in RFS, and possibly improves 5 yr OS. Benefits not seen when high-dose IFN∝ compared with low-dose [ECOG 1680] or GM2 ganglioside vaccine [ECOG 1694]
- Melanoma vaccines: No randomized phase III trials demonstrate a survival benefit, but multiple trials pending

Adjuvant RT:
- Ang (*Arch Otolaryngol Head Neck Surg* 1990). 83 pts with >1.5 mm thick primary or cN+ received 24–30 Gy in 4–5 fx with improved LC over historic controls treated with surgery alone
- Ang (*IJROBP* 1994). Phase II trial of adjuvant RT in H&N melanoma pts with a projected LRR rate 50%. 79 pts had WLE of a ≥1.5 mm primary or Clark's IV–V, 32 pts had WLE & elective LND, & 63 pts had LND after neck relapse. RT was 6 Gy/fx given bi-weekly to 30 Gy over 2.5 wks. Results: 5 yr LRC 88%, OS 47%. 5 yr OS by pathologic parameters: ≤1.5 mm 100%, 1.6–4 mm 72%, >4 mm

30%, >3 LN+ 23%, 1–3 LN+ 39%. Minimal acute/late toxicity

Hyperthermia:

- Overgaard (*Lancet* 1995). 70 pts with metastatic/recurrent melanoma randomized to 24 Gy or 27 Gy in 3 fx over 8 days alone or followed by hyperthermia (43°C for 60 min). HT improved LC (26→48%), as did 27 Gy LC (25→56%)

RADIATION DOSE

- No data to support the commonly held idea that melanoma is radioresistant
- Early radiobiologic data did suggest that human melanoma cell lines have a large shoulder on the dose-response curve necessitating hypofractionation
- RTOG 8305 (Sause *IJROBP* 1991) showed no difference between 32 Gy in 4 fx vs 50 Gy in 20 fx
- Thus the dose recommendations for SCC/BCC can be followed for treating melanoma definitively
- However, many people extrapolate doses used in the Ang trial for use even outside of H&N sites for adjuvant RT due to the excellent LC

FOLLOW-UP (Adapted From NCCN 2005 RECOMMENDATIONS)

- Stage IA – annual skin exam for life (directed H&P <1 yr as clinically indicated)
- Stage IB-III – q 3–6 mo × 3 yrs, q 4–12 mo × 2 yrs, then annually for life

REFERENCES

Ang KK, Morrison W, Garden A. Cutaneous carcinoma and melanoma. In: Gunderson L, Tepper J, editors. Clinical Radiation Oncology, 1st ed. Philadelphia: Churchill Livingstone; 2000. pp. 563–576.

Ang KK, Byers RM, Peters LJ. Regional radiotherapy as adjuvant treatment for head and neck malignant melanoma. Arch Otolaryngol Head Neck Surg. 1990;116(2):169–172.

Ang KK, Peters LJ, Weber RS. Postoperative radiotherapy for cutaneous melanoma of the head and neck region. Int J Radiat Oncol Biol Phys. 1994;30(4):795–798.

Dana-Farber Cancer Institute. Merkel Cell Carcinoma: Information for Patients and Their Physicians. Available at: http://www.merkelcell.org. Accessed on January 12, 2005.

Greene FL. American Joint Committee on Cancer, American Cancer Society. AJCC Cancer Staging Manual. 6th ed. New York: Springer Verlag; 2002.

Kirkwood JM, Ibrahim JG, Sondak VK, et al. High- and low-dose alfa-2b in high-risk melanoma: First analysis of intergroup trial E1690/S9111/C9190. J Clin Oncol 2000;18:2444–2458.

Kirkwood JM, Ibrahim JG, Sosman JA, et al. High-dose interferon alfa-2b significantly prolongs relapse-free and overall survival compared with the GM2-KLH/QS-21 vaccine in patients with resected stage IIB–III melanoma: Results of intergroup trial E1694/S9512/C509801. J Clin Oncol 2001;19:2370–2380.

Kirkwood JM, Strawderman MH, Ernstoff MS, et al. Interferon alfa-2b adjuvant therapy of high-risk resected cutaneous melanoma: The Eastern Cooperative Oncology Group trial EST 1684. 1996; 14:7–17.

Margolin KA, Sondak VK. Melanoma and other skin cancers. In: Pazdur R, Coia L, Hoskins W, Wagman L, editors. Cancer Management: A Multidisciplinary Approach. 8th ed. New York: CMP Healthcare Media; 2004. pp. 509–538.

Martinez A. Ovarian cancer. In: Gunderson L, Tepper J, editors. Clinical Radiation Oncology, 1st ed. Philadelphia: Churchill Livingstone; 2000. pp. 939–957.

National Comprehensive Cancer Network. Clinical Practice Guidelines in Oncology: Basal Cell and Squamous Skin Cancer. Available at: http://www.nccn.org/professionals/physician_gls/PDF/nmsc.pdf. Accessed on January 12, 2005.

National Comprehensive Cancer Network. Clinical Practice Guidelines in Oncology: Merkel Cell Carcinoma. Available at: http://www.nccn. org/professionals/physician_gls/PDF/mcc.pdf. Accessed on January 12, 2005.

National Comprehensive Cancer Network. Clinical Practice Guidelines in Oncology: Melanoma. Available at: http://www.nccn.org/profes-sionals/physician_gls/PDF/melanoma.pdf. Accessed on January 12, 2005.

Overgaard J, Gonzalez D, Hulshof MC. Randomised trial of hyperther-mia as adjuvant to radiotherapy for recurrent or metastatic malig-nant melanoma. European Society for Hyperthermic Oncology. Lancet 1995;345(8949):540–543.

Solan M, Brady L. Skin cancer. In: Perez CA, Brady LW, Halperin EC, et al., editors. Principles and Practice of Radiation Oncology. 4th ed. Philadelphia: Lippincott Williams and Wilkins; 2004. pp. 757–775.

Wilder RB, Margolis LW. Cancer of the skin. In: Leibel SA, Phiilips TL, editors. Textbook of Radiation Oncology. 2nd ed. Philadelphia: Saunders; 2004. pp. 1483–1501.

Chapter 2
Central Nervous System

Charlotte Y. Dai, Jean L. Nakamura, Daphne Haas-Kogan, and David A. Larson

INTRODUCTION

- This chapter will discuss malignant glioma, low-grade glioma, brainstem glioma, optic glioma, CNS lymphoma, ependymoma, choroid plexus tumor, meningioma, acoustic neuroma, craniopharyngioma, pituitary tumor, pineal tumor, medulloblastoma, primary spinal cord tumor, arteriovenous malformation, and trigeminal neuralgia

ANATOMY

- Meninges (outer to inner) = dura mater → arachnoid mater → subarachnoid space → pia mater
- Precentral gyrus = primary motor strip; postcentral gyrus = primary somatosensory cortex. Medial = body, lower extremities, feet. Lateral = trunk, arms, head
- Brain gray matter is peripheral and white matter is central
- Broca's (motor) area = dominant frontal lobe just superior to lateral sulcus (Sylvian fissure) = site of expressive aphasia (comprehend but not fluent)
- Wernicke's (sensory) area = dominant temporal lobe at posterior end of lateral sulcus = site of receptive aphasia (fluent but not comprehend)
- Diencephalon = thalamaus, hypothalamus, and pineal gland
- Telencephalon = olfactory lobes, cerebral hemispheres, basal ganglia, amygdalae
- Mesencephalon = tectum, crus cerebri, superior & inferior colliculi, cerebral aqueduct
- Only CN IV exits from dorsal surface of midbrain
- CSF: Choroid plexus produces → lateral ventricles → foramen of Monroe → 3rd ventricle → cerebral aqueduct of Sylvius → 4th ventricle → foramen of Magendie & 2 lateral foramina of Lushka

- Caverous sinus contains CN III, IV, V1, V2, VI and the internal carotid artery. Cavernous involvement commonly produces CN VI palsy
- CN exits:
  - Superior orbital fissure = CN III, IV, VI, V1
  - Foramen rotundum = V2
  - Foramen ovale = V3
  - Foramen spinosum = middle meningeal artery & vein
  - Internal auditory meatus = CN VII, VIII
  - Jugular foramen = CN IX, X, XI
  - Hypoglossal canal = CN XII
- Lateral plain film
  - Hypothalamus = 1 cm superior to sellar floor
  - Optic canal = 1 cm superior & 1 cm anterior to the hypothalamus
  - Pineal body (supratentorial notch) = 1 cm posterior & 3 cm superior to external acoustic meatus
  - Lens = 1 cm posterior to anterior eyelid, 8 mm posterior to line connecting lateral canthus. Median globe size = 2.5 cm
  - Location of cribiform plate cannot always be correctly identified with lateral plain film alone (Gripp, *IJROBP* 2004)
- Spinal cord
  - 31 pairs of spinal nerves: 8 cervical, 12 thoracic, 5 lumbar, 5 sacral, 1 coccygeal
  - Spinal cord white matter is peripheral & gray matter is central
  - Pia mater covers cord and condenses into dentate ligaments
  - Arachnoid contains CSF (normal pressure 70–200 mm H_2O lying down, 100–300 mm H_2O sitting or standing, ~150 cc total volume)
  - Dura ends at S2
  - Cord ends at L1 in adults, conus ends at ~L2 in adults, cord ends ~L3–4 in newborns

EPIDEMIOLOGY

- 18,300 new primary brain tumors and 13,100 deaths in the U.S. in 2003
- Brain metastases are the most common neoplastic process involving the CNS (incidence ~170,000/yr in U.S.)

- Approximately 20–40% of all cancer patients develop brain metastases
- Adult primary CNS tumors: 30% GBM, 10% AA, 10% low-grade astrocytomas, 15% meningioma, 10% pituitary, 5–10% schwannoma, <5% oligodendroglioma
- Of adult gliomas, 75% are high grade and 25% are low grade
- Children: 20% of all pediatric tumors (2nd to ALL). 30–50% astrocytoma, 25% medulloblastoma, 20% malignant astrocytoma/GBM, 10% ependymoma, <5% optic nerve glioma
- Possible etiologic associations: rubber compounds, polyvinyl chloride, N-nitroso compounds, and polycyclic hydrocarbons
- Prior ionizing RT has been associated with new meningiomas, gliomas, and sarcomas (~2% at 20 yrs)

GENETICS

- NF-1: von Recklinghausen, Chromosome 17q11.2, 1/3500 live births, *NF1* encodes neurofibromin, autosomal dominant, 50% germline, 50% new mutations, peripheral nerve sheath neurofibromas, café au lait spots, optic & intracranial gliomas, and bone abnormalities
- NF-2: chromosome 22, 1/50,000 live births, *NF2* encodes merlin, autosomal dominant, bilateral acoustic neuromas, gliomas, ependymomas, and meningiomas
- von Hippel-Lindau: chromosome 3, autosomal dominant, renal clear cell carcinoma, pheochromocytoma, hemangioblastoma, pancreatic tumors, and renal cysts
- Tuberous sclerosis: TSC1 on chromosome 9, TSC2 on CH6, autosomal dominant, subependymal giant cell astrocytoma, and retinal and rectal hamartomas
- Retinoblastoma: Rb tumor suppressor gene, chromosome 13
- Li-Fraumeni symdrome: germline p53 mutation = breast, sarcoma, and brain CA
- Turcot's syndrome: primary brain tumors with colorectal CA
- Neuroblastoma: N-myc amplication commonly seen and serves as a prognostic factor

IMAGING

- MRI: T1 pre- & post-gadolinium, T2, & FLAIR (fluid attenuation inversion recovery, removes increased CSF signal on T2)

- Enhancement with gadolinium correlates with breakdown of the blood-brain barrier (BBB)
- Tumor: high grade – increased signal on T1 post-gadolinium and T2 (T2 also shows edema). Low grade – increased signal on T2/FLAIR
- Acute blood = increased signal on T1 pre-gadolinium
- Post-op MRI should be performed within 48 h to document any residual disease after surgical intervention
- At UCSF, triple dose gadolinium is used at the time of Gamma Knife SRS to improve the sensitivity of detection of brain metastases
- JPA: enhancing nodule, highly vascular, 50% associated with cysts, high uptake on PET
- Grade 2 glioma: non-enhancing, hypointense on T1, hyperintense on T2/FLAIR, well-circumscribed, solid, round, calcifications associated with oligodendroglioma
- Grade 3 glioma: enhancing with gadolinium, infiltrative, less well-defined borders, mass effect (sulcal effacement, midline shift, ventricular dilatation, and vasogenic edema)
- GBM: rim enhancing, central necrosis, irregular borders, and mass effect
- Dural tail sign: linear meningeal thickening and enhancement adjacent to a peripherally located cranial mass, reported in 60% of meningioma, also seen in chloroma, lymphoma, and sarcoidosis
- MR spectroscopy: NAA = neuronal marker, choline = marker of cellularity and cellular integrity, creatine = marker of cellular energy, lactate = marker of anaerobic metabolism. Tumor = increased choline, decreased creatine, decreased NAA. Necrosis = increased lactate, decreased choline, creatine and NAA

PATHOLOGY

- Histologies particularly prone to CSF spread = medulloblastomas, ependymoblastomas, pineoblastomas, CNS lymphomas, choroid plexus tumors, germ cell tumors, and metastases
- World Health Organization grading system of gliomas: WHO grade 1 = JPA, grade 2 = fibrillary astrocytoma, grade 3 = anaplastic astrocytoma, grade 4 = glioblastoma multiform
- Astrocytoma grading (AMEN) = nuclear atypia, mitoses, endothelial proliferation, necrosis

- Pearls: pseudopalisading & necrosis = GBM, Rosenthal fibers = JPA, psammoma bodies = meningioma, Verocay body = schwannoma, Schiller-Duval body = yolk-sac tumor, fried-egg = oligodendroglioma, pseudorossette = ependymoma, Homer-Wright rosettes = medulloblastoma, pineoblastoma, Flexner-Wintersteiner rosettes = pineoblastoma

RADIATION TECHNIQUES
Fractionated EBRT
- Simulate patient with head mask
- Opposed laterals for whole brain
- Individualize tumor volume based on propensity to infiltrate, follow disease extension along the white matter tracts (e.g., internal capsule and corpus collosum) and use non-uniform margin
- 3DCRT or IMRT for most lesions. 3DCRT provides better dose homogeneity, fewer hot spots. Inverse planning may allow greater sparing of critical structures and/or deliver hot spots in center of (hypoxic) tumor. Must be determined on a case-by-case basis
- Fuse planning CT and MRI (pre-op vs post-op) to help delineate target volume. Post-op MRs are better than pre-op MRs in some cases and we may not need to extend tumor volume across midline

General guidelines for target volumes
- High-grade gliomas:
  GTV1 = T1 enhancement + T2/FLAIR. CTV1 = GTV1 + 2 cm margin
  > Boost: GTV2 = T1 enhancement. CTV2 = GTV2 + 2 cm
  > PTV = Add 0.5 cm
- Low-grade gliomas:
  These tumors are often non-enhancing & tumor may be best visualized on FLAIR
  > GTV = T1 enhancement or FLAIR for oligodendrogliomas:
  > CTV = GTV + 1–2 cm margin

DOSE TOLERANCE GUIDELINES
Individual patient dose constrains should be determined based on physicians' clinical judgment and experience.

EBRT using 1.8–2.0 Gy/fx	SRS max point dose
Whole brain 50 Gy	Brainstem 12 Gy
Partial brain 60 Gy	Optic nerve and chiasm 8 Gy
Brainstem 54 Gy	Visual pathway 12 Gy
Spinal cord 45 Gy	
Chiasm 50–54 Gy	
Retina 45 Gy	
Lens 10 Gy	
Inner ear 30 Gy (increasing risk of hearing deficit with increasing dose)	
Epilation 20–30 Gy	
Lacrimal gland: 30 Gy transient, 60 Gy permanent	

- Fetal dose for cranial RT = 0.05–0.1% of total dose (<0.1 Gy)

POSSIBLE RADIATION COMPLICATIONS

- **Acute**: Alopecia, radiation dermatitis, fatigue, transient worsening of symptoms due to edema, nausea, and vomiting (particularly with brainstem and posterior fossa radiation), and otitis externa. Mucositis, esophagitis, and myelosuppression are associated with cranial spinal irradiation. Subside within 4 to 6 wks after radiation. Dose-related
- **Subacute** (6–12 wks after RT): Somnolence (mainly in children, infrequently in adults), perhaps caused by changes in capillary permeability and transient demyelination
- **Late** (3 mo to 3 yrs after RT): Radiation necrosis, diffuse leukoencephalopathy (especially with chemo, but not necessarily correlated with clinical symptoms), hearing loss, retinopathy, cataract, visual changes, endocrine abnormalities (if hypothalamic–pituitary axis is irradiated), vasculopathy moyamoya syndrome, decreased new learning ability, short-term memory, and problem-solving skills

FUNCTIONAL STATUS: SEE APPENDIX A

MALIGNANT GLIOMAS

PEARLS

- 35–45% of primary brain tumors
- 85% are GBM

- Multicentric tumors in <5% of cases
- Incidence rises with age, peaks at 45–55 yrs (bimodal based on primary vs transformation)
- Presentation: #1 headache (50%), #2 seizures (20%)
- Prognostic factors: age, histology, KPS, extent of surgery, duration of symptoms (see RPA below)

RTOG RPA classes for malignant glioma

I & II:	Anaplastic astrocytoma, age ≤50, normal mental status, or age >50, KPS >70, symptoms >3 mo	MS: 40–60 mo
III & IV:	Anaplastic astrocytoma, age ≤50, abnormal MS, or age >50, symptoms <3 mo; Glioblastoma age <50 or age >50 & KPS ≥70	MS: 11–18 mo
V & VI:	Glioblastoma, age >50, KPS <70 or abnormal mental status	MS: 5–9 mo

TREATMENT RECOMMENDATIONS

General management	■ Dexamethasone before/after surgery when clinically indicated; taper gradually ■ Surgical decompression for increased ICP ■ Anti-seizure medications as indicated, ensure therapeutic levels
Resectable, or partially resectable, operable	■ GTR/STR → RT (60 Gy) + concurrent temozolamide qd → temozolamide × 6c monthly [Stupp NEJM 2005] ■ Or 40 Gy/15 fx for age ≥60 and KPS >50 [Roa, JCO 2004]

	■ Or 30 Gy/10 fx for age ≥65 and KPS <50 [Bauman, IJROBP 1994]
Inoperable	RT (60 Gy) + concurrent temozolamide qd → temozolamide × 6c monthly [Stupp NEJM 2005]
Recurrence	■ Steroids ■ If local & resectable &/or symptomatic: surgery → chemo ■ If local & unresectable: chemo &/or highly conformal RT or SRS ■ If diffuse: chemo + best supportive care ■ If poor KPS: best supportive care

STUDIES

Post-op RT

■ Walker BTSG 6901 (*J Neurosurg* 1978). Phase III. 222 pts (90% GBM, 10% AA) → surgery → randomized to observation vs BCNU alone vs WBRT 50–60 Gy alone vs WBRT + BCNU. RT was WB to 50 Gy, then boost to 60 Gy. RT +/– BCNU improved MS

Dose and fractionation

■ Walker BTSG (*IJROBP* 1979). Pooled 3 randomized trials. Compared observation vs WBRT 45 Gy vs 50 Gy vs 55 Gy vs 60 Gy. MS increased with higher doses, 4 mo → 7 mo → 9 mo → 10 mo

■ Roa (*JCO* 2004). Phase III. 100 pts with GBM age ≥60 and KPS ≥50 randomized to 60 Gy/30 fx vs 40 Gy/15 fx. No difference in MS (5.1 vs 5.6 mo). Fewer patients in the short course RT arm required increased steroids (23 vs 49%)

■ Bauman (*IJROBP* 1994). Single arm prospective study. 29 pts with GBM age ≥65 & KPS ≤50 treated with WBRT (30 Gy/10 fx). RT increased MS vs best supportive care (10 vs 1 mo)

■ MRC (Bleehen, *Br J Cancer* 1991). Randomized 474 pts to 45 Gy/20 fx vs 60 Gy/30 fx. No adjuvant chemo. MS 12 mo (60 Gy) vs 9 mo (45 Gy, p = 0.007)

■ Multiple altered fractionation trials, no survival benefit

Post-op chemo-RT

- EORTC/NCIC (Stupp, *NEJM* 2005). Phase III. 573 pts with newly diagnosed glioblastoma (16% biopsy only, 40% GTR, 44% STR) randomized to RT alone vs RT + concurrent and adjuvant temozolamide. RT was 60 Gy/30 fx. Temozolamide was concurrent daily (75 mg/m^2/d) and adjuvant (150–200 mg/m^2/d × 5 days) q 4 wks × 6 mo. Concurrent & adjuvant temozolamide significantly improved MS (14.6 vs 12.1 mo) & 2 yr OS (26.5% vs 10.4%, p < 0.001). Only 7% Grade 3 or 4 hematologic toxicity in the combined chemo-RT arm
- RTOG 94-02 (ASCO abstr. 2004). Phase III. 291 pts with pure or mixed anaplastic oligodendroglioma → surgery → randomized to PCV chemo ×4c → RT vs RT alone. RT was 50.4 Gy → boost to 59.4 Gy. No difference in MS (4.8 vs 4.5 yr), but PCV chemo improved PFS (2.5 vs 1.9 yr, p = 0.018). Loss of 1p/19q predicted excellent sensitivity to PCV chemo & better prognosis
- Walker BTSG 7201 (NEJM 1980) Phase III. 476 pts (84% GBM, 11% AA) → surgery → randomized to MeCCNU alone vs RT alone vs RT + MeCCNU vs RT + BCNU. RT was WB 60 Gy/30–35 fx. RT +/– chemo increased MS compared to chemo alone (37–43 vs 31 wks). No difference between MeCCNU & BCNU

DOSE

- EBRT: 1.8 Gy/fx to 59.4 Gy or 2 Gy/fx to 60 Gy

FOLLOW-UP

- MRI 2–6 wks after RT and then every 2 mo

LOW-GRADE GLIOMA

PEARLS

- 10% of primary intracranial tumors, 20% of gliomas
- Oligodendrogliomas account for 5% of intracranial tumors
- Age of onset: 30–40 yrs for WHO grade II & 10–20 yrs for JPA
- Presentation: seizures (60–70%, better prognosis) > headache > paresis
- Favorable prognostic factors: age <40 yr, good KPS, oligo subtype, GTR, low proliferative indices, 1p/19q deletions for oligodendroglioma

- MS: low-grade pure oligodendroglioma (120 mo) > low-grade mixed oligoastrocytoma > low-grade astrocytoma (60 mo) ≥ anaplastic oligodendroglioma (60 mo) > anaplastic astrocytoma (36 mo) > GBM (12 mo)

TREATMENT RECOMMENDATIONS

JPA	GTR → observation STR → consider observation vs chemo vs RT vs SRS, depending on location of tumor, symptoms, age of pt
Oligodendroglioma, oligoastrocytoma, astrocytoma (adults)	Maximal safe resection (GTR or STR) → ■ Observation if age <40 yrs, oligodendroglioma, GTR, good function. Serial MRIs, if progresses → RT 50–54 Gy (UCSF standard dose for low-grade gliomas is 54 Gy) ■ Or, immediate post-op RT to 54 Gy. No survival benefit, but RT delays time to relapse ■ QOL gained by delaying recurrence must be weighted against QOL lost due to late toxicities of RT
Oligodendroglioma, oligoastrocytoma, astrocytoma (children)	Maximal safe resection (GTR or STR) → observation & serial MRIs. Adjuvant chemo may prolong DFS & delay need for RT. Adjuvant RT may improve DFS but not recommended for children <3 yrs. Consider 2nd surgery for operable progression and RT for inoperable progression (doses 45–54 Gy)

STUDIES
Retrospective

- <u>Shaw</u> (*J Neurosurg* 1989). 5/10yr OS surgery alone = 30/10%, surgery + <53 Gy = 50/20%, surgery + >53 Gy = 67/40%

Timing of RT

- EORTC 22845 (Karim, *IJROBP* 2002, van den Bent, *Lancet* 2005). Phase III. 311 pts (WHO 1–2, 51% astro., 14% oligo., 13% mixed oligo-astro) treated with surgery (42% GTR, 19% STR, 35% biopsy) randomized to observation vs post-op RT to 54 Gy. RT improved median progression-free survival (5.3 yrs vs 3.4 yrs), 5 yr PFS (55% vs 35%) but not OS (68% vs 66%). 65% of pts in the observation arm received salvage RT

Dose

- EORTC 22844 (Karim, *IJROBP* 1996). Phase III. 343 pts (WHO 1–2, astro., oligo., and mixed) treated with surgery (25% GTR, 30% STR, 40% biopsy) randomized to post-op RT 45 Gy vs 59.4 Gy (shrinking fields). No difference in OS (59%) or PFS (49%). 5 yrs OS oligo vs astro = 75% vs 55%, <40 yrs vs ≥40 yrs = 80% vs 60%. Age <40 yrs, oligo histology, low T-stage, GTR, and good neurologic status are important prognostic factors
- INT/NCCTG (Shaw, *JCO* 2002). Phase III. 203 pts (WHO 1–2, astro., oligo., mixed) treated with surgery (14% GTR, 35% STR, 51% Bx) randomized to post-op RT 50.4 Gy vs 64.8 Gy. No difference in 5 yr OS (72% low dose vs 64% high dose). Best survival in pts <40 yrs, tumor <5 cm, oligo histology & GTR. Increased Grade 3–5 toxicity (2.5 vs 5%) with higher dose. Pattern of failure: 92% in field, 3% within 2 cm of RT field

Role of chemotherapy

- INT/RTOG 9802 (closed, results pending). Phase II/III of low-grade gliomas. Low-risk (<40 yrs + GTR) observed until symptoms. High-risk (>40 yrs or STR or biopsy) randomized to RT alone vs RT → PCV ×6 cycles q 8 wks. RT 54 Gy to FLAIR + 2 cm margin. No boost

DOSE

- EBRT: 1.8 Gy/fx to 50.4–54 Gy

FOLLOW-UP

- MRI 2–6 wks after RT, then every 6 mo for 5 years, then annually

BRAINSTEM GLIOMA

PEARLS

- Most common in young patients
- Accounts for 5% of adult, and 10% of pediatric CNS tumors
- Incidence peaks between age 4–6 yrs
- 70–80% are high-grade astrocytomas, remaining are low-grade astrocytomas & ependymomas
- Biopsy associated with high mortality and morbidity
- MRI & presentation to determine grade
- High-grade tumors = infiltrative, often originate in the Pons, extend alone white matter tracts into the cerebellum or diencephalon, diffusely expand the brainstem, younger age, rapid onset of symptoms, multiple neurological deficits
- Low-grade tumors = focal lesions in the midbrain or thalamus, or dorsally exophytic lesions, older age, and indolent course
- Differential diagnosis (non-diffuse): abscess, demyelinating AVM, encephalitis
- 5 yr OS in adults 20–50%. MS 10 mo for high-grade gliomas

TREATMENT RECOMMENDATIONS

- **Steroids**: can help to stabilize neurologic symptoms
- **Shunts**: may be necessary in severe hydrocephalus
- **Surgery**: role is limited, generally not indicated in diffuse pontine lesions. Dorsally exophytic tumors and cervico-medullary tumors may be surgically resected
- **Radiation**
  - Conventional fractionation to 54–60 Gy. Recommend 3DCRT
  - For diffuse lesions, cover the tumor with 2 cm margin or the entire brainstem (diencephalon to C2) and any cerebellar extension with margin
  - No benefit of dose escalation above 72 Gy at 1 Gy bid
  - No benefit of hyperfractionation (Pediatric Oncology Group)
- **Chemotherapy**
  - No benefit of adjuvant CCNU, vincristine, prednisone vs RT
  - No survival benefit of neoadjuvant chemotherapy

- High-dose chemo with stem-cell rescue showed no benefit in Phase I/II trials

OPTIC GLIOMA

PEARLS

- 5% of all CNS tumors in the pediatric age group
- Subdivided into: anterior/optic nerve gliomas, chiasmatic gliomas, and chiasmatic/hypothalamic gliomas (bulky lesions)
- Bilateral involvement in up to 20% NF-1 patients
- Presentation: long-standing proptosis, optic atrophy, impaired visual acuity, and temporal field defects
- MRI: small and well circumscribed, homogenous enhancement
- Biopsy not necessary for diagnosis

TREATMENT RECOMMENDATIONS

Optic nerve + chiasmatic tumors	Chemo first for all pts and reserve RT for chemo failures
Chiasmatic/ hypothalamic tumors	CSF diversion if indicated. Maximal safe surgical resection. Chemo. Reserve RT (45–50 Gy) for pts who progress on or after chemo

SURVIVAL

- Long-term OS 90–100%
- Long-term PFS 60–90%
- For chiasmatic/hypothalamic gliomas: LC 40–60% & long-term OS 50–80%

CNS LYMPHOMA

PEARLS

- ~2% of intracranial tumors
- Rapidly rising incidence (3–10×) in the last two decades in both immunocompetent and immunodeficient populations
- EBV present in 60–70% of immunodeficient & 15% immunocompetent patients
- Median age: 55 yrs in immunocompetent & 31 yrs in immunocompromised pts

- Multifocal tumors: 25–50% of immunocompetent & 60–80% of immunodeficient pts
- MRI: single or multiple periventricular masses, intensely enhancing
- In AIDS patients, smaller lesions may demonstrate ring enhancement. Differential diagnosis includes toxoplasmosis
- Leptomeningeal involvement in $\frac{1}{3}$ of pts
- Retinal & vitreous seeding in 15–20% of pts
- In primary intraocular lymphoma, 80% develop CNS involvement within 9 mo
- Histology: majority are B-cell origin, high grade large cell or small non-cleaved cell lymphomas. Intermediate or low-grade lymphomas are rare
- Presentation: focal deficits, seizures, headache, lethargy, confusion. Neck or back pain (spinal cord involvement). Blurred vision or floaters (ocular involvement)
- Workup: MRI brain & spine, biopsy, ophthalmologic exam, CXR, CSF cytology, CBC, EBV titer, HIV testing. If B symptoms → CT chest, abdomen, pelvis, & bone marrow biopsy
- Systemic or intrathecal methotrexate given with RT has synergistic neurotoxicity

TREATMENT RECOMMENDATIONS

Surgery	Biopsy for tissue diagnosis. Extensive resection does not improve OS
Steroids	Should be withheld until after biopsy. 90% have clinical response. 40% have shrinkage. 10% have complete resolution on imaging. Response is short-lived and tumor recurs within wks to mo after steroids and stopped
General management	▪ Chemo (high-dose methotrexate-based) → WBRT 45 Gy → chemo [RTOG 93–10]. For pts >50 yrs, may omit WBRT if CR to chemo & reserve RT for recurrence ▪ For leptomeningeal spread, use intrathecal chemo or CSI to 39.6 Gy with additional 5.4–10.8 Gy to gross disease

	■ For ocular lymphoma with CNS lymphoma, treat eye to 36 Gy concurrently with WB to 45 Gy ■ For isolated ocular lymphoma, treat to 36 Gy ■ Use of anti-CD20 antibody is under investigation

STUDIES

■ RTOG 83-15 (Nelson, *IJROBP* 1992). Phase II. 41 pts with CNS lymphoma treated with 40 Gy WBRT + 20 Gy boost to tumor bed. 88% of recurrences were within the boost field. MS 12.2 mo. 2 yr OS 28%. Better survival in pts with KPS >70 and age <60

■ RTOG 88-06 (Schultz, *JCO* 1996). Phase I/II. 51 pts with HIV-negative CNS lymphoma treated with CHODx2 (cytoxan, adriamycin, vincristine, dexamethasone) → WB to 41.4 Gy and boost to 59.4 Gy. No difference in MS when compared with RTOG 83-15

■ RTOG 93-10 (DeAngelis, *JCO* 2002). Phase II. 102 HIV-negative CNS lymphoma pts treated with chemo x5 (IV/IT MTX, vincristine, procarbozine) → WBRT 45 Gy → high dose cytarabine. 58% CR, 36% PR, MPFS 24 mo, MS 36.9 mo. 15% pts with severe delayed neuro-toxicity. Better survival in pts <60 yrs (50 vs 22 mo, p < 0.001)

SURVIVAL

■ RT alone MS 12 mo, 2 yr OS 20–30%
■ Chemo (high-dose MTX-based) + WBRT MS 30–60 mo, 2 yr OS 55–75%

EPENDYMOMA

PEARLS

■ Ependymal cells form the lining of the ventricular system & the central spinal canal
■ <5% of adult brain tumors, incidence peaks at 35 yrs
■ 10% of pediatric brain tumors, incidence peaks at 5 yrs
■ Most intracranial lesions are located in the posterior fossa and arise from floor of the 4th ventricle
■ Increased frequency of spinal cord ependymomas in pts with NF2

- up to 15% ultimately, rare without local progression
- CSF relapse 5–15%. More common with LF, infratentorial and high-grade tumors
- Overexpression of EGF receptors erbB-2 and erbB-4 are associated with worse survival
- Complete resection of posterior fossa tumors is difficult due to proximity to 4th ventricle, CNS, and major vessels
- Complete resection is the single most important prognostic factor
- Other good prognostic factors: low grade and age >2–4 yrs

TREATMENT RECOMMENDATIONS

General management	Hydrocephalus: steroids and/or CSF diversion
Ependymoma resectable	Maximal safe surgical resection Negative CSF GTR → observe or limited field RT (54–60 Gy) STR → limited field RT Positive CSF → CSI (36 Gy, boost gross disease 54–60 Gy)
Anaplastic ependymoma resectable	Maximal safe surgical resection Negative CSF GTR or STR → limited field RT (54–60 Gy) Positive CSF → CSI (36 Gy, boost gross disease 54–60 Gy)
Unresectable	Negative CSF → limited field RT (54–60 Gy) Positive CSF → CSI (36 Gy, boost gross disease 54–60 Gy)
Recurrence	Maximal surgical resection Post-op RT if no prior RT, consider SRS Chemotherapy, best supportive care
Children <4 yrs	Maximal safe surgical resection. If STR → chemo (platinum-based compounds and cyclophosphamide) & delay RT to avoid toxicities

SURVIVAL

- 5 yr OS: low grade 60–80%, high grade 10–40%

FOLLOW-UP

- MRI brain & spine every 3–6 mo for the 1st year, every 6 mo for the 2nd yr, then annually

CHOROID PLEXUS TUMORS

PEARLS

- <2% of all glial tumors
- Most common location: lateral ventricles in children, the 4th ventricle in adults
- Benign (WHO grade I) = choroid plexus papilloma, 60–80%, papillary formation, lack of mitosis and normal tissue invasion
- Malignant (WHO grade III) = choroid plexus carcinoma, 20–40%, nuclear atypia, pleomorphism, frequent mitoses, and invasion of subependymal brain tissue
- Mostly commonly present with hydrocephalus due to CSF overproduction and flow obstruction
- Up to 30% of children present with metastatic disease at diagnosis
- Workup: MRI brain & spine, CSF cytology

TREATMENT RECOMMENDATIONS

General management	Maximal safe resection is first-line therapy for both choroid plexus papilloma and carcinoma
Choroid plexus papilloma	GTR & spine negative → observation
	STR & spine negative → RT to post-op bed 50–54 Gy
	STR & spine positive (rare!) → CSI 36 Gy + LF boost 54 Gy & boost to mets 45–54 Gy
	No role for chemotherapy
Choroid plexus carcinoma	GTR & spine negative → observation, consider RT
	STR & spine negative → RT to post-op bed to 54 Gy
	STR & spine positive → CSI 36 Gy + LF boost 54 Gy & boost to mets 45–54 Gy
	Consider chemotherapy

SURVIVAL

- Choroid plexus papilloma 5 yrs OS 90–100%
- Choroid plexus carcinoma 5 yrs OS 20–30%

MENINGIOMA

PEARLS

- 15–20% of primary intracranial neoplasms
- 8600 new cases in the U.S. in 2002
- Incidence increases with age, peaks in the 7th decade
- F:M = 2:1 for all meningiomas and 1:1 for anaplastic meningiomas
- Locations: cerebral convexities, falx cerebri, tentorium cerebelli, cerebellopontine angle, sphenoid ridge, and spine
- Possible risk factors: ionizing radiation, viral infection, sex hormone receptors, NF2, loss of chromosome 22q

WORKUP

- H&P: most common presentation headaches > personality change/confusion > paresis. Symptoms correlate with location: cranial neuropathy (cerebellopontine angle), headaches or seizures (convexities, falx), visual loss (sphenoid ridge wing or optic nerve involvement)
- CT: extraaxial, well circumscribed and smooth, with moderate to intense homogenous enhancement with contrast, often minimal edema (consistent with slow growth). Bony changes (destruction or hyperostosis) in 15–20%. Malignant meningiomas may frequently invade the brain
- MRI: isointense on T1 and T2, intensely enhance with gadolinium
- Dural tail sign: linear meningeal thickening and enhancement adjacent to a peripherally located cranial mass, reported in 60% of meningiomas, also seen in chloroma, lymphoma and sarcoidosis
- Slower tumor growth has been linked to calcification, homogeneous enhancement, and iso to hypointense T2 signal

TREATMENT RECOMMENDATIONS

Resectable, operable	GTR (often facilitated by pre-op angiography +/– embolization) → observation & serial MRIs. If recurrence → RT.

	Alternative, definitive RT or SRS
Unresectable, operable	STR → RT or RT alone. Alternative, definitive RT or SRS
Inoperable	RT alone or SRS alone
Malignant meningioma	GTR or STR → RT to 60 Gy with 2–3 cm margin
Recurrence	RT or SRS as salvage therapy

STUDIES
Post-op EBRT
- Goldsmith (*J Neurosurg* 1994). 140 pts from USCF with STR + post-op RT for benign (84%) and malignant (16%) meningiomas. 5 yr OS 85% for benign, 60% for malignant. Improved PFS in patients who received >52 Gy (95% vs 65% benign, 65% vs 15% malignant). No benefit of aggressive STR vs biopsy alone if post-op RT given

SRS
- Kondziolka (*J Neurosurg* 1999). 99 pts from U. Pittsburgh, 43% SRS alone, 57% surgery + SRS, median tumor margin dose 16 Gy, max dose 32 Gy, median tumor volume 4.7 cc. LC 95%, PFS 93% at 5–10 yrs

DOSES
- EBRT: 54 Gy for benign, 60 Gy for malignant
- SRS: individual dose chosen based on tumor volume, location, surgical history, and radiosensitivity of nearby structures

SURVIVAL
- WHO I: 5 yr PFS for GTR 88–98%, for STR alone 43–83%, & for STR + RT 88–98%. 5/10/15 yr OS 85/75/70%
- Malignant: surgery + RT, 40–50% PFS at 5 yrs

FOLLOW-UP
- MRI every 4 months for 1 year, every 6 months for 2 years, then annually

ACOUSTIC NEUROMA

PEARLS
- 6% of intracranial tumors

- Arise from Schwann cells of myelin sheath of peripheral nerves
- Sporadic (unilateral, age 40–50 yrs) or associated with NF 2 (bilateral)
- Slow growing, well circumscribed, expansile, displace adjacent nerves
- Symptoms: progressive sensorineuronal hearing loss and vestibular deficits. May affect CN VII function. Expansion into cerebellopontine angle may lead to CN V symptoms. Hydrocephalus may occur
- Screening: pure tone and speech audiometry (selective loss of speech discrimination common)
- Thin slice, gadolinium enhanced MRI through the cerebello-pontine angle. Thin slice contrasted enhanced CT is acceptable
- Suspected NF should have neuraxis imaging

TREATMENT RECOMMENDATIONS

- **Surgery**: 90% are total or near total resection (<10% LF). STR without post-op RT (45% LF) vs STR with post-op RT (6% LF). Preservation of CN VII function >60%. Preservation of useful hearing 30–50%, depending on lesion size and surgical technique
- **SRS**: >90% LC. Dose 12–13 Gy single fraction, increased complications with >14 Gy. Similar outcome with fractionated and single fraction SRS. Preservation of CN VII function >90%. Preservation of useful hearing ~75%. Preservation of CN V function >90%
- **EBRT**: Dose 54 Gy/1.8 Gy fx. Preservation of CN VII function >95%. Preservation of useful hearing ~75%. Preservation of CN V function >95%

CRANIOPHARYNGIOMA

PEARLS

- Benign, partially cystic, epithelial tumors
- Arise from Rathke's pouch in the sellar region
- 5–10% of pediatric intracranial tumors, ages 5–14 yrs
- Bimodal distribution: 55% occur in children and 45% are over age 20 yrs
- Present with neuroendocrine deficits such as diabetes insipidus or growth failure, visual field cuts, decreased acuity, increased ICP, cognitive and behavioral changes

- MRI: solid nodule (calcified and contrast enhancing) with cystic component filled lipoid, cholesterol-laden fluid
- May develop invaginations into adjacent brain, causing a glial reaction

TREATMENT

- Maximal safe resection. GTR accomplished in 70% of cases
- If GTR → observation
- If STR → post-op EBRT to 54 Gy at 1.8 Gy/fx or observation
- Cyst decompression for non-resectable lesions
- SRS: for small primaries or recurrent tumors
- Chemo: intralesional bleomycin effective in shrinking and fibrosing cysts
- For children <3 yrs, limited surgery and close follow-up, defer RT

SURVIVAL

- Long-term event-free survival 80–100%

PITUITARY TUMORS

PEARLS

- 10–15% of primary brain tumors
- The pituitary gland is surrounded by anterior & posterior clinoids; superiorly by anterior cerebral arteries, the optic nerves and chiasm; laterally by cavernous sinuses (CN III, IV, V1, V2, VI, internal carotid artery); inferiorly by sphenoid sinus
- Nearly all pituitary tumors arise from the anterior lobe, which is derived from Rathke's pouch (an evagination of ectodermal tissue from NPX)
- Anterior lobe produces GH, PRL, ACTH, TSH, FSH, LH, controlled by hypothalamic portal system hormones
- Posterior lobe produces ADH and oxytocin
- 75% functional, 25% non-functional
- Tumors secreting prolactin are the most common of the secreting tumors (30%), followed by GH (25%) → ACTH → TSH (rare)
- Macroadenomas: ≥1 cm; microadenomas: <1 cm
- MEN-1: autosomal dominant, pituitary, parathyroid, pancreatic island cell tumors

- Mass effect on stalk (infundibulum) causes increased PRL because loss of inhibition from hypothalamus
- Immunohistochemistry to identify subtype

WORKUP

- H&P: headache, visual field testing (bitemporal hemianopsia, superior temporal deficits, homonymous hemianopsia, central scotoma, etc.), CN deficits (involvement of cavernous sinus), sleep/appetite/behavior changes (compression of hypothalamus), growth abnormalities, and cold or heat intolerance
- Imaging: MRI (thin cuts with contrast) or CT if MR not available, skeletal survey when indicated
- Complete endocrine evaluation
  - Prolactin
  - Basal GH, somatomedin-C, glucose suppression, insulin tolerance, TRH stimulation
  - Serum ACTH, urine 17-hydroxycorticosteroids, free cortisol, dexamethasone suppression
  - Gonadal: LH, FSH, plasma estrodial, testosterone
  - Thyroid: TSH, T3, T4
- Acromegaly = headache, changes in facial/skull/hand bones, heat intolerance, wt gain. Dx = GH >10, not suppressed by glucose, or elevated IGF-1
- Prolactinoma = amenorrhea, infertility, decreased libido, galactorrhea. PRL >20
- Cushing's disease = bilateral adrenal hyperplasia, central obesity, HTN, glucose intolerance, hirsutism, easy bruising, osteoporosis. Diagnosis = elevated cortisol, not suppressed with low-dose dexamethasone, partially suppressed with high-dose dexamethasone, normal or moderately elevated plasma ACTH. In adrenal tumors, ACTH is depressed

TREATMENT
Treatment modalities

Medical management	Bromocriptine for prolactinomas, somatostatin for GH secreting tumors, & ketoconazole for ACTH secreting tumors may be used Frequent relapse when discontinued temporary control of remission while awaiting response to RT

Surgery	Immediate decompression Microadenomas Maximal safe resection for large tumors
Radiation	Indications: Medically inoperable (especially with hypopituitarism), STR with persistent post-op hypersecretion, or large tumor with extrasellar extension

Treatment and outcome by tumor type

Nonfunctioning pituitary tumors	Surgery → observation or RT vs definitive RT alone 10 yr DFS 90% (S + RT) vs 80% (RT alone)
GH-secreting	Surgery → observation → RT 45–50 Gy for recurrent GH elevation. Or, RT alone 45–50 Gy for inoperable pts 10 yr DFS 70–80% (S + RT) vs 60–70% (RT alone)
Prolactin-secreting	Observation vs medical management vs surgery vs RT, individualize treatment based on symptoms, side effect profile, and pt preferences. 10 yr DFS 80–90%
ACTH-secreting	Surgery → observation → RT 45–50 Gy for recurrent ACTH elevation. RT alone 45–50 Gy for inoperable pts. Surgery results in more rapid normalization of hormones than RT alone. 10 yr remission rate 50–60%
TSH-secreting	Aggressive, always treat with post-op RT
Histiocytosis X	6–10 Gy

DOSE

- 1.8 Gy/fx to 45–50 Gy for non-functioning or 50.4–54 Gy for functioning
- No more than 5% of dose inhomogeneity in tumor volume

■ 1.8 Gy to 54 Gy for TSH, and to 50.4 Gy for ACTH secreting tumors

SURVIVAL

■ No difference in OS between surgery, surgery + RT, or RT alone

FOLLOW-UP

■ Post-RT contrast-enhanced MRI every 6 mo ×1 yr, then annually

■ Endocrine testing every 6 mo to 1 yr. GH < 10 ng/ml = good response to therapy, gonadal, thyroid, and adrenal function to monitor hypopituitarism

■ Formal visual field testing before RT for baseline & annually

PINEAL TUMORS

PEARLS

■ Adults: 1% of adult brain CA. 30–40% are germ-cell tumors & 10–20% NGGCTs

■ Children: 5% of pediatric brain CA. 50% are germ-cell tumors & 25–33% pineal parenchymal tumors. 15% of pediatric brain CA in Asia. Incidence peaks at age 10–12 yrs. M : F 3 : 1

■ Non-germinomatous germ cell tumors (NGGCTs) include embryonal carcinoma, endodermal sinus tumor (elevated AFP), choriocarcinoma (elevated β-HCG), and malignant teratoma

■ Pineoblastoma & NGGCTs more commonly have CSF dissemination

■ Presenting symptoms: sellar (visual field cut), suprasellar (endocrinopathies), and pineal (hydrocephalus, Parinaud's [see below])

■ Classic triad = diabetes insipidus, precocious or delayed sexual development, visual deficits

■ Workup = MRI brain & spine, baseline ophthalmologic exam, CSF & serum markers (β-HCG and AFP)

Pineoblastoma

■ Highly malignant primitive embryonal tumor, variant of PNET, WHO grade IV

■ Associated with bilateral retinoblastoma = trilateral retinoblastoma

- Presents with rapidly raised ICP and enlarged head circumference
- MRI: multilobulated, heterogeneous enhancement with areas of necrosis and/or hemorrhage
- Leptomeningeal spread at diagnosis in up to 50% cases

Pineocytoma

- Slow growing tumor. WHO grade II
- Most common in teens. Present with raised ICP
- Parinaud's syndrome: limited upward gaze, lid retraction, retraction nystagmus, pupils that react more poorly to light than to accommodation
- MRI: spherical, well-circumscribed, homogeneous enhancement, hypo on T1, hyper on T2

Pineal parenchymal tumor of intermediate differentiation

- Moderately high cellularity, mild nuclear atypia, occasional mitoses
- No pineocytomatous rosettes
- Rare tumor, optimal treatment need to be decided on an individual basis

Germinomas

- Germinoma = like seminoma in men, dysgerminoma in women
- MRI: hypodense, well circumscribed, homogeneous enhancement
- Mildly elevated β-HCG but not AFP

NGGCT

- Elevated serum or CSF AFP and marked elevated β-HCG
- Less radiosensitive than germinoma

TREATMENT RECOMMENDATIONS AND OUTCOME

Histology	Recommended Treatment
Pineoblastoma	Treat like medulloblastoma: Maximal safe resection (to determine risk category) → CSI (35–40 Gy) + local boost to 54 Gy + chemo (5 yr OS 50–70%). Radiosurgery boost possible for gross residual. If no CSI, poor outcome (MPFS 11–14 mo)

Pineocytoma	Treat like low-grade glioma: Surgery when possible. If GTR, observe. If STR → post-op RT (residual + 1–1.5 cm margin; 50–55 Gy). 5 yr OS 60–90%
Germinoma	Triple-dose gadolinium MRI of neuraxis. RT alone or chemo with RT. Prophylactic neuraxis RT is controversial, not done at UCSF. Consider partial cranial field → whole ventricular irradiation to 30 Gy, boost to primary to 50 Gy. If there is neuraxis or subependymal spread, or multiple midline tumors → CSI 30–36 Gy + primary disease to 50 Gy. 5 yr OS 80–90% with RT, spinal relapse 10–20%
NGGCT	Maximal safe resection → platinum based chemo. Triple dose gadolinium MRI and lumbar puncture. If negative neuraxis, consolidative local RT. If positive neuraxis, CSI 30–36 Gy + primary disease 50 Gy. 5 yr OS <30%

MEDULLOBLASTOMA

PEARLS

- 20% of pediatric CNS tumors, 40% of all posterior fossa tumors
- The 2nd most common pediatric CNS tumor: low-grade glioma 35–50%, medulloblastoma 20%, brainstem glioma 10–15%, high-grade glioma 10%
- M:F = 2:1
- Median age 7 yrs in children and 25 yrs in adults
- 30–40% of patients have CSF spread at the time of diagnosis
- Bad prognostic factors: male, age <5 yrs, M1 disease
- At diagnosis, $\frac{2}{3}$ of pts are standard risk & $\frac{1}{3}$ are high risk

- Common presentation: vomiting, nausea, ataxia, headaches, papilledema, CN palsy, and motor weakness
- Differential diagnosis of posterior fossa mass: medulloblastoma, ependymoma, astrocytoma, brainstem glioma, JPA, and metastasis
- Posterior fossa syndrome = difficulty swallowing, truncal ataxia, mutism, respiratory failure in 10–15% of children after posterior fossa craniotomy for medulloblastoma
- PCV chemo = cisplatin, CCNU, vincristine

WORKUP

- H&P
- MRI of the brain (pre-op and post-op within 24–48 hrs after surgery)
- MRI of the spine to rule out leptomeningeal spread
- CSF cytology
- Bilateral bone marrow biopsy
- Consider bone scan and CXR
- Baseline audiometry, IQ, TSH, CBC, and growth measurements

STAGING

Chang System (Radiology 1969):

T1: ≤ 3 cm, confined to cerebellum, vermis, roof of 4th ventricle
T2: >3 cm, invading 1 adjacent structure or partially filling 4th ventricle
T3a: Invading 2 adjacent structures, complete filling 4th ventricle with proximal or distal extension
T3b: Arising from floor of 4th ventricle and/or brainstem and filling the 4th ventricle
T4:   Involving 3rd ventricle/midbrain/upper cervical cord

M0   No metastases
M1   Microscopic cells in CSF
M2   Nodular seeding in cerebellar, cerebral subarachnoid space, 3rd or lateral ventricles
M3   Nodular seeding in spinal subarachnoid space
M4   Extraneuraxial metastasis

Risk categories:
Standard risk: Age >3 yrs & GTR/STR with <1.5 cm^2 residual & M0
High risk: Age <3 yrs or >1.5 cm^2 residual, or M+

Survival:
Standard risk DFS = 60–90%
High-risk DFS = 20–40%, increased to 50–85% with adjuvant chemo

TREATMENT RECOMMENDATIONS

General management	Hydrocephalus and increased ICP: Steroids and VP shunt before attempting resection
Standard risk	Surgical resection → reduced dose CSI + chemo [Packer, CCG9892]. Post-op CSI 23.4 Gy at 1.8 Gy/fx with posterior fossa boost to 54 Gy with concurrent vincristine → PCV chemo
High risk Residual >1.5 cm² M+	Surgical resection → post-op CSI 36–39 Gy at 1.8 Gy/fx, with entire posterior fossa & mets >1 cm boosted to 54 Gy with concurrent vincristine → PCV chemo
Infants < 3 yo	Surgery → intensive chemo. Reserve RT for salvage [Duffner POG, NEJM 1993; Rutkoski, NEJM 2005]

STUDIES

Role of chemotherapy

- Evans, CCSG/RTOG (*J Neurosurg* 1990). Phase III. 233 pts with medulloblastoma → surgery → randomized to post-op RT vs post-op chemo-RT followed by chemo × 1 yr. RT was CSI 35–40 Gy with posterior fossa (PF) boost to 50–55 Gy + spinal mets to 50 Gy. Chemo was concurrent vincristine, adjuvant vincristine, CCNU, and prednisone × 1 yr. 5 yr OS 65% in both arms. Chemo improved EFS in T3–4, M1–3 (46% for chemo-RT vs 0% for RT alone)
- Tait, SIOP I (*Eur J Cancer* 1990). Phase III. 286 pts with medulloblastoma → surgery → randomized to post-op RT vs post-op chemo-RT followed by chemo × 1 yr. RT was CSI 30–35 Gy/PF boost to 50–55 Gy. 5 yr/10 yr OS 53/45%. Initial DFS & OS benefit of chemo disappeared with longer F/U secondary to late failures in chemo arm. Subgroups T3–4 & gross residual disease still benefited from chemo

Timing of chemotherapy

- Bailey SIOP II (*Med Ped Onc* 1995). 364 pts with low-risk (GTR/STR, no brainstem involvement, M0) and high-risk (gross residual, brainstem invasion, or M+) medulloblastoma. All low-risk pts randomized to surgery + chemo → RT vs surgery → RT. Chemo was vincristine, procarbazine, and methotrexate. RT was randomized to either standard dose 35 Gy CSI + 20 Gy PF boost vs low dose 25 Gy CSI + 30 Gy PF boost. All high-risk pts received 35 Gy CSI + adjuvant vincristine & CCNU. Results: pre-RT chemo did not improve 5 yr EFS (58% with chemo and 60% without chemo). For low risk, no difference with RT alone for 35 Gy vs 25 Gy (5 yr EFS 75% vs 69%)

Standard/average/low risk

- Packer CCG 9892 (*JCO* 1999). Phase II. 65 pts (Age 3–10, M0) → surgery
  → treated with CSI 23.4 Gy/PF 55.8 Gy with concurrent vincristine qwk ×8 → vincristine, CCNU, cisplatin ×8c. 3 yr/5 yr PFS 86/79%. 1/3 developed hearing loss
- Thomas POG8631/CCG923 (*JCO* 2000). 88 low-risk (age 3–21, Chang T1–3a, residual <1.5 cm, M0) medulloblastoma → randomized to CSI 23.4 Gy/PF 54 Gy vs CSI 36 Gy/PF 54 Gy. No chemo. A trend toward improved outcome with 36 Gy. However, overall EFS is suboptimal in the absence of chemo
- POG A9961 (trial closed, result pending). Average-risk medulloblastoma → CSI 23.4 Gy/PF 55.8 Gy randomized one of two adjuvant chemotherapy regimens (CCNU, cisplatin, vincristine vs CPM, cisplatin, vincristine)

High risk

- Zeltzer CCG 921 (*JCO* 1999). High risk pts (age 1.5–21, or M1–4, or T3–4, or residual >1.5 cm^2) randomized to CSI 36 Gy/PF 54 Gy/spinal mets 50.4–54 Gy (age <3 received CSI 23.4 Gy/PF 45 Gy) + vincristine → VCP ×8 vs "8 in 1" chemo ×2 → RT → "8 in 1" chemo ×8. "8 in 1" chemo was vincristine, prednisone, lomustine, hydroxyurea, procarbazine, cisplatin, cyclophosphamide, & cytarabine. Better 5 yr PFS with VCP (63% vs 45%, p = 0.006). 78% 5 yr PFS for M0, >3 yo, ≤1.5 cm^2 residual
- Tarbell POG 9031 (*IJROBP* 2000). 226 high-risk pts. randomized to chemo1 → RT → chemo2 vs RT → chemo1 →

chemo2. Chemo1 was cisplatin/etoposide × 7 wks. Chemo2 was vincristine/cyclophosphamide. RT was CSI 35.2–44 Gy/PF 53.2–56.8 Gy. Results: no difference in 5 yr EFS (70% RT first vs 66% chemo first)

Infants

- Duffner POG (*NEJM* 1993). This study addressed whether RT can be delayed by giving chemo post-op & delay RT until >3 yrs age. Pts <3 yrs with malignant brain tumors (including medulloblastoma, malignant glioma, brainstem glioma, ependymoma, PNET, etc.) underwent surgery → age <2 yrs, 24 mo of chemo; age >2 yrs, 12 mo of chemo → if disease progression → re-resect or RT. Chemo was cyclophosphamide + vincristine ×2 → cisplatin + etoposide ×1. RT was CSI 35.2 Gy/PF 54 Gy (reduced to 24 Gy/50 Gy if complete response after surgery/chemo). 39% CR after the 1st 2 cycles of chemo. No difference in 2 yr PFS (39% vs 33%) and OS (53% vs 55%) between two groups (<2 yrs vs >2 yrs). 34% PFS and 46% OS for medulloblastoma at 2 yrs. These results suggest that it is safe to delay RT until age >3 yrs

- Rutkowski (*NEJM* 2005). Phase II. 43 pts (age <3) with medulloblastoma → surgery (40% GTR, 32% STR, 28% macro mets) → intensive chemo ×3c (cyclophosphamide, vincristine, methotrexate, carboplatin, and etoposide) and intrathecal methotrexate. 5 yr PFS was 82% vs 50% vs 33% & 5 yr OS was 93% vs 56% vs 38% for GTR vs STR vs macro mets. For M0 pts, 5 yr PFS & OS were 68% and 77%. 62% chemo response rate in pts with measurable disease after surgery. Age >2, desmoplastic histology & M0 were good prognostic factors. Mean IQ after treatment was lower than healthy controls but higher than those who received RT. This study shows that lengthy remission can be obtained with intensive post-op chemo in children <3 yrs, reserving RT for salvage

Other trials

- P9934. A phase I/II study evaluating the safety and efficacy of systemic chemo, second-look surgery & IFRT for children ≥8 mo and ≤36 mo with non-metastatic (M0) medulloblastoma
- ACNS0331. A phase III randomized study comparing limited target volume boost irradiation and reduced dose

CSI to 18 Gy to standard dose RT in children with newly diagnosed standard risk medulloblastoma

TREATMENT PLANNING

- Simulate patient prone,hyperextend the neck to avoid PA beam exiting through mouth. Head mask for immobilization. Anesthesia may be required for patients unable to cooperate
- Simulate the spine field first. Superior border: C2 without exiting through mouth (slight neck hyperextension may help minimize exit through mouth). Inferior border: bottom of S2 or lowest level of the thecal sac as seen on MRI. Lateral borders: 1 cm lateral to the lateral edge of pedicles, increase by 1–2 cm in sacrum to cover spreading of neural foramen inferiorly. Field length <35 cm, use 100 cm SSD; >35 cm, use 120 cm SSD. In some patients, two adjacent spinal fields may be required to encompassed the spine. When two spinal fields are used, match at depth of mid spinal cord. Use MRI to determine depth of spinal cord. Alternatively, put lead tape on skin over the spine, and take lateral X-ray film, the distance from skin to the posterior border of vertebral body = depth of spinal cord
- Simulate the cranial field second. Two parallel-opposed lateral fields. Superior border flash the skin. Inferior border 0.5–1 cm on cribiform plate, 1 cm on middle cranial fossa. 1 cm anterior to the vertebral bodies, 2–2.5 cm posterior to eye markers. May angle gantry to align eyelid markers to avoid radiation to the lens
- Collimator angle (of the cranial field) to match diverging spinal fields = [arctan(1/2 length superior spine field/SSD)]
- Couch angle (of the spinal field) to match diverging cranial fields = [arctan(1/2 length cranial field/SSD)]. The foot of couch is rotated towards the side treated. Alternative to couch angle is to beam split lower border of the cranial field to avoid any overlaps at any depth with upper border of the spinal field
- Various beamsplit techniques may be utilized to avoid overlaps at depth (see Figure 2.1)
- Gap shift = Increase cranial field by 2 cm & shift both spinal fields inferiorly by 1 cm every 9 Gy. Need to recalculate couch angle each time
- PF boost: Use CT/MRI for planning

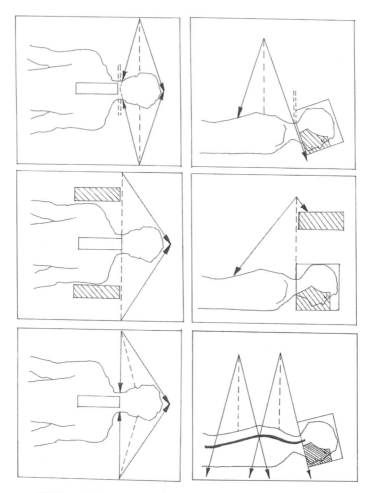

FIGURE 2.1. Various techniques of craniospinal irradiation

PRIMARY SPINAL CORD TUMORS

PEARLS

- Primary spinal cord tumors account for 15% of CNS tumors
- $2/3$ extramedullary, $1/3$ intramedullary
- Intramedullary = astrocytoma (most common), ependymoma, and oligodendroglioma

- Intradural-extramedullary = meningioma, ependymoma, nerve sheath tumors
- Extradural = metastasis, bone osteogenic sarcoma, chondrosarcoma, chordoma, myeloma, epidural hemangiomas, lipomas, extradural meningiomas, and lymphomas
- Astrocytomas are more common in C/T spine and frequently associated with cysts
- Ependymomas are more common in L/S spine
- Presentation: focal pain, segmental or nerve root weakness, sensory deficit in dermatomal distribution, incontinence
- Brown-Séquard syndrome = ipsilateral loss of motor function and fine touch sensation, and contralateral loss of pain and temperature sensation
- Workup: MRI spine, CSF cytology, MRI brain for ependymoma, lymphoma, AA, metastases and GBM, CT chest for sarcomas, no LP before MRI
- MRI: nearly all spinal cord tumors enhance with gadolinium, including low grade gliomas
- CSF: increased protein, possible xanthochromia (with extradural compression)

TREATMENT RECOMMENDATIONS

All tumors Resectable, operable	Maximal safe surgical resection
Low-grade glioma, GTR	Observation
Low-grade glioma, STR	RT 50–54 Gy
High-grade glioma	RT to 54 Gy
Ependymoma	RT to 50–54 Gy ± CSI
Meningioma, GTR	Observation
Meningioma, STR	Observation, or RT to 50–54 Gy
Spinal cord sarcomas, vertebral body chondrosarcomas, chordomas, osteogenic sarcomas	Stereotactic body radiotherapy Charged particle beams
Recurrent tumor	Surgical resection or re-irradiation

SURVIVAL

- Low-grade astrocytoma (S + RT): 5 yr OS 60–90%, 10 yr OS 40–90%
- High-grade astrocytoma (S + RT): MS 6 mo–2 yrs
- Soft tissue sarcoma (S + RT): 4 yr OS 60–70%

ARTERIOVENOUS MALFORMATION

PEARLS

- Average age 30 yrs
- Annual rate of spontaneous hemorrhage ~2–4% with morbidity 20–30% per bleed & mortality 1%/yr or 10–15% per bleed
- There is a period of decreased risk of hemorrhage during latent interval after SRS treatment before complete angiographic resolution
- After angiographic obliteration, risk of hemorrhage is ≤1%
- SRS produces progressive thickening of the vascular wall & luminal thrombosis
- Obliteration takes several years
- Microsurgical resection or SRS
  - Microsurgical resection and STR are both options
  - Treat entire nidus, but not feeding arteries or draining veins
  - Tailor dose according to volume & location
- <u>Maruyama</u> (*NEJM* 2005). Reviewed 500 pts treated with SRS who were followed with serial exams, MRI &/or angiography. Mean dose 21 Gy. Cumulative 4 yr obliteration rate 81%, 5 yr 91%. Hemorrhage risk reduced by 54% during latency period & by 88% after obliteration compared to before SRS
- Obliteration rate at 2 yrs for lesions <2 cm is 90–100% & for >2 cm is 50–70%
- F/U: MRI every 6 mo × 1–3 yrs, then annually. Once MRI obliteration, obtain angiogram to confirm (gold standard)

TRIGEMINAL NEURALGIA

PEARLS

- Disorder of the sensory nucleus of CN V causing episodic, paroxysmal, severe pain lasting seconds to minutes followed by a pain-free period in the distribution of one or more of its divisions
- Peak age 60 yrs. F:M 2:1
- Often precipitated by stimulation (e.g., shaving, brushing teeth, wind)
- Obtain MRI to rule-out neoplasm in cerebellopontine angle

- Medical management is standard treatment (carbamazepine, gabapentin, anti-depressants, etc.)
- Surgical options include nerve blocks, partial sensory rhizotomy, balloon decompression of the Gasserian ganglion, microvascular decompression, & peripheral nerve ablation (radiofrequency, neurectomy, cryotherapy)
- SRS may also be used with dose of ~80 Gy
- Median time to pain relief with SRS is ~1 mo. ~50–60% become pain-free, ~10–20% have decreased severity or frequency of pain, & ~5–10% have slight improvement only

REFERENCES

Bailey CC, Gnekow A, Wellek S, et al. Prospective randomised trial of chemotherapy given before radiotherapy in childhood medulloblastoma. International Society of Paediatric Oncology (SIOP) and the (German) Society of Paediatric Oncology (GPO): SIOP II. Med Pediatr Oncol 1995;25:166–178.

Bauman GS, Gaspar LE, Fisher BJ, et al. A prospective study of short-course radiotherapy in poor prognosis glioblastoma multiforme. Int J Radiat Oncol Biol Phys 1994;29:835–839.

Berger C, Thiesse P, Lellouch-Tubiana A, et al. Choroid plexus carcinomas in childhood: clinical features and prognostic factors. Neurosurgery 1998;42:470–475.

Bleehen NM, Stenning SP. A Medical Research Council trial of two radiotherapy doses in the treatment of grades 3 and 4 astrocytoma. The Medical Research Council Brain Tumour Working Party. Br J Cancer 1991;64:769–774.

Carter M, Nicholson J, Ross F, et al. Genetic abnormalities detected in ependymomas by comparative genomic hybridisation. Br J Cancer 2002;86:929–939.

Chung HT, Ma R, Toyota B, et al. Audiologic and treatment outcomes after linear accelerator-based stereotactic irradiation for acoustic neuroma. Int J Radiat Oncol Biol Phys 2004;59:1116–1121.

DeAngelis LM, Seiferheld W, Schold SC, et al. Combination chemotherapy and radiotherapy for primary central nervous system lymphoma: Radiation Therapy Oncology Group Study 93-10. J Clin Oncol 2002;20:4643–4648.

Duffner PK, Horowitz ME, Krischer JP, et al. Postoperative chemotherapy and delayed radiation in children less than three years of age with malignant brain tumors. N Engl J Med 1993;328:1725–1731.

Evans AE, Jenkin RD, Sposto R, et al. The treatment of medulloblastoma. Results of a prospective randomized trial of radiation therapy with and without CCNU, vincristine, and prednisone. J Neurosurg 1990;72:572–582.

Freeman CR, Farmer J, Taylor RE. Central nervous system tumors in children. In: Perez CA, Brady LW, Halperin EC, et al., editors. Principles and Practice of Radiation Oncology. 4th ed. Lippincott Williams and Wilkins; 2004. pp. 2206–2237.

Freire JE, Brady LW, Shields JA, et al. Eye and orbit. In: Perez CA, Brady LW, Halperin EC, et al., editors. Principles and Practice of Radiation Oncology. 4th ed. Lippincott Williams and Wilkins; 2004. pp. 876–896.

Fulton DS, Urtasun RC, Scott-Brown I, et al. Increasing radiation dose intensity using hyperfractionation in patients with malignant glioma. Final report of a prospective phase I-II dose response study. J Neurooncol 1992;14:63–72.

Gilbertson RJ, Bentley L, Hernan R, et al. ERBB receptor signaling promotes ependymoma cell proliferation and represents a potential novel therapeutic target for this disease. Clin Cancer Res 2002;8:3054–3064.

Goldsmith BJ, Wara WM, Wilson CB, et al. Postoperative irradiation for subtotally resected meningiomas. A retrospective analysis of 140 patients treated from 1967 to 1990. J Neurosurg 1994;80:195–201.

Goldsmith BJ. Meningeal tumors. In: Leibel SA, Phillips TL, editors. Textbook of Radiation Oncology. 2nd ed. Saunders; 2004. pp. 497–514.

Gripp S, Kambergs J, Wittkamp M, et al. Coverage of anterior fossa in whole-brain irradiation. Int J Radiat Oncol Biol Phys 2004;59:515–520.

Gupta N. Choroid plexus tumors in children. Neurosurg Clin N Am 2003;14:621–631.

Gururangan S, Friedman HS. Recent advances in the treatment of pediatric brain tumors. Oncology (Huntingt) 2004;18:1649–1661; discussion 1662, 1665–1646, 1668.

Huang D, Halberg FE. Pituitary tumors. In: Leibel SA, Phillips TL, editors. Textbook of Radiation Oncology. 2nd ed. Saunders; 2004. pp. 533–548.

Karim AB, Maat B, Hatlevoll R, et al. A randomized trial on dose-response in radiation therapy of low-grade cerebral glioma: European Organization for Research and Treatment of Cancer (EORTC) Study 22844. Int J Radiat Oncol Biol Phys 1996;36:549–556.

Karim AB, Afra D, Cornu P, et al. Randomized trial on the efficacy of radiotherapy for cerebral low-grade glioma in the adult: European Organization for Research and Treatment of Cancer Study 22845 with the Medical Research Council study BRO4: an interim analysis. Int J Radiat Oncol Biol Phys 2002;52:316–324.

Kondziolka D, Levy EI, Niranjan A, et al. Long-term outcomes after meningioma radiosurgery: physician and patient perspectives. J Neurosurg 1999;91:44–50.

Kondziolka D, Lunsford LD, Flickinger JC. Stereotactic radiosurgery for the treatment of trigeminal neuralgia. Clin J Pain 2002;18:42–47.

Kun LE, Tarbell NJ. Astro Education Session: Current Treatment and Controversies in Childhood Brain Tumors. Atlanta, GA; 2004.

Lunsford LD, Niranjan A, Flickinger JC, et al. Radiosurgery of vestibular schwannomas: summary of experience in 829 cases. J Neurosurg 2005;102(Suppl):195–199.

Maire JP, Caudry M, Darrouzet V, et al. Fractionated radiation therapy in the treatment of stage III and IV cerebello-pontine angle neurinomas: long-term results in 24 cases. Int J Radiat Oncol Biol Phys 1995;32:1137–1143.

Maire JP, Caudry M, Guerin J, et al. Fractionated radiation therapy in the treatment of intracranial meningiomas: local control, functional efficacy, and tolerance in 91 patients. Int J Radiat Oncol Biol Phys 1995;33:315–321.

Maruyama K, Kawahara N, Shin M, et al. The risk of hemorrhage after radiosurgery for cerebral arteriovenous malformations. N Engl J Med 2005;352:146–153.

Mehta M, Rogers L. Astro Education Session: Adult Brain Tumors. Atlanta, GA; 2004.

Michalski JM. Spinal canal. In: Perez CA, Brady LW, Halperin EC, et al., editors. Principles and Practice of Radiation Oncology. 4th ed. Lippincott Williams and Wilkins; 2004. pp. 860–875.

Narayana A, Leibel SA. Primary and metastatic brain tumors in adults. In: Leibel SA, Phillips TL, editors. Textbook of Radiation Oncology. 2nd ed. Saunders; 2004. pp. 463–497.

National Comprehensive Cancer Network. Clinical Practice Guidelines in Oncology: Central Nervous System Tumors. Available at: http://www.nccn.org/professionals/physician_gls/PDF/cns.pdf. Accessed on May 10, 2005.

Nelson DF, Martz KL, Bonner H, et al. Non-Hodgkin's lymphoma of the brain: can high dose, large volume radiation therapy improve survival? Report on a prospective trial by the Radiation Therapy Oncology Group (RTOG): RTOG 8315. Int J Radiat Oncol Biol Phys 1992;23:9–17.

Packer RJ, Goldwein J, Nicholson HS, et al. Treatment of children with medulloblastomas with reduced-dose craniospinal radiation therapy and adjuvant chemotherapy: A Children's Cancer Group Study. J Clin Oncol 1999;17:2127–2136.

Roa W, Brasher PM, Bauman G, et al. Abbreviated course of radiation therapy in older patients with glioblastoma multiforme: a prospective randomized clinical trial. J Clin Oncol 2004;22:1583–1588.

Rutkowski S, Bode U, Deinlein F, et al. Treatment of early childhood medulloblastoma by postoperative chemotherapy alone. N Engl J Med 2005;352:978–986.

Scally LT, Lin C, Beriwal S, et al. Brain, brain stem, and cerebellum. In: Perez CA, Brady LW, Halperin EC, et al., editors. Principles and Practice of Radiation Oncology. 4th ed. Lippincott Williams and Wilkins; 2004. pp. 791–838.

Schultz C, Scott C, Sherman W, et al. Preirradiation chemotherapy with cyclophosphamide, doxorubicin, vincristine, and dexamethasone for primary CNS lymphomas: initial report of radiation therapy oncology group protocol 88-06. J Clin Oncol 1996;14: 556–564.

Shaw EG, Daumas-Duport C, Scheithauer BW, et al. Radiation therapy in the management of low-grade supratentorial astrocytomas. J Neurosurg 1989;70:853–861.

Shaw E, Arusell R, Scheithauer B, et al. Prospective randomized trial of low-versus high-dose radiation therapy in adults with supratentorial low-grade glioma: initial report of a North Central Cancer Treatment Group/Radiation Therapy Oncology Group/Eastern Cooperative Oncology Group study. J Clin Oncol 2002;20: 2267–2276.

Shaw E, Sneed PK. Astro Education Session: Intracranial Stereotactic Radiosurgery: Benign/Malignant Tumors and Functional Disorders. Atlanta, GA; 2004.

Sheehan J, Pan HC, Stroila M, et al. Gamma knife surgery for trigeminal neuralgia: outcomes and prognostic factors. J Neurosurg 2005;102: 434–441.

Shrieve DC, Larson DA, Loeffler JS. Radiosurgery. In: Leibel SA, Phillips TL, editors. Textbook of Radiation Oncology. 2nd ed. Saunders; 2004. pp. 549–564.

Silvani A, Eoli M, Salmaggi A, et al. Combined chemotherapy and radiotherapy for intracranial germinomas in adult patients: a single-institution study. J Neurooncol 2005;71:271–276.

Stupp R, Dietrich PY, Ostermann Kraljevic S, et al. Promising survival for patients with newly diagnosed glioblastoma multiforme treated with concomitant radiation plus temozolomide followed by adjuvant temozolomide. J Clin Oncol 2002;20:1375–1382.

Tait DM, Thornton-Jones H, Bloom HJ, et al. Adjuvant chemotherapy for medulloblastoma: the first multi-centre control trial of the International Society of Paediatric Oncology (SIOP I). Eur J Cancer 1990;26:464–469.

Tarbell NJ, Smith AR, Adams J, et al. The challenge of conformal radiotherapy in the curative treatment of medulloblastoma. Int J Radiat Oncol Biol Phys 2000;46:265–266.

Thomas PR, Deutsch M, Kepner JL, et al. Low-stage medulloblastoma: final analysis of trial comparing standard-dose with reduced-dose neuraxis irradiation. J Clin Oncol 2000;18:3004–3011.

Van den Bent MJ, de Witte O, Hassel MB, et al. Long-term efficacy of early versus delayed radiotherapy for low-grade astrocytoma and oligodendroglioma in adults: the EORTC 22845 randomized trial. Lancet 2005;366:985–990.

Walker MD, Alexander E, Jr., Hunt WE, et al. Evaluation of BCNU and/or radiotherapy in the treatment of anaplastic gliomas. A cooperative clinical trial. J Neurosurg 1978;49:333–343.

Walker MD, Strike TA, Sheline GE. An analysis of dose-effect relationship in the radiotherapy of malignant gliomas. Int J Radiat Oncol Biol Phys 1979;5:1725–1731.

Walker MD, Green SB, Byar DP, et al. Randomized comparisons of radiotherapy and nitrosoureas for the treatment of malignant glioma after surgery. N Engl J Med 1980;303:1323–1329.

Weil MD, Hass-Kogan DA, Wara WM. Pediatric central nervous system tumors. In: Leibel SA, Phillips TL, editors. Textbook of Radiation Oncology. 2nd ed. Saunders; 2004. pp. 1199–1214.

Zeltzer PM, Boyett JM, Finlay JL, et al. Metastasis stage, adjuvant treatment, and residual tumor are prognostic factors for medulloblastoma in children: conclusions from the Children's Cancer Group 921 randomized phase III study. J Clin Oncol 1999;17:832–845.

NOTES

Chapter 3
Cancer and Benign Diseases of the Eye and Orbit

Alice Wang-Chesebro and Jeanne Marie Quivey

GENERAL PEARLS

- All eye/orbit malignancies uncommon: per ACS, approximately 2200 new cases/yr
- Percentage of malignant tumors increases with age, due to increases in lymphoma and metastatic lesions in elderly (both in choroid and the orbit)
- Most common intraocular malignancy in adults: choroidal metastasis, usually adenocarcinoma, especially from lung, breast, and prostate
- Most common primary eye malignancy in adults: uveal melanoma (ME)
- Most common primary eye malignancy in children: retinoblastoma (RB)
- Most common primary orbital malignancy in adults: lymphoma
- Most common primary orbital malignancy in children: rhabdomyosarcoma
- This chapter will discuss uveal melanoma, orbital lymphoma, intraocular lymphoma, thyroid ophthalmopathy, and orbital lymphoid hyperplasia

I. UVEAL MELANOMA

PEARLS

- Risk factors: light eyes, melanocytosis in affected eye, welding, history of sun/snow burn
- Presentation: $\sim^1/_3$ asymptomatic, found on exam; visual distortion, field loss, floaters, scotomas, flashing lights, unilateral cataract, pain
- Patterns of spread: 1) intraocular spread, including vitreous seeding, 2) extrascleral extension (15% of pts), 3) hema-

togenous; may occur after prolonged disease free interval; first to liver (~90%), also skin, lung; brain mets are rare
- Prognostic factors for increased metastases: mixed/epithelioid type, larger tumor size, ciliary body invasion, monosomy of chromosome 3, scleral penetration, high mitotic rate, Ki-67, pleomorphic nucleoli, high Mib-1 index, optic nerve invasion, vascular networks of closed vascular loops

WORKUP

- H&P includes measurement of tumor diameter/thickness, location, geometry, and tumor coloration
- Labs: CBC, LFTs, LDH
- Imaging: fundus photography, ocular ultrasound (Kretz A&B), & MRI depending on extent. CT of chest/abdomen if LFTs are elevated

STAGING

Primary tumor
All Uveal Melanomas
TX: Primary tumor cannot be assessed
T0: No evidence of primary tumor
Tis: Carcinoma in situ
Iris
T1: Tumor limited to iris
T1a: Tumor limited to iris not more than 3 clock hours in size
T1b: Tumor limited to iris more than 3 clock hours in size
T1c: Tumor limited to iris with melanomalytic glaucoma
T2: Tumor confluent with or extending into the ciliary body and/or choroid
T2a: Tumor confluent with or extending into the ciliary body and/or choroids with melanomalytic glaucoma
T3: Tumor confluent with or extending into the ciliary body and/or choroid with scleral extension
T3a: Tumor confluent with or extending into the ciliary body with scleral extension and melanomalytic glaucoma
T4: Tumor with extraocular extension
Ciliary Body and Choroid
T1: Tumor 10mm or less in greatest diameter and 2.5mm or less in greatest height (thickness)
T1a: Tumor 10mm or less in greatest diameter and 2.5mm or less in greatest height (thickness) without microscopic extraocular extension
T1b: Tumor 10mm or less in greatest diameter and 2.5mm or less in greatest height (thickness) with microscopic extraocular extension

T1c: Tumor 10 mm or less in greatest diameter and 2.5 mm or less in greatest height (thickness) with macroscopic extraocular extension

T2*: Tumor greater than 10 mm but not more than 16 mm in greatest basal diameter and between 2.5 and 10 mm in maximum height (thickness)

T2a: Tumor greater than 10 mm but not more than 16 mm in greatest basal diameter and between 2.5 and 10 mm in maximum height (thickness) without microscopic extraocular extension

T2b: Tumor 10 mm to 16 mm in greatest basal diameter and between 2.5 and 10 mm in maximum height (thickness) with microscopic extraocular extension

T2c: Tumor 10 mm to 16 mm in greatest basal diameter and between 2.5 and 10 mm in maximum height (thickness) with macroscopic extraocular extension

T3*: Tumor more than 16 mm in greatest diameter and/or greater than 10 mm in maximum height (thickness) without extraocular extension

T4: Tumor more than 16 mm in greatest diameter and/or greater than 10 mm in maximum height (thickness) with extraocular extension

Note: When basal dimension and apical height do not fit this classification, the largest tumor diameter should be used for classification.

Regional lymph nodes
NX: No regional lymph node metastasis cannot be assessed
N0: No regional lymph node metastasis
N1: Regional lymph node metastasis

Distant metastasis
MX: Distant metastasis cannot be assessed
M0: No distant metastasis
M1: Distant metastasis

Stage Grouping		10 yr OS by Stage	
I:	T1N0M0, T1a-1cN0M0	I:	~80%
II:	T2N0M0, T2a-2cN0M0	II:	~60%
III:	T3N0M0, T4N0M0	III:	~30–40%
IV:	Any T N1 M0	IV:	<7 months (*Cancer* 1993)
	Any T Any N M1		

TREATMENT RECOMMENDATIONS

Stage	Recommended Treatment
Small, indeterminate pigmented lesions	Serial observation (COMS showed no difference in survival with early treatment, & vision preserved longer with observation)
Medium-sized lesions (T2)	Options (no difference in survival) ■ Surgery: enucleation ■ I-125 brachytherapy (other isotopes used) with episcleral plaque to apex dose of 70–85 Gy ■ Proton radiotherapy
Large-sized lesions(T3+)	Enucleation

STUDIES

- Only randomized study of plaques vs particles: <u>UCSF/ Berkeley</u> (*Ophthal* 1993). 184 pts with T2/T3 lesions randomized to 70 Gy with helium (5 fx in 5–7 d, <2 min fx) vs I-125 plaque (0.7–0.75 Gy/hr at apex). LC was 100% He vs 83% I-125; subsequent enucleation He 9.3% vs I-125 17.3%. No survival differences. Different toxicities: more dry eye, epiphora, neovascular glaucoma with He vs temporary strabismus unique to brachytherapy
- <u>UCSF</u> (*IJROBP* 1993). 449 pts treated with I-125; ~13% recurred locally; increased local failure with smaller tumor height, closer proximity to fovea/disc and optic nerve, larger diameter, lower radiation dose
- <u>COMS</u> (Arch Ophth 2001, Am J Ophth 1998). 3-part multi-center randomized study
  - Small tumors: 204 pts with small/T1 non-progresive tumors enrolled for observational study with treatment only if progression documented. 5 yr OS 94%, 8 yr OS 85%; 5 yr DSS 99%; 8 yr DSS 96%. No apparent loss of survival & good preservation of vision with close f/u of small lesions
  - Medium tumors/T2: 1317 pts with selected T2 tumors (not abutting optic disc) randomized to brachytherapy (n = 657) vs enucleation (n = 660). No difference in 5 yr OS (81–82%). ~60% pts who died had DM at death. Visual acuity declined over time with brachytherapy. Plaque pts 5 y LF 10%, 5 y eye retention 85%

- Large tumors: 1003 pts with large-sized tumors randomized to enucleation vs pre-op 20 Gy EBRT + enucleation. No improvement in survival for preoperatively irradiated pts (5 yr OS 60%, 5 yr DSS 73%)
- Metastasis screening – COMS 23 (*JCO* 2004)
  - Evaluation of COMS study efficacy of at least one abnormal LFT for metastasis screening in follow-up. Low sensitivity (14.7%) & PPV (45%) supports use of ultrasound of liver (as in Europe) or CT of chest & abdomen

RADIATION TECHNIQUES
Episcleral plaque
- Field design: tumor + margin to include scleral thickness (1 mm) + 1–2 mm around tumor diameter as defined by ophthalmologist
- 1 mm spacer (or contact lens) used to minimize hot spots over individual seeds
- Surgical placement with general or local anesthesia. 360° perilimbal incision made and rectus muscles isolated with suture slings. Localize melanoma with transillumination, suture dummy plaque into place, and verify position. Then suture radioactive plaque, irrigated eye with antibiotic solution, and close conjunctiva, place lead eye shield
- Dose prescription: 70–85 Gy to tumor apex; dose rate 0.7–1.0 Gy/hr
- Patient usually discharged in 24 hrs, return for plaque removal in 4–7 d

Proton/charged particle therapy
- Standard dose 56 Gy in 4 fractions with LC in most series 96–98%

COMPLICATIONS
- Episcleral plaque: RT retinopathy up to 43% (depends on length of f/u), optic atrophy, cystoid macular edema, cataracts, vitreous hemorrhage, secondary glaucoma, central retinal vein occlusion, scleral necrosis, secondary strabismus (5%)
- Proton/helium: increased anterior complications from entrance beam including epiphora, lash loss, neovascular glaucoma, maculopathy (75% if tumor <1 disc diameter of fovea, 40% >1 disc diameter from fovea)

FOLLOW-UP

- H&P including ocular ultrasound every 3 mo for 1 yr, every 4 mo for 2nd yr, every 6 mo for 3rd & 4th yr, then annually. Chest X-ray annually for 5 yr

II. ORBITAL LYMPHOMA

PEARLS

- Includes lymphoid malignancies of the conjunctiva, lacrimal apparatus, eyelids, uvea, and intraconal and extraconal retrobulbar areas
- In contrast to intraocular lymphoma (IOL), orbital lymphoma (OL) is a generally an indolent disease
- Most lesions are low-grade B-cell lymphomas
- Most common histology: extranodal marginal zone B-cell lymphoma of mucosa-associated lymphoid tissue (MALT)
- Common presentations: orbital mass, proptosis, eye swelling, redness, increased tearing
- Most patients present in seventh decade of life

WORKUP

- H&P includes fundoscopy, measurement of tumor including exophthalmometer if proptosis
- Labs: CBC, LFTs
- Imaging: Orbit CT and MRI. Rule out systemic lymphoma with CT chest, abdomen, & pelvis
- Tissue diagnosis: biopsy of lesion with immunohistochemistry and flow cytometry analysis; also bone marrow biopsy for systemic work-up

STAGING

- Ann Arbor staging system (see Chapter 33)
- Working formulation and REAL classifications of NHL used to characterize low-grade versus intermediate/high grade lesions for management decisions

TREATMENT RECOMMENDATIONS

Extent of Disease	Treatment Options
Low grade, limited disease	Best results seen with RT alone, dose 30–30.6 Gy, in 1.5–1.8 Gy fractions
Intermediate/high grade, or systemic disease with orbital involvement	Combined systemic chemo (e.g., CHOP) and RT to orbit (40 Gy). For CD20+, add rituximab

STUDIES

- Esik (*Radiother Oncol* 1996). review of 37 pts with OL treated with RT after biopsy (17 pts), surgery alone (13 pts), or chemo (7 pts). Median RT dose 34.8 Gy. 10 y local RFS was 100% with RT, 0% with surgery alone, & 42% with chemo. 20 yr CSS was 100% with RT, 67% with surgery alone, & 0% with chemo

- Stanford (Le, *IJROBP* 2002). series of 31 pts with MALT lymphoma treated with 30–40 Gy (mean 34 Gy) using 9–20 MeV electrons for conjunctival lesions, 6 MV photons for retrobulbar; lens shielded. 10 yr OS 73%, LC 100%. 10 yr FF relapse 71% with most failures extranodal mucosa. No difference with dose ≤34 Gy vs >34 Gy. 2 pts had retinal damage >34 Gy

- Bolek (*IJROBP* 1999). series of 38 pts, 20 with limited disease treated with curative intent, 18 with extensive disease. Median dose 25 Gy. LC achieved in 37/38 pts. For pts treated curatively, 5 yr CSS was 89% for low grade, & 33% for intermediate/high grade. Cataracts: 7/21 pts without shielding, 0/17 with shielding

RADIATION TECHNIQUES
EBRT

- Set up patient supine, immobilize head with thermoplastic mask
- Place radiopaque markers at lateral canthus or radiopaque contact lens to help define fields
- For anterior lesions involving eyelid or bulbar conjunctiva, use electron beam 6–9 MeV with 0.5–1.0 cm bolus
- Lens shield used if doesn't compromise tumor coverage. Lens block can be placed directly on the cornea after topical anesthetic if mounted on a Lucite conformer. Daily placement of block should carefully place it within limbus. Hanging blocks provide less reliable shielding when using electron beams
- Lacrimal lesions as well as those involving intra or extraconal spread benefit from more sophisticated planning techniques: obtain CT for 3D CRT/IMRT planning
- Dose prescription: 30 Gy in 1.8–2 Gy fractions with CT/MRI planning

COMPLICATIONS

- Acute: mild skin erythema

- Late: depends on technique and shielding; includes cataracts, vitreous hemorrhage, retinopathy, second tumors in field of irradiation, dry eye, glaucoma

FOLLOW-UP
- H&P every 3 mo for 1 yr, every 4 mo for 2nd yr, every 6 mo for 3rd & 4th yr, then annually

III. INTRAOCULAR LYMPHOMA

PEARLS
- Very rare: a subset of primary CNS lymphomas, which account for 1–2% extranodal lymphomas
- Confined to neural structures; distinguished from orbital lymphomas that involve the uvea and ocular adnexa of the orbit, lacrimal gland, and conjunctiva
- Histology: usually diffuse large B-cell non-Hodgkin's lymphoma
- Median age of onset in immunocompetent pts late 50s–60s
- Of pts who develop primary intraocular lymphoma (PIOL), 60–80% will go on to develop CNS disease within 3 years. Conversely, 25% of pts with primary CNS lymphoma without initial eye involvement will develop intraocular lymphoma
- Common presentations: blurred vision, floaters; less common: red eye, photophobia, ocular pain, uveitis; ocular disease is bilateral in ~80% cases
- Recurs in 50% cases
- No universal staging system
- Optimum treatment remains unclear

WORKUP
- H&P includes fundoscopy, slit-lamp examination, measurement of tumor; thorough CNS evaluation
- Labs: CBC, LFTs, ESR, lumbar puncture – CSF for cytology, chemistry, cytokine analysis; immunohistochemistry and flow cytometry of lymphoma cells from CSF/vitrectomy/biopsy
- Brain/orbit MRI. Consider stereotactic brain biopsy for suspicious brain lesions, fluorescein angiography, ocular ultrasound
- Systemic workup (CT chest, abdomen, pelvis, & bone marrow biopsy)

- Tissue diagnosis: diagnostic vitrectomy, vitreous aspiration needle tap. Pts suspected of having IOL with no lesion on imaging should have diagnostic vitrectomy on eye with more severe vitreitis/worse visual acuity
- If vitrectomy non-diagnostic, consider chorioretinal biopsy or enucleation

TREATMENT RECOMMENDATIONS

Extent of Disease	Treatment Options
Limited to eye	Combined chemo-RT: use high-dose systemic chemo ± intrathecal chemo + RT (ocular + brain) or chemo alone
Eye disease with primary CNS lymphoma	Combined chemo-RT. Ocular RT ± whole brain or chemo alone RT, from 20–45Gy in 1.8–2Gy fractions
Refractory/recurrent	Chemo alone or high dose chemo & stem cell rescue

STUDIES

- Hoffman (*Eye* 2003). Series of 14 HIV negative pts with IOL. Most had lymphoma elsewhere; 64% had bilateral disease; 29% had prior systemic lymphoma; 57% had PCNSL; 29% non-B cell. 10/14 (71%) received combined chemo-RT (most common 40Gy in 20–25fx). 4/14 received chemo alone. 79% of pts died of lymphoma with 16mo median survival. Pts without CNS involvement had improved survival (50% vs 10%). RT complications included cataracts (50%), dry eye (40%), punctuate keratopathy (20%), retinopathy (20%), & optic atrophy (10%)

IV. THYROID OPHTHALMOPATHY

PEARLS

- Usually in association with Graves' disease, but can arise in association with Hashimoto's thyroiditis
- Histopathology: T-cell predominant lymphocytic infiltration of orbital tissues; also glycosaminoglycans in periorbital fat, extraocular muscles
- Present with exophthalmos, impaired extraocular muscle involvement, diplopia, periorbital edema, lid retraction

WORKUP

- H&P includes measurement with Hertel exophthalmometer
- Labs: CBC, chemistries, and thyroid function tests
- Imaging: Orbit CT, MRI

TREATMENT RECOMMENDATIONS

- If stable, no threat of impending visual loss, begin with treatment of underlying thyroid disorder
- If moderate symptomatic/progressive/refractory to thyroid treatment, options include: orbital RT (preferred, less toxicity) ± systemic immunosuppressive agents (corticosteroids, cyclosporine, others)
- For visual loss unresponsive to corticosteroids (loss of color vision a key symptom): decompressive surgery
- EBRT: 20 Gy in 10 fx, see 50–80% response rate

STUDIES

- <u>UPenn Study</u> (Prummel, *Lancet* 1993). 56 pts with moderately severe Graves' ophthalmopathy (no corneal involvement or loss of visual acuity) euthyroid for at least 2 months, randomized to 3 months oral prednisone + sham RT vs retrobulbar RT to 20 Gy + placebo capsules. Results: Same rate of responders/no change/failures (RT 46/40/14%, prednisone 50/36/14%), but steroid therapy had much higher minor, moderate, & major complications rates. Note that 75% of all pts (71% RT, 79% prednisone) ultimately needed decompressive/squint/rehabilitation surgery regardless of treatment
- <u>Stanford series</u> (*IJROBP* 1990). 311 pts treated from 1968 to 1988, most with 20 Gy. Some pts treated from 1979 to 1983 received 30 Gy, but no benefit was noted from increased dose. Results: improved or complete resolution of soft tissue changes 80%, proptosis 51%, eye muscle impairment 61%, visual acuity 61%. Of 1/3 pts who were on steroids when starting RT, 76% were able to discontinue use. Treatment well-tolerated with 10% acute toxicity

RADIATION TECHNIQUES
Simulation and field design

- Set up patient supine, immobilize head with thermoplastic mask. Highly recommend cutting out around eyes to allow verification of clinical setup

- Place radiopaque markers at lateral canthus or radiopaque contact lens to define fields
- Place the beam split anterior field border 11–12 mm behind cornea to spare lens
- Fields: generally lateral opposed, extending from just behind the lens of the globe to the anterior clinoids with superior and inferior margins defined by the bony orbit; general range of 4×4 cm to 5.5×5.5 cm with appropriate shielding
- Techniques to minimize divergence into contralateral lens
  - Half beam block anterior edge of field
  - Alternatively, angle lateral fields 5 degrees posteriorly (Can use CT scan to ensure the optimal beam angle is selected.)
- Dose prescription: 20 Gy in 2 Gy fx
- Dose limitation: Lens <10 Gy

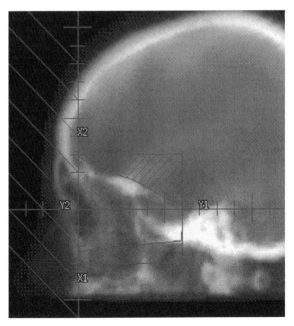

FIGURE 3.1. Lateral DRR of a field used to treat thyroid ophthalmopathy.

V. ORBITAL PSEUDOTUMOR/LYMPHOID HYPERPLASIA/PSEUDOLYMPHOMA

PEARLS

- Very rare benign orbital mass lesions in which mature lymphocytes (polyclonal) are noted
- Usually present with soft tissue swelling, orbital pain, proptosis, extraocular muscle involvement, and less common decreased visual acuity

WORKUP

- A diagnosis of exclusion: need to rule out lymphoma and infectious causes of orbital inflammation
- H&P exam includes measurement of tumor diameter, location, and geometry
- Labs: CBC, LFTs, ESR, lumbar puncture – CSF for cytology, chemistry, and cytokine analysis
- Imaging: brain/orbit CT, MRI
- Tissue diagnosis: biopsy to rule out malignancy; may analyze with flow cytometry for clonality, immunohistochemistry

TREATMENT RECOMMENDATIONS

- First line: corticosteroids; ~50% patients have durable complete response
- If contraindications to steroid therapy, unacceptable toxicities with steroids, or refractory/recurrent: EBRT most commonly 20 Gy in 10 fx

TRIALS/STUDIES

- Lanciano (*IJROBP* 1990). Series of 26 orbits in 23 pts with orbital pseudotumor, of whom 87% had trial of corticosteroids before RT treated with 20 Gy in 10 fx. Results: 66% durable complete response; 11% had local relapse and went on to achieve CR with more treatment or spontaneously. 11% had PR; only 11% no response

RADIATION TECHNIQUES

- Simulation and field design: as per thyroid ophthalmopathy
- Dose prescription: 20 Gy in 2 Gy fxs

COMPLICATIONS

- Acute: mild skin erythema
- Late: depends on technique and shielding; includes cataracts, vitreous hemorrhage, retinopathy, hypopituitarism, and second tumors in field of irradiation, especially with and >60 Gy

FOLLOW-UP

- H&P every 3 mo for 1 yr, every 4 mo for 2nd yr, every 6 mo for 3rd & 4th yrs, then annually

REFERENCES

Akpek E, et al. Intraocular-central nervous system lymphoma: clinical features, diagnosis, and outcomes. Ophthalmology 1999;106: 1805–1810.

Bell D, et al. Choroidal melanoma: natural history and management options. Cancer Control 2004;11(5):296–303.

Bhatia S, et al. Curative radiotherapy for primary orbital lymphoma. IJROBP 2002;54:818–821.

Bolek T, et al. Radiotherapy in the management of orbital lymphoma. IJROBP 1999;44:31–36.

Chan C, Wallace D. Intraocular lymphoma: update on diagnosis and management. Cancer Control 2004;11(5):285–295.

Char D, Quivey J, et al. Helium ions versus I-125 brachytherapy in management of uveal melanoma. A prospective, dynamically balanced trial. Ophthalmology 1993;100:1547–1554.

Char D, et al. Primary intraocular lymphoma (ocular reticulum cell sarcoma) diagnosis and management. Ophthalmology 1988;95: 625–630.

COMS. The COMS randomized trial of pre-enucleation radiation of large choroidal melanoma II: initial mortality findings: COMS Report No. 10. Am J Ophth 1998;124:779–996.

COMS. The COMS randomized trial of iodine 125 brachytherapy for choroidal melanoma III: initial mortality findings: COMS Report No. 18. Arch Ophthalmol 2001;119:969–982.

Diener-West M, et al. Screening for metastasis from choroidal melanoma: the COMS Group Report 23. JCO 2004;22:2438–2444.

Esik O, et al. Retrospective analysis of different modalities for treatment of primary orbital non-Hodgkin's lymphomas. Radiother Oncol 1996;38:13–18.

Hoffman PM, et al. Intraocular lymphoma: a series of 14 patients with clinicopathological features and treatment outcomes. Eye 2003; 17:513–521.

Kath R, et al. Prognosis and treatment of disseminated uveal melanoma. Cancer 1993;72(7):2219–2223.

Kujala E, et al. Very long term prognosis of patients with malignant uveal melanoma. Investigative Ophthalmol Visual Sci 2003;44: 4651–4659.

Lanciano R, et al. The results of radiotherapy for orbital pseudotumor. IJROBP 1990;18:407.

Le Q, et al. Primary radiotherapy for localized orbital malt lymphoma. IJROBP 2002;52:657–663.

Nguyen LN, Ang K. The orbit. In: Cox J, Ang K, editors. Radiation Oncology. 8th ed. St. Louis: Mosby; 2003. pp 282–292.

Pelloski CE, et al. Clinical stage IEA-IIEA orbital lymphomas: outcomes in the era of modern staging and treatment, Radiother Oncol 2001;59:145–151.

Peterson IA, et al. Prognostic factors in the radiotherapy of Graves' ophthalmopathy. IJROBP 1990;19:259–264.

Peterson K, et al. The clinical spectrum of ocular lymphoma. Cancer 1993;72:843–849.

Prummel M, et al. Randomized double-blind trial of prednisone versus radiotherapy in Graves' ophthalmopathy. Lancet 1993;342: 949–954.

Quivey J, Char D, et al. High intensity 125-iodine (125I) plaque treatment of uveal melanoma. IJROBP 1993;26(4):613–618.

Quivey J, et al. Uveal melanoma. In: Leibel SA, Phillips TL, editors. Textbook of Radiation Oncology. 2nd ed. Philadelphia: Saunders; 2004. pp. 1443–1461.

Rosenthal S. Benign disease. In: Leibel SA, Phillips TL, editors. Textbook of Radiation Oncology. 2nd ed. Philadelphia: Saunders; 2004. pp. 1525–1543.

Shields C, Shields J. Diagnosis and management of retinoblastoma. Cancer Control 2004;11(5):317–327.

Shields J, et al. Survey of 1264 patients with orbital tumors and simulating lesions. Ophthalmology 2004;111:997–1008.

Stafford SL, et al. Orbital lymphoma: radiotherapy outcome and complications. Radiother Oncol 2001;59:139–144.

NOTES

Chapter 4
Cancer of the Ear

Eric K. Hansen and M. Kara Bucci

PEARLS

- The ear consists of the pinna (auricle), the external auditory canal, the tympanic membrane, the middle ear (containing the auditory ossicles), & the inner ear in the petrous portion of the temporal bone (consisting of the bony & membranous labyrinth)
- Lymphatic drainage is to parotid, retroauricular, & cervical nodes
- Tumors of the ear are rare. BCC is more common than SCC for the external ear, but SCC accounts for 85% of auditory canal, middle ear, & mastoid tumors. Nodal metastases occur in <15%

WORKUP

- H&P with otoscopy & careful LN exam. CBC, chemistries, BUN/Cr. CT, MRI. Biopsy. Audiology testing

STAGING

- No site-specific AJCC/UICC staging system for the ear exists; use histology appropriate staging (e.g., skin)

TREATMENT RECOMMENDATIONS

- Tumors of the external ear may be treated with surgery or RT (either EBRT or IS brachytherapy). Surgery is used if the lesion has invaded the cartilage or extends medially into the auditory canal. Advanced lesions or close/+ margins require post-op RT. Treatment of the lymphatics may be indicated for tumors >4 cm or for cartilage invasion.
- Tumors of the middle ear or temporal bone may be treated with surgery or RT. Surgery may require mastoidectomy or subtotal or total temporal bone resection. Post-op RT is generally required to increase LRC
- LC depends on extent of disease, and ranges from 40–100%

RADIATION TECHNIQUES
Simulation and field design
- Tumors of the pinna may be treated with electrons or orthovoltage photons. For small tumors, 1 cm margins are adequate, but for larger lesions, 2–3 cm margins are required
- Treatment volumes for tumors of the external auditory canal include the entire ear canal & temporal bone with 2–3 cm margin, & the ipsilateral preauricular, postauricular, & upper level II nodes
- Advanced or unresectable tumors may be treated with high energy electrons (energy appropriate to tumor depth) alone or mixed with photons
- Immobilization with a thermoplastic mask will be necessary
- Use bolus to fill external auditory canal & surrounding concha for pinna tumors to decease complications & improve superficial dose delivery

Dose prescriptions
- Tumors of the pinna may be treated with 1.8–2 Gy per fraction to 50 Gy for small, thin lesions <1.5 cm, 55 Gy for larger tumors, 60 Gy for minimal or suspected cartilage or bone invasion, or 65 Gy for large lesions with bone or cartilage invasion
- Tumors of the auditory canal or temporal bone should be treated to 60–70 Gy

Dose limitations
- Limit temporal bone to ≤70 Gy to minimize risk of osteoradionecrosis (~10% for doses >65 Gy)

COMPLICATIONS
- Cartilage necrosis of the pinna and/or temporal bone necrosis is possible if careful planning is not used
- Hearing compromise or loss
- Chronic otitis
- Xerostomia

FOLLOW-UP
- Frequent H&P with otoscopy every 3–4 mo for 1–2 yr, then every 6 mo for 1–2 yr, then annually

REFERENCES

Chao KSC, Devineni VR. Ear. In: Perez CA, Brady LW, Halperin EC, et al., editors. Principles and Practice of Radiation Oncology. 4th ed. Philadelphia: Lippincott Williams & Wilkins; 2004. pp. 897–904.

Hussey DH, Wen B-C. The temporal bone, ear, and paraganglia. In: Cox JD, Ang KK, editors. Radiation Oncology: Rationale, Technique, Results. 8th ed. St. Louis: Mosby; 2003. pp. 293–309.

Pfreundner L, Schwager K, Willner J, et al. Carcinoma of the external auditory canal and middle ear. Int J Radiat Oncol Biol Phys 1999;44:777–788.

NOTES

Chapter 5
Nasopharyngeal Cancer

Eric K. Hansen, James Rembert, and M. Kara Bucci

PEARLS

- Uncommon in U.S., but WHO III (undifferentiated) common in Southern China & Hong Kong (e.g., 3rd most common cancer among men in Hong Kong)
- Strongly associated with EBV (70% of pts have + titers)
- Two peak ages: 15–25 yrs & 50–60 yrs. More common among men (2 : 1)
- Alcohol & tobacco are associated with WHO type I (keratinizing SCC)
- Borders of the nasopharynx: anterior = posterior end of nasal septum & choanae; posterior = clivus & C1-2 vertebral bodies; superior = sphenoid bone/sinus; inferior = roof of soft palate
- The parapharyngeal & masticator spaces are lateral to the nasopharynx. Extension to the parapharyngeal space can cause symptoms relating to involvement of CN IX-XII. Involvement of the masticator space causes trismus
- The Eustachian tubes enter the lateral nasopharynx, & the posterior aspect of the orifice creates a protuberance (torus tubarius). Rosenmueller's fossa is posterior to the torus tubarius and is the #1 location for nasopharyngeal cancer
- Tumors spread along the walls of nasopharynx, & can occlude the Eustachian tube, erode into bone, & involve CN V2 (foramen rotundum) or CN V3 (foramen ovale). Tumors can also invade the foramen lacerum to the cavernous sinus (containing CN III, IV, V1, V2, VI) & the middle cranial fossa
- 90% of tumors are SCC: WHO type 1 (keratinizing SCC, 20% of cases in the U.S.), WHO type 2 (non-keratinizing SCC), & WHO type 3 (undifferentiated carcinoma, 99% of cases where endemic)
- Lymphoepithelioma = SCC with lymphoid component. It has higher LRC, but the same OS due to an increased rate of DM

- Other tumors include lymphoma, minor salivary gland tumors, plasmacytomas, melanomas, chordomas, & rhabdomyosarcomas
- <10% of tumors have intracranial extension
- 70% of pts have clinically involved lymph nodes, 90% have subclinical nodes, & 40–50% have bilateral nodes
- Metastases correlate with N stage (but not T stage): N0-N1 = 10–20% DM, N2 = 30–40% DM, & N3 = 40–70% DM
- Before IMRT, recurrence was predominantly local, but with IMRT, distant recurrence is more common than LR

WORKUP

- H&P. Common signs/symptoms include hearing loss, otitis media, neck mass, nasal obstruction, epistaxis, headache, diplopia, trismus. Perform fiberoptic nasopharyngolaryngoscopy & thorough oropharyngeal & neck exam. Also perform otoscopy. Thorough CN exam is critical
- Labs: CBC, LFTs, BUN/Cr, baseline TSH, EBV IgA/DNA titer
- MRI head/neck with contrast; +/– CT head/neck with contrast. CT optimally demonstrates cortical bone, & MRI, medullary bone. A normal-appearing basisphenoid (clivus) on CT may demonstrate marked tumor infiltration on MRI
- CXR. For Stage III/IV, consider CT of chest & abdomen ± bone scan
- Consider PET scan
- All pts should have a pre-RT dental evaluation & audiology testing

STAGING

Primary tumor	
TX:	Primary tumor cannot be assessed
T0:	No evidence of primary tumor
Tis:	Carcinoma in situ
T1:	Tumor confined to the nasopharynx
T2:	Tumor extends to soft tissues
	T2a: Tumor extends to the oropharynx and/or nasal cavity without parapharyngeal extension*
	T2b: Any tumor with parapharyngeal extension*
T3:	Tumor involves bony structures and/or paranasal sinuses
T4:	Tumor with intracranial extension, and/or involvement of cranial nerves, infratemporal fossa, hypopharynx, orbit, or masticator space

* Parapharyngeal extension denotes posterolateral infiltration of tumor beyond the pharyngobasilar fascia

STAGING

Regional lymph nodes	
NX:	No regional lymph node metastasis cannot be assessed
N0:	No regional lymph node metastasis
N1:	Unilateral metastasis in lymph node(s), 6 cm or less in greatest dimension, above the supraclavicular fossa
N2:	Bilateral metastasis in lymph node(s), 6 cm or less in greatest dimension, above the supraclavicular fossa
N3:	Metastasis in lymph node(s) >6 cm and/or to supraclavicular fossa
	N3a: Greater than 6 cm in dimension
	N3b: Extension to the supraclavicular fossa

Distant metastasis	
MX:	Distant metastasis cannot be assessed
M0:	No distant metastasis
M1:	Distant metastasis

Stage Grouping		~3yr OS by Stage	
0:	TisN0M0		
I :	T1N0M0	I:	70–100%
IIA:	T2aN0M0	II:	65–100%
IIB:	T2bN0M0, T1-2N1M0		
III:	T3N0M0, T3N1M0, T1-3N2M0	III:	60–90%
IVA:	T4N0-2M0	IV	50–70%
IVB:	Any T, N3, M0		
IVC:	Any T, any N, M1		

Used with the permission of the American Joint Committee on Cancer (AJCC), Chicago, Illinois. The original source for this material is the AJCC Cancer Staging Manual, Sixth Edition (2002) published by Springer-Verlag New York, www.springeronline.com.

TREATMENT RECOMMENDATIONS

Stage	Recommended Treatment
Stage I-IIA	RT alone (2/70 Gy)
Stage IIB-IVB	Concurrent chemo-RT followed by adjuvant chemo ■ 2/70 Gy + cisplatin 100 mg/m^2 on days 1, 21, 42 → cisplatin/5-FU ×3c ■ Neck dissection for persistent/recurrent neck nodes
Stage IVC	Platinum-based combination chemo
Local recurrence	Re-irradiation with IMRT, SRS, or brachytherapy. Cumulative dose is limited to respect surrounding normal tissue tolerance(s). Alternative, surgery

STUDIES

- Al-Sarraf, Int 0099 (*JCO* 1998). 147 pts with Stage III-IV disease randomized to RT (2/70 Gy) vs chemo-RT (2/70 Gy + concurrent cisplatin → adjuvant cisplatin/5-FU × 3 cycles). Used old staging, so many stage II would now be included. Chemo-RT improved 3 yr OS (47→78%) & PFS (24→69%). Trial stopped early due to OS benefit. Criticized because poor LRC & OS for RT alone group, & high % of WHO I tumors (rare outside U.S.)
- Wee (*JCO* 2005). Confirmed Int 0099 with 221 pts from Singapore with stage III-IV disease & same randomization as Int 0099. Chemo-RT improved 2 yr OS (78→85%), DFS (57→75%), & DM (30→13%)
- Chan (*J Natl Cancer Inst* 2005). 350 pts from Hong Kong with Ho's N2/3 or N1 >4 cm randomized to RT alone vs RT + weekly cisplatin 40 mg/m^2. Chemo-RT increased 5 yr OS (59→70%) & PFS (52→60%)
- Lin (*NEJM* 2004). 99 pts with III-IV disease had EBV titer followed. EBV titer <1500 copies/ml had increased OS & RFS. Persistently elevated EBV titer 1 wk after completion of sequential chemo-RT had worse OS, RFS
- Lee, UCSF (*IJROBP* 2002, 2003). 67 pts treated with IMRT to 70 Gy. Excellent 4 yr OS (88%) & LRC (97%)

RADIATION TECHNIQUES
Simulation and field design

- Patient set-up supine and immobilized with head & neck thermoplastic mask or equivalent device
- Planning CT scan obtained with IV contrast if available. A pre-chemo MRI is critical for definition of GTV. Use CT-MRI fusion if available
- In every case, the entire GTV must be treated to the entire prescription dose. Except in the case of very early T1-T2N0 tumors, it is not possible to accomplish this without exceeding normal tissue tolerances with conventional 2D planning. 3DCRT or IMRT is necessary for the final cone down
- IMRT volumes: GTV = gross disease. CTV1 includes the entire nasopharynx, sphenoid sinus, cavernous sinus, base of skull, posterior 1/2 of nasal cavity (~2 cm), posterior 1/3 of maxillary sinuses, posterior ethmoid sinus, pterygoid fossa, lateral & posterior pharyngeal walls to the level of the mid-tonsillar fossa, the retropharyngeal nodes, & bilateral cervical nodes including level V &

supraclavicular nodes. CTV2 includes low-risk nodal regions as determined by the clinician per case

- Conventional setup = 3 fields (lateral opposed for primary & upper neck, matched to a low neck field). Use a central larynx block on low neck field
- Conventional borders: superior = cover sphenoid sinus & base of skull. Inferior = match plane above true vocal cord (to block larynx in AP field). Posterior = spinous processes. Anterior = 2–3 cm anterior to GTV (& include pterygoid plates and posterior 1/3 of maxillary sinuses)
- If supraclavicular nodes +, then use a mediastinal 8 cm wide T-field with inferior border 5 cm below the head of the clavicle
- Use wedges and compensators as needed

Dose prescriptions

- Conventional: 2 Gy/fx to 44 Gy → off cord boost to 50 Gy with a posterior neck electron field → conedown to GTV + 2 cm margin to 70 Gy. For the neck, N0 = 50 Gy, nodes <3 cm = 66 Gy, & nodes ≥3 cm = 70 Gy
- IMRT: GTV = 2.12/70 Gy, CTV1 = 1.8/59.4 Gy, CTV2 = 1.64/54 Gy in 33 fx
- Rotterdam NPX applicator: optional boost after 66–70 Gy to gross disease. Use 1 wk after EBRT (T1-T3 60 Gy EBRT → HDR 3 Gy ×6; T4 70 Gy EBRT → HDR 3 Gy ×4)

Dose limitations

- EBRT: partial brain 60 Gy, brainstem 50–54 Gy (60 Gy point dose), cord 45–50 Gy, optic chiasm 50–54 Gy, retina 45 Gy, lens 10 Gy, lacrimal gland 30 Gy, ear (sensorineuronal hearing loss) 45–50 Gy, parotid V24 <50%, TMJ <70 Gy
- SRS: brainstem 12 Gy, optic nerves or chiasm 8 Gy

COMPLICATIONS

- Acute: mucositis, dermatitis, xerostomia
- Late: soft tissue fibrosis, trismus, xerostomia, hearing loss, osteoradionecrosis, hypothyroidism, and hypopituitarism (if included)

FOLLOW-UP

- H&P every 1–3 mo 1st yr, every 2–4 mo 2nd yr, every 4–6 mo yrs 3–5, then every 6–12 mo

- MRI at 2 & 4 mo post-RT, then every 6 mo or as clinically indicated
- TSH every 6–12 mo

REFERENCES

Al-Sarraf M, LeBlanc M, Giri PG, et al. Chemoradiotherapy versus radio-therapy in patients with advanced nasopharyngeal cancer: phase III randomized Intergroup study 0099. J Clin Oncol 1998;16:1310–1317.

Chan AT, Leung SF, Ngan RK, et al. Overall survival after concurrent cisplatin-radiotherapy compared with radiotherapy alone in locore-gionally advanced nasopharyngeal carcinoma. J Natl Cancer Inst 2005;97:536–539.

Chao KC, Perez CA. Nasopharynx. In: Perez CA, Brady LW, Halperin EC, et al., editors. Principles and Practice of Radiation Oncology. 4th ed. Philadelphia: Lippincott Williams & Wilkins; 2004. pp. 918–961.

Garden AS. The nasopharynx. In: Cox JD, Ang KK, editors. Radiation Oncology: Rationale, Technique, Results. 8th ed. St. Louis: Mosby; 2003. pp. 178–195.

Greene FL, American Joint Committee on Cancer., American Cancer Society. AJCC Cancer Staging Manual. 6th ed. New York: Springer-Verlag; 2002.

Lee N, Xia P, Quivey JM, et al. Intensity-modulated radiotherapy in the treatment of nasopharyngeal carcinoma: an update of the UCSF experience. Int J Radiat Oncol Biol Phys 2002;53:12–22.

Lee N, Xia P, Fischbein NJ, et al. Intensity-modulated radiation therapy for head-and-neck cancer: the UCSF experience focusing on target volume delineation. Int J Radiat Oncol Biol Phys 2003;57:49–60.

Lee N, Fu K. Cancer of the nasopharynx. In: Leibel SA, Phillips TL, editors. Textbook of Radiation Oncology. 2nd ed. Philadelphia: Saunders; 2004. pp. 579–600.

Lin JC, Wang WY, Chen KY, et al. Quantification of plasma Epstein-Barr virus DNA in patients with advanced nasopharyngeal carcinoma. N Engl J Med 2004;350:2461–2470.

National Comprehensive Cancer Network. Clinical Practice Guidelines in Oncology: Head and Neck Cancers. Available at: http://www.nccn.org/professionals/physician_gls/PDF/head-and-neck.pdf. Accessed on January 19, 2005.

National Cancer Institute. Nasopharyngeal Cancer (PDQ): Treatment. Available at: http://cancer.gov/cancertopics/pdq/treatment/nasopha-ryngeal/healthprofessional/. Accessed on January 19, 2005.

Wee J, Tan EH, Tai BC, et al. Randomized trial of radiotherapy versus concurrent chemo-radiotherapy followed by adjuvant chemotherapy in patients with American Joint Committee on Cancer/International Union Against Cancer Stage III and IV nasopharyngeal cancer of the endemic variety. J Clin Oncol 2005;23:6730–6738.

Chapter 6
Nasal Cavity and Paranasal Sinus Cancer

Brian Missett and M. Kara Bucci

PEARLS

- Maxillary cancers are most common (70%)
- Incidence higher in Japan and South Africa
- More common in males (4:1)
- Ohngren's line runs from the medial canthus to the angle of the mandible
- Tumors superior-posterior to Ohngren's line have a poorer prognosis
- Histology: most common is SCC. Adenoid cystic, esthesioneuroblastoma, plasmacytoma, lymphoma, melanoma and sarcoma also seen
- See Chapter 12, "Unusual Neoplasms of the Head & Neck," for more information on esthesioneuroblastoma

WORKUP

- H&P, nasal endoscopy, CT/MRI, biopsy, CXR

STAGING

Primary tumor – Maxillary Sinus	
Tis:	Carcinoma in situ
T1:	Tumor limited to maxillary sinus mucosa with no erosion or destruction of bone
T2:	Tumor causing bone erosion or destruction including extension into the hard palate &/or middle nasal meatus, except extension to posterior wall of the maxillary sinus & pterygoid plates
T3:	Tumor invades any of the following: posterior wall of maxillary sinus, subcutaneous tissues, floor or medial wall of orbit, pterygoid fossa, &/or ethmoid sinuses
T4a:	Tumor invades anterior orbital contents, skin of cheek, pterygoid plates, infratemporal fossa, cribriform plate, sphenoid or frontal sinuses

T4b: Tumor invades any of the following: orbital apex, dura, brain, middle cranial fossa, cranial nerves other than maxillary division of trigerminal verve (V2), nasopharynx, or clivus

Primary tumor – Ethmoid Sinus & Nasal Cavity
Ethmoid Sinus Subsites: Right, Left
Nasal Cavity Subsites: Septum, Wall, Floor, Vestibule
Tis: Carcinoma in situ
T1: Tumor restricted to any one subsite, with or without bony invasion
T2: Tumor invading two subsites in single region or extending to involve an adjacent region within the nasothemoidal complex, with or without bony invasion
T3: Tumor extends to invade the medial wall or floor of orbit, maxillary sinus, palate, or cribriform plate
T4a: Tumor invades any of the following: anterior orbital contents, skin of nose or cheek, minimal extension to anterior cranial fossa, pterygoid plates, sphenoid or frontal sinuses
T4b: Tumor invades any of the following: orbital apex, dura, brain, middle cranial fossa, cranial nerves other than V2, nasopharynx, or clivus

Regional lymph nodes
Nx: Regional lymph nodes cannot be assessed
N1: Metastasis in a single ipsilateral lymph node, 3 cm or less in greatest dimension
N2a: Metastasis in a single ipsilateral lymph node more than 3 cm but not more than 6 cm in greatest dimension
N2b: Metastasis in multiple ipsilateral lymph nodes, none more than 6 cm in greatest dimension
N2c: Metastasis in bilateral or contralateral lymph nodes, none more than 6 cm in greatest dimension
N3: Metastasis in a lymph node, more than 6 cm in greatest dimension

Metastases
Mx: Distant metastasis cannot be assessed
M0: No distant metastasis
M1: Distant metastasis

Stage Grouping		~2/5 yr OS (Maxillary Sinus)	
0	TisN0M0	I:	80/55%
I	T1N0M0	II:	67/44%
II	T2N0M0	III:	60/40%
III	T3N0, T1-3N1M0	IV:	51/27%
IVA	T4aN0-1, T1-4aN2M0		
IVB	T4b any N, Any T N3M0		
IVC	Any M1		

TREATMENT RECOMMENDATIONS

Stage	Recommended Treatment
Nasal cavity & ethmoid sinus	■ T1-2N0: Resection → post-op RT for close/+ margins or PNI. Alternatively, definitive RT. Choice depends on size, location & expected cosmetic outcome ■ T3-4N0: resectable: Resection → post-op RT ■ Unresectable or inoperable: Definitive RT or chemo-RT ■ N+: Resection + neck dissection → post-op RT or chemo-RT. Alternatively, definitive chemo-RT
Maxillary sinus	■ T1-2N0: Resection → post-op RT for close margin, PNI, adenoidcystic. For + margin, re-resect (if possible) → post-op RT ■ T3-4N0 resectable: Resection → post-op RT or chemo-RT ■ Unresectable or inoperable: Definitive RT or chemo-RT ■ N+: Resection + neck dissection → post-op RT or chemo-RT. Alternatively, definitive chemo-RT

STUDIES

- Le (*IJROBP* 2000). 97 pts with maxillary sinus tumors. 12% LN relapse at 5 yrs. Initial SCC N0 pts treated with RT did not have neck failures
- Although not included in the studies, some physicians extrapolate from the Bernier and Cooper studies (*NEJM* 2004) to support using post-op concurrent chemo and RT in patients with SCC of the paranasal sinuses

RADIATION TECHNIQUES
Simulation and field design
- Simulate supine with thermoplastic mask immobilization
- Eyes open, straight ahead to keep posterior pole away from high dose region
- Tongue blade/cork to depress tongue out of fields
- Fill surgical defects with tissue equivalents
- Recommend 3DCRT or IMRT planning to increase sparing of normal structures
- GTV = clinical &/or radiographic gross disease. CTV1 = 0.5–2 cm margin on primary &/or nodal GTV (depending on presence or absence of anatomic boundaries to microscopic spread). CTV2 = elective neck. Individualized planning target volumes are used for the GTV, CTV1, & CTV2
- Generally no elective nodal RT for nasal cavity tumors

Dose prescriptions
- EBRT 1.8–2 Gy/fx
- Definitive RT or chemo-RT: GTV to 66–70 Gy, CTV1 to 60 Gy, CTV2 to 50–54 Gy
- Post-op RT: CTV1 to 60 Gy with optional boost to 66 Gy to high-risk areas (close/+ margins, ECE, PNI). CTV2 to 50–54 Gy
- For selected nasal cavity tumors, brachytherapy may be appropriate. Use equivalent doses

Dose limitations
- Lens <10 Gy (cataracts)
- Retina <45 Gy (vision). May go higher if treating bid or partial volume
- Mandible <60 Gy (osteoradionecrosis)
- Brain <70 Gy (necrosis)
- Parotid mean dose <26 Gy (xerostomia)
- Optic chiasm and nerves <54 Gy at standard fractionation
- Lacrimal gland <30–40 Gy

COMPLICATIONS
- Acute = mucositis, skin erythema, nasal dryness, xerostomia
- Late = xerostomia, chronic keratitis & iritis, optic pathway injury, soft tissue or osteoradionecrosis, cataracts

FOLLOW-UP

- H&P, labs, & CXR every 3 mo for 1st yr, every 4 mo for 2nd yr, every 6 mo for 3rd yr, then annually. Imaging of the H&N at 3 mo post-treatment, then as indicated

REFERENCES

Barker J, Ang KK. Nasal cavity and paranasal sinuses. In: Perez CA, Brady LW, Halperin EC, et al., editors. Principles and Practice of Radiation Oncology. 4th ed. Philadelphia: Lippincott Williams & Wilkins; 2004. pp. 962–975.

Le QT, Fu KK, Kaplan MJ, et al. Lymph node metastasis in maxillary sinus carcinoma. Int J Radiat Oncol Biol Phys 2000;46:541–549.

National Comprehensive Cancer Network. Clinical Practice Guidelines in Oncology: Head and Neck Cancers. Available at: http://www.nccn. org/professionals/physician_gls/PDF/head-and-neck.pdf. Accessed on January 19, 2005.

National Cancer Institute. Paranasal Sinus and Nasal Cavity Cancer (PDQ): Treatment. Available at: http://cancer.gov/cancertopics/pdq/ treatment/paranasalsinus/healthprofessional/. Accessed on January 19, 2005.

Nguyen L, Ang KK. The nasal fossa and paranasal sinuses. In: Cox JD, Ang KK, editors. Radiation Oncology: Rationale, Technique, Results. 8th ed. St. Louis: Mosby; 2003. pp. 160–177.

Ryu JK. Cancer of the nasal cavity and paranasal sinuses. In: Leibel SA, Phillips TL, editors. Textbook of Radiation Oncology. 2nd ed. Philadelphia: Saunders; 2004. pp. 731–756.

NOTES

Chapter 7
Oropharyngeal Cancer

Kim Huang and Jeanne Marie Quivey

PEARLS

- ~8500 cases/year in U.S. with male predominance (3:1)
- Etiologies include consumption of alcohol, tobacco, betal and areca nuts, and HPV infection
- Second primary tumors in the upper aerodigestive tract and lung occur in ~25% of pts due to risk factors & lifestyle
- Subsites: soft palate, tonsils, tonsillar pillars, base of tongue, pharyngeal wall
- Anatomic boundaries: superior = plane of superior surface of soft palate; inferior = superior surface of hyoid bone (or floor of vallecula)
- Ear pain may be referred via the tympanic nerve of Jacobson (CN IX) via the petrosal ganglion
- Histology: 95% SCC, others = adenocarcinoma, mucoepidermoid, adenoid cystic, melanoma, small cell carcinoma of tonsil, non-Hodgkin's lymphoma of tonsil
- Presentation: sore throat, dysphagia, otalgia, odynophagia, hot potato voice (with base of tongue invasion), hoarseness (with larynx invasion)

WORKUP

- H&P. Palpation, indirect mirror exam, flexible endoscopy
- Panendoscopy with biopsy
- Labs: CBC, chemistries, BUN, Cr, LFTs including alkaline phosphatase
- Imaging: MRI with contrast ± CT scan with contrast of head and neck. PET scan. CXR or CT chest. Panorex as indicated
- Preventive dental care with extractions 10–14 days before RT
- Speech & swallow evaluation as indicated

STAGING

<u>Primary tumor</u>

TX:	Primary tumor cannot be assessed
T0:	No evidence of primary tumor
Tis:	Carcinoma in situ
T1:	Tumor 2 cm or less in greatest dimension
T2:	Tumor more than 2 cm but not more than 4 cm in greatest dimension
T3:	Tumor more than 4 cm in greatest dimension
T4a:	Tumor invades the larynx, deep/extrinsic muscle of tongue, medial pterygoid, hard palate, or mandible
T4b:	Tumor invades lateral pterygoid muscle, pterygoid plates, lateral nasopharynx, or skull base or encases internal carotid artery

<u>Regional lymph nodes</u>

NX:	Regional lymph nodes cannot be assessed
N0:	No regional lymph node metastasis
N1:	Metastasis in a single ipsilateral lymph node, 3 cm or less in greatest dimension
N2a:	Metastasis in a single ipsilateral lymph node, more than 3 cm but not more than 6 cm in greatest dimension
N2b:	Metastasis in multiple ipsilateral lymph nodes, none more than 6 cm in greatest dimension
N2c:	Metastasis in bilateral or contralateral lymph nodes, none more than 6 cm in greatest dimension
N3:	Metastasis in a lymph node more than 6 cm in greatest dimension

<u>Distant Metastases</u>

MX:	Distant metastasis cannot be assessed
M0:	No distant metastasis
M1:	Distant metastasis

Stage Grouping		~2 yr Survival	
0:	TisN0M0	I:	75%
I:	T1N0M0	II:	70%
II:	T2N0M0	III:	55%
III:	T3N0M0, T1-3N1M0	IVA:	40%
IVA:	T4aN0-1M0, T1-4aN2M0	IVB:	20%
IVB:	Any T, N3M0; T4b, any N, M0	IVC:	10%
IVC:	Any T, any N, M1		

Used with the permission of the American Joint Committee on Cancer (AJCC), Chicago, Illinois. The original source for this material is the AJCC Cancer Staging Manual, Sixth Edition (2002) published by Springer-Verlag New York, www.springeronline.com.

TREATMENT RECOMMENDATIONS

Stage	Recommended Treatment
I–II	Definitive RT to 66–72 Gy. Alternative, surgery with post-op RT as indicated
III–IV	Concurrent chemo-RT (preferred). Alternative, surgery with post-op (chemo-)RT as indicated. For pts not considered candidates for standard chemo-RT (e.g., with cisplatin), consider RT + cetuximab. If unable to tolerate concurrent chemo, altered fractionation RT may be used

Surgery
- For T3-4 primaries, tonsillar lesions require radical tonsillectomy often with partial mandibulectomy; base of tongue lesions require partial or total glossectomy & myocutaneous flap reconstruction. Patients requiring removal of more than 1/2 of tongue or elderly patients with poor pulmonary function often require total laryngectomy to prevent subsequent aspiration. Therefore, for locally advanced oropharyngeal primary, organ preservation approach with chemo-RT is preferred

Types of neck dissection
- Radical neck dissection (RND) removes levels I-V, sternocleidomastoid muscle, omohyoid muscle, internal and external jugular veins, CN XI, & the submandibular gland
- Modified RND leaves ≥1 of sternocleidomastoid muscle, internal jugular vein, or CN XI
- Selective neck dissection does not remove ≥1 level of levels I–V
- Supraomohyoid neck dissection only removes levels I–III
- Lateral neck dissection only removes levels II–IV

Post-op RT or chemo-RT
- Post-op chemo-RT indications (major risk factors): extracapsular nodal spread, + margins
- Post-op RT indications (minor risk factors): close margin, multiple LN+, PNI, LVSI

STUDIES
Pre-op vs post-op RT

- RTOG 73-03 (*Head Neck Surg* 1987, *IJROBP* 1991). 354 pts with advanced H&N cancer randomized to 2/50 Gy pre-op vs 2/50/60 Gy post-op. Post-op RT improved LRC (48→65%), & OS for oropharynx lesions (26→38%). Complications not different

Altered fractionation

- RTOG 90-03 (Fu, *IJROBP* 2000). 268 pts with locally-advanced H&N cancer randomized to 2/70 Gy vs 1.2 bid/81.6 Gy vs split-course 1.6 bid/67.2 Gy (with a 2 wk break) vs concomitant boost RT to 72 Gy [with bid RT for last 12 fractions (1.8 Gy & 1.5 Gy)]. Concomitant boost & hyperfractionated RT improved 2 yr LRC (54%), DFS (39%), & OS (53%) compared to standard or split-course accelerated RT. Altered fractionation increased acute side effects
- EORTC (Horiot, *Radiother Oncol* 1992). 325 pts with T2-3 oropharyngeal cancer randomized to 2/70 Gy vs 1.15 bid/80.5 Gy. BID RT increased 5 yr LC (40→59%) & OS (31→47%) with benefit primarily for T3 tumors

Chemo-RT +/− altered fractionation

- GORTEC 94-01 (Calais/Denis, *JCO* 2004). 226 pts with stage III/IV oropharyngeal cancer randomized to 2/70 Gy vs 2/70 Gy + carboplatin/5-FU ×3 cycles. Chemo-RT improved LC (25→48%), DFS (15→27%), & OS (16→23, p = 0.13), but increased acute toxicity. Trend for increased late toxicity
- Adelstein, Intergroup (*JCO* 2003). 295 pts with unresectable H&N cancer, randomized to 2/70 Gy vs 2/70 Gy + cisplatin (100 mg/m^2) ×3 cycles vs split-course RT (2/30 Gy + 2/30–40 Gy) + cisplatin/5-FU ×3 cycles. Results: Chemo-RT improved 3 yr OS (23 vs 37 vs 27%) & DFS (33 vs 51 vs 41%), but did not change DM & it increased toxicity
- Brizel Duke (*NEJM* 1998). 116 pts w/advanced H&N cancer randomized to 1.25 bid/75 Gy vs 1.25 bid/70 Gy (with 1 wk break at 40 Gy) + concurrent cisplatin/5-FU ×2 cycles. Both arms received adjuvant cisplatin/5-FU ×2 cycles. Chemo-RT improved LC (44→70%), DFS (41→61%), & OS (34→55%). No change DM or toxicity
- Bonner (*NEJM* 2006). 424 pts with locoregionally advanced resectable or unresectable stage III–IV SCC of

oropharynx, larynx, or hypopharynx randomized to RT or RT + cetuximab given 1 wk before RT & weekly during RT. RT options included 2/70 Gy, 1.2 bid/72–76.8 Gy, or concomitant boost 72 Gy. Cetuximab increased 3 yr LRC (34 → 47%) & OS (45 → 55%). With the exception of acneiform rash & infusion reactions with cetuximab, toxicity was similar

Post-op chemo-RT

- <u>EORTC 22931</u> (*IJROBP* 2001, *NEJM* 2004). 334 pts with operable stage III/IV H&N cancer randomized to post-op 2/66 Gy vs post-op 2/66 Gy + concurrent cisplatin (100 mg/m^2) on days 1, 22, & 43. Eligibility: oral cavity, oropharynx, hypopharynx, & larynx with pT3-4N0/+, T1-2N2-3, or T1-2N0-1 with ECE, +margin, or PNI. Chemo-RT improved 3/5 yr DFS (41/36→59/47%) OS (49/40→ 65/53%), & 5 yr LRC (69→82%). No difference in DM (21–25%) or 2nd primaries (12%). Chemo-RT increased grade 3/4 toxicities (21→41%)
- <u>RTOG 95-01</u> (*NEJM* 2004). 459 pts with operable H&N cancer who had ≥2 LN, ECE, or + margin randomized to post-op RT (2/60–66 Gy) vs post-op chemo-RT (2/60–66 + cisplatin ×3 cycles same as EORTC). Chemo-RT improved 2 yr DFS (43→54%), LRC (72→82%), & had trend for improved OS (57→63%). No difference in DM (20–23%). Chemo-RT increased grade 3/4 toxicities (34→77%)

Meta-analysis for chemo

- <u>Pignon meta-analysis</u> (*Lancet* 2000). No significant benefit with adjuvant or neoadjuvant chemo, but concomitant chemo-RT provided a 7% absolute 2–5 yr OS benefit. Also, benefit to cisplatin & 5-FU vs other regimens

TECHNIQUES
Simulation and field design

- Simulate patient supine with head hyperextended. Wire neck scars & consider wiring commissure of lips. Shoulders may be pulled down with straps. Immobilize with a thermoplastic mask. Use a bite block. Bolus may be needed
- CT planning with MRI fusion may be used
- 3DCRT or IMRT provides improved normal tissue sparing & is used most frequently

■ Conventional volumes cover the skull base & mastoid to the supraclavicular nodes with a 3-field technique (opposed laterals matched to AP lower neck field). Beam-split above larynx at thyroid notch if possible

■ The spinal cord is shielded on lateral fields at the match-line if no nodes present, or on the AP field if larynx not involved. If cN0, a 1.5–2 cm midline block may spare larynx and cord on AP field

■ The anterior border includes a 2 cm margin on the tumor & includes the faucial arch, & a portion of the buccal mucosa and oral tongue. Include level IB if buccal mucosa or N+

■ Treat bilateral neck unless T1-2 tonsil or small faucial arch. For T1N0 tonsil, may leave out levels IV–V

■ For BOT, may leave out hard palate superiorly

■ Lymph node coverage: N0 include levels II–IV & retropharyngeal nodes. N1 include levels IB–IV & retropharyngeal nodes; N2-3 include IB–V & retropharyngeal nodes

■ Compensating filters required

■ After 45 Gy, the posterior neck is blocked and boosted with electrons

■ Ipsilateral wedged pair may be used for tonsil primaries to reduce dose to contralateral salivary glands

■ Base of tongue implants may be done, but controversial as to whether adds to LRC or decrease in morbidity

Dose prescriptions

■ Definitive (chemo-)RT: 1.8–2 Gy/fx to 70 Gy for primary & gross LN, 60 Gy to high-risk neck, & 50–54 Gy to low-risk neck. Post-op RT: 60–66 Gy to primary & high-risk neck, 50–54 Gy to low-risk neck

■ Concomitant boost: 1.8 Gy/fx × 18 (to 32.4 Gy) → 1.8 Gy to the large volume in the AM + 1.5 Gy to the boost volume ≥6 hrs later in the PM for last 12 days to 72 Gy total dose

■ UCSF IMRT: GTV = clinical &/or radiographic gross disease (primary & nodal). CTV1 = 0.5–2 cm margin on the primary & nodal GTV (with margin size depending on presence or absence of anatomic boundaries to microscopic spread). CTV2 = elective neck. Dose: GTV 2.12/69.96 Gy, CTV1 1.8/59.4 Gy, CTV2 1.64/54 Gy in 33 fx

Dose limitations

■ Spinal cord <45 Gy, brainstem <54 Gy, parotid glands mean dose < 26 Gy &/or attempt to keep 50% volume of each parotid ≤20 Gy (if possible), mandible <70 Gy, retina <45 Gy

COMPLICATIONS

- Acute & chronic mucositis, xerostomia
- Skin reaction treated with Aquafor, Radiacare, Domeboro's solution
- Preventive dental care with extractions before XRT, intensive fluoride treatment, mouth washing, & gargling with antiseptics
- Severe nutritional problems occur in 10% of pts. Need minimum 2000 cal/d diet. Use Ensure or Boost prn. Feeding tube controversial
- Risk of pharyngocutaneous fistula related to surgery, not RT
- Flap reconstruction decreases complications
- Mandibular necrosis uncommon, carotid a rupture <1%
- Amifostine can be used to decrease acute and late xerostomia

FOLLOW-UP

- Every 1–2 mo for 1 yr, every 3 mo for yrs 2–3, every 6 mo for yrs 4–5, then annually
- If recurrence suspected but biopsy is negative, follow-up monthly until resolved
- 85–90% of LRR occur within 3 yrs

REFERENCES

Adelstein DJ, Li Y, Adams GL, et al. An intergroup phase III comparison of standard radiation therapy and two schedules of concurrent chemoradiotherapy in patients with unresectable squamous cell head and neck cancer. J Clin Oncol 2003;21:92–98.

Bernier J, Domenge C, Ozsahin M, et al. Postoperative irradiation with or without concomitant chemotherapy for locally advanced head and neck cancer. N Engl J Med 2004;350:1945–1952.

Bonner JA, Harari PM, Giralt J, et al. Radiotherapy plus cetuximab for squamous-cell carcinoma of the head and neck. N Engl J Med 2006;354:567–578.

Brizel DM, Albers ME, Fisher SR, et al. Hyperfractionated irradiation with or without concurrent chemotherapy for locally advanced head and neck cancer. N Engl J Med 1998;338:1798–1804.

Calais G, Alfonsi M, Bardet E, et al. Randomized trial of radiation therapy versus concomitant chemotherapy and radiation therapy for advanced-stage oropharynx carcinoma. J Natl Cancer Inst 1999; 91:2081–2086.

Cooper JS, Pajak TF, Forastiere AA, et al. Postoperative concurrent radiotherapy and chemotherapy for high-risk squamous-cell carcinoma of the head and neck. N Engl J Med 2004;350:1937–1944.

Denis F, Garaud P, Bardet E, et al. Final results of the 94-01 French Head and Neck Oncology and Radiotherapy Group randomized trial comparing radiotherapy alone with concomitant radiochemotherapy in advanced-stage oropharynx carcinoma. J Clin Oncol 2004; 22:69–76.

Fu KK, Pajak TF, Trotti A, et al. A Radiation Therapy Oncology Group (RTOG) phase III randomized study to compare hyperfractionation and two variants of accelerated fractionation to standard fractionation radiotherapy for head and neck squamous cell carcinomas: first report of RTOG 9003. Int J Radiat Oncol Biol Phys 2000; 48:7–16.

Horiot JC, Le Fur R, N'Guyen T, et al. Hyperfractionation versus conventional fractionation in oropharyngeal carcinoma: final analysis of a randomized trial of the EORTC cooperative group of radiotherapy. Radiother Oncol 1992;25:231–241.

Kramer S, Gelber RD, Snow JB, et al. Combined radiation therapy and surgery in the management of advanced head and neck cancer: final report of study 73-03 of the Radiation Therapy Oncology Group. Head Neck Surg 1987;10:19–30.

Perez CA, Chao KS, Simpson JR, et al. Oropharynx (tonsillar fossa, faucial arch, and base of tongue). In: Perez CA, Brady LW, Halperin EC, et al., editors. Principles and Practice of Radiation Oncology. 4th ed. Philadelphia: Lippincott Williams & Wilkins; 2004. pp. 1022–1070.

Pignon JP, Bourhis J, Domenge C, et al. Chemotherapy added to locoregional treatment for head and neck squamous-cell carcinoma: three meta-analyses of updated individual data. MACH-NC Collaborative Group. Meta-Analysis of Chemotherapy on Head and Neck Cancer. Lancet 2000;355:949–955.

Tupchong L, Scott CB, Blitzer PH, et al. Randomized study of preoperative versus postoperative radiation therapy in advanced head and neck carcinoma: long-term follow-up of RTOG study 73-03. Int J Radiat Oncol Biol Phys 1991;20:21–28.

NOTES

Chapter 8
Cancer of the Lip and Oral Cavity

Eric K. Hansen and Naomi R. Schechter

PEARLS

- The oral cavity consists of the upper & lower lips, gingivobuccal sulcus, buccal mucosa, upper & lower gingiva (including alveolar ridge), retromolar trigone, hard palate, floor of mouth, & anterior $^2/_3$ of tongue
- CN XII provides motor innervation of the tongue, & the lingual nerve (CN V) provides sensory innervation. Taste is mediated by the chorda tympani branch of CN VII for the anterior 2/3 of the tongue & CN IX for the posterior $^1/_3$
- Risk factors for oral cavity cancer include tobacco, alcohol, poor oral hygiene, betel and areca nuts. Oral leukoplakia can proceed to cancer (4–18%) as can erythroplakia (30%)
- Neck LN levels: IA (submental), IB (submandibular), II (upper jugular, extending from the skull base superiorly to the hyoid bone inferiorly), III (middle jugular, extending from the hyoid to the lower border of the cricoid), IV (lower jugular, extending from the lower border of the cricoid to the clavicle), V (posterior triangle spinal accessory nodes), VI [paratracheal, pretracheal, prelaryngeal (Delphian), and tracheoesophageal nodes]
- LN drainage
  - Upper lip: periauricular and periparotid nodes & level IB
  - Floor of mouth, lower lip & lower gingiva: levels I, II, & III
  - Anterior oral tongue: IA, IB, & II & also directly to levels III–IV
  - Bilateral node drainage is frequent
- Depth of invasion, increasing T size, & grade increase risk of involved LN
- Risk of LN involvement
  - Lip: T1/2 ~5%, T3/4 ~33%
  - Floor of mouth: T1/2 ~10–20%, T3/4 ~33–67%

95

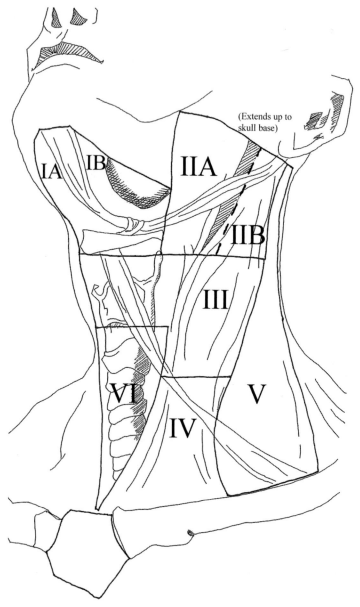

FIGURE 8.1. Lymph node levels in the neck.

- Oral tongue: T1/2 ~20%, T3/4 ~33–67%
- Buccal mucosa: T1/2 ~10–20%, T3/4 ~33–67%
- 90% of tumors are SCC. Less common tumors include minor salivary gland cancers (common in the hard palate & include adenoid cystic carcinoma, mucoepidermoid carcinoma, adenocarcinoma). Rarely, lymphoma, melanoma, or sarcoma

WORKUP

- H&P with palpation. Direct nasopharyngolaryngoscopy. EUA, if indicated
- Biopsy tumor &/or lymph node(s)
- Labs include CBC, chemistries, BUN/Cr, LFTs
- Imaging includes CT &/or MRI of the head & neck. Panorex of mandible for advanced lesions (also helps to rule-out extension through the mental foramen). PET scans may be informative for stage III–IV. CXR
- Preventive dental care & extractions should occur 10–14 days before RT & should include custom fluoride trays
- Speech & swallowing consultation

STAGING

Primary tumor
TX: Primary tumo cannot be assessed
T0:   No evidence of primary tumor
Tis: Carcinoma in situ
T1:   Tumor 2 cm or less in greatest dimension
T2:   Tumor more than 2 cm but not more than 4 cm in greatest dimension
T3:   Tumor more than 4 cm in greatest dimension
T4 (lip):   Tumor invades through cortical bone, inferior alveolar nerve, floor of mouth, or skin of face, i.e., chin or nose
T4a (oral cavity):   Tumor invades adjacent structures (e.g., through cortical bone, into deep [extrinxic] muscle of tongue [genioglossus, hyoglossus, palatoglossus & styloglossus], maxillary sinus, skin of face)
T4b: Tumor invades masticator space, pterygoid plates, or skull base and/or encases internal carotid artery

Note: Superficial erosion alone of bone/tooth socket by gingival primary is not sufficient to classify a tumor as T4

Regional lymph nodes
NX: Regional lymph nodes cannot be assessed
N0:   No regional lymph node metastasis

N1:   Metastasis in a single ipsilateral lymph node, 3 cm or less in greatest dimension

N2a: Metastasis in a single ipsilateral lymph node, more than 3 cm but not more than 6 cm in greatest dimension

N2b: Metastasis in multiple ipsilateral lymph nodes, none more than 6 cm in greatest dimension

N2c: Metastasis in bilateral or contralateral lymph nodes, none more than 6 cm in greatest dimension

N3:   Metastasis in a lymph node more than 6 cm in greatest dimension

Distant Metastases
MX: Distant metastasis cannot be assessed
M0:   No distant metastasis
M1:   Distant metastasis

Stage Grouping		~5 yr OS		~LC with EBRT &/or brachy	
0:	TisN0M0	I:	60–90%	T1:	85–100%
I:	T1N0M0	II:	40–70%	T2:	70–95%
II:	T2N0M0	III:	30–40%	T3:	50–90%
III:	T3N0M0, T1-3N1M0	IV:	20–30%	T4:	10–50%
IVA:	T4aN0-1M0, T1-4aN2M0				
IVB:	Any T, N3M0; T4b, any N, M0	(Varies by site)		(Varies by site)	
IVC:	Any T, any N, M1				

Used with the permission of the American Joint Committee on Cancer (AJCC), Chicago, Illinois. The original source for this material is the AJCC Cancer Staging Manual, Sixth Edition (2002) published by Springer-Verlag New York, www.springeronline.com.

TREATMENT RECOMMENDATIONS

Stage	Lip
T1N0	Surgery or RT (for commissure involvement or poorlydifferentiated tumors). Post-op RT with treatment of the neck (dissection or RT) for + margins or PNI. RT may consist of EBRT, brachytherapy, or both
T2N0	Surgery or RT (EBRT, brachytherapy, or both). If + margins or PNI → post-op RT with treatment of the neck (dissection or RT)

Stage	Lip
T3-4N0	Excision of primary & unilateral or bilateral neck dissection (if crosses midline). Reconstruction as indicated. Surgery preferred especially if bone invasion. Post-op chemo-RT for + margin; post-op RT for close margin, PNI, &/or LVSI Alternatively, concomitant chemo-RT. If primary has <CR to chemo-RT, salvage surgery & neck dissection
T1-4N+	Excision of primary & ipsilateral comprehensive neck dissection ± contralateral selective neck dissection (if crosses midline) or bilateral neck dissection (for N2c). Post-op chemo-RT for + margin or nodal ECE; post-op RT or chemo-RT for close margin, PNI, LVSI, &/or multiple + LN Alternatively, concomitant chemo-RT. If residual neck mass, post-RT neck dissection considered. If primary has <CR to chemo-RT, salvage surgery & neck dissection remain considerations

Stage	Floor of Mouth
T1 & superficial T2N0	Surgery or RT. Neck treatment (dissection or RT) required for lesions >1.5 mm thick. Post-op RT for close/+ margins (brachytherapy or intraoral cone)
Resectable large T2N0 & T3-4N0	Excision of primary & unilateral or bilateral neck dissection (if crosses midline). Reconstruction as indicated. Post-op chemo-RT for + margin; post-op RT for close margin, PNI, &/or LVSI

Stage	Floor of Mouth
T1-4N+	Excision of primary & ipsilateral comprehensive neck dissection ± contralateral selective neck dissection (if crosses midline) or bilateral neck dissection (for N2c). Post-op chemo-RT for + margin or nodal ECE; post-op RT or chemo-RT for close margin, PNI, LVSI, &/or multiple + LN
Unresectable T2-4N0/+	Concomitant chemo-RT. If residual neck mass, post-RT neck dissection considered. If primary has <CR to chemo-RT, salvage surgery & neck dissection remain considerations

Stage	Oral Tongue
T1 & superficial T2N0	Surgery or RT. Neck treatment (dissection or RT) required for lesions >2 mm thick. Post-op RT indicated for close/+ margins, PNI, LVSI
Large T2N0	Wide local excision of primary ± unilateral or bilateral selective neck dissection (depending on depth of invasion & location). Post-op chemo-RT for + margin; post-op RT for close margin, PNI, &/or LVSI. If inoperable, definitive RT (EBRT ± brachytherapy or oral cone)
T3-4N0 & T1-4N+	Excision of primary & ipsilateral comprehensive neck dissection ± contralateral selective neck dissection (if crosses midline) or bilateral neck dissection (for N2c).

Stage	Oral Tongue
	Post-op chemo-RT for + margin or nodal ECE; post-op RT or chemo-RT for close margin, PNI, LVSI, &/or multiple + LN Alternatively, concomitant chemo-RT. If residual neck mass, post-RT neck dissection considered. If primary has <CR to chemo-RT, salvage surgery & neck dissection remain considerations

Stage	Buccal Mucosa
T1 & superficial T2N0	Surgery or RT (especially for commissure involvement). Post-op RT with treatment of the neck (dissection or RT) for + margins, tumor thickness >6mm, depth of invasion >3mm, or PNI. T2 lesions require treatment of the neck. RT may consist of EBRT, brachytherapy alone, or both
Large T2 & T3-4N0	Wide local excision of primary & unilateral or bilateral selective neck dissection (depending on depth of invasion & location). Post-op chemo-RT for + margin; post-op RT for close margin, PNI, &/or LVSI If inoperable or superficial, definitive RT (EBRT ± brachytherapy) ± concomitant chemotherapy (for T3-4 tumors)

Stage	Buccal Mucosa
T1-4N+	Excision of primary & ipsilateral comprehensive neck dissection ± contralateral selective neck dissection or bilateral neck dissection (for N2c). Post-op chemo-RT for + margin or nodal ECE; post-op RT or chemo-RT for close margin, PNI, LVSI, &/or multiple + LN Alternatively, concomitant chemo-RT. If residual neck mass, post-RT neck dissection considered. If primary has <CR to chemo-RT, salvage surgery & neck dissection remain considerations

Stage	Gingiva and Hard Palate
T1 & superficial T2N0	Surgery. Upper neck treatment (dissection or RT). Post-op RT for close/+ margins
Large T2 & T3-4N0	Excision of primary & unilateral or bilateral selective neck dissection (depending on stage & location). Post-op chemo-RT for + margin; post-op RT for close margin, PNI, &/or LVSI If inoperable or superficial, definitive RT ± concomitant chemotherapy (for T3-4 tumors)
T1-4N+	Excision of primary & ipsilateral comprehensive neck dissection ± contralateral selective neck dissection or bilateral neck dissection (for N2c). Post-op chemo-RT for + margin or nodal ECE; post-op RT or chemo-RT for close margin, PNI, LVSI, &/or multiple + LN

Stage	Gingiva and Hard Palate
	Alternatively, concomitant chemo-RT. If residual neck mass, post-RT neck dissection considered. If primary has <CR to chemo-RT, salvage surgery & neck dissection remain considerations

Stage	Retromolar Trigone
T1-T2N0	Surgery or RT (especially for involvement of tonsillar pillar, buccal mucosa, or soft palate). Upper neck treatment (dissection or RT). Post-op RT for close/+ margins
T3-4N0	Excision of primary & unilateral or bilateral selective neck dissection (depending on stage & location). Post-op chemo-RT for + margin; post-op RT for close margin, PNI, &/or LVSI If inoperable, definitive RT ± concomitant chemotherapy
T1-4N+	Excision of primary & ipsilateral comprehensive neck dissection ± contralateral selective neck dissection or bilateral neck dissection (for N2c). Post-op chemo-RT for + margin or nodal ECE; post-op RT or chemo-RT for close margin, PNI, LVSI, &/or multiple + LN Alternatively, concomitant chemo-RT. If residual neck mass, post-RT neck dissection considered. If primary has <CR to chemo-RT, salvage surgery & neck dissection remain considerations

STUDIES
Chemoradiation and altered fractionation

- <u>RTOG 90-03</u> (Fu, *IJROBP* 2000). 268 pts with locally-advanced cancer of the oral cavity, oropharynx, supra-glottic larynx, or hypopharynx randomized to 2/70 Gy vs 1.2 bid/81.6 Gy vs split-course 1.6 bid/67.2 Gy (with 2 wk break) vs concomitant boost RT to 72 Gy (1.8 Gy/fraction with a 1.5 Gy boost on the last 12 treatment days). Concomitant boost & continuous bid RT improved the 2 year LRC (54%), DFS (38–39%), & OS (51–54%) vs standard or split-course bid RT. Altered fractionation increased the acute side effects

- <u>Adelstein</u> (*JCO* 2003). 295 pts with unresectable cancer of the oral cavity, oropharynx, larynx, or hypopharynx randomized to RT (2/70 Gy) vs chemo-RT (2/70 Gy & cisplatin ×3c) vs split-course chemo-RT (2/30 Gy → 2/30–40 Gy with cisplatin/5-FU ×3c). Continuous chemo-RT with cisplatin improved 3 yr OS (37% vs RT 23% vs split C-RT 27%) & DFS (51% vs RT 33% vs split C-RT 41%), but increased grade 3–4 toxicity (89% vs RT 52% vs split C-RT 77%)

- <u>Brizel</u> (*NEJM* 1998). 116 pts with T3-T4N0/+ or T2N0 (base of tongue) cancers of the oral cavity, oropharynx, hypopharynx, larynx, nasopharynx, & paranasal sinus randomized to RT (1.25 bid/75 Gy) vs concurrent chemo-RT (1.25 bid/70 Gy with 1 wk break at 40 Gy with cisplatin/5-FU weeks 1 & 6). Most pts received 2 cycles of adjuvant cisplatin/5-FU. Chemo-RT improved 3 yr LC (44→70%), DFS (41→61%), & OS (34→55%) but did not significantly increase toxicity

Post-op RT and post-op chemo-RT

- <u>Ang</u> (*IJROBP* 2001). 213 pts with locally-advanced oral cavity, oropharynx, larynx, & hypopharynx cancers treated with surgery randomized by risk factors to post-op RT. Risk factors included >1 node group, ≥2 nodes, nodes >3 cm, microscopic +margins, PNI, oral cavity site, & nodal extracapsular extension. Low-risk = no risk factors → no RT. Intermediate risk = 1 risk factor (but not ECE) → 1.8/57.6 Gy. High-risk = ECE or ≥2 risk factors → 1.8/63 Gy in 7 weeks or in 5 weeks with a concomitant boost. The 5 yr LRC/OS for low-risk was 90/83%, for intermediate risk 94/66%, & for high-risk 68/42%. Overall treatment time <11 weeks increased LRC, and concomitant boost had a trend for improved OS

- EORTC 22931 (Bernier, *NEJM* 2004). 334 pts with operable stage III/IV oral cavity, oropharynx, larynx, & hypopharynx cancer randomized to post-op RT (2/66 Gy) vs post-op chemo-RT (2/66 Gy & cisplatin 100 mg/m^2 on days 1, 22, 43). All patients received 54 Gy to the low risk neck. Eligible stages included pT3-4N0/+, T1-2N2-3, & T1-2N0-1 with ECE, +margin, or PNI. Chemo-RT improved 3/5 yr DFS (41/36→59/47%), 3/5 yr OS (49/40→65/53%), & 5 yr LRC (69→82%), but increased grade 3–4 toxicity (21→41%)
- RTOG 95-01 (Cooper, *NEJM* 2004). 459 pts with operable cancer of the oral cavity, oropharynx, larynx, or hypopharynx who had ≥2 involved lymph nodes, nodal extracapsular extension, or a + margin randomized to post-op RT (2/60–66 Gy) vs post-op chemo-RT (2/60–66 Gy & cisplatin ×3c as in EORTC 22931). Chemo-RT improved 2 yr DFS (43→54%), LRC (72→82%), & had a trend for improved OS (57→63%), but increased grade 3–4 toxicity (34→77%)

RADIATION TECHNIQUES
Simulation and field design
- In general, simulate the patient supine with the head on a head rest device. Wire nodes, scars, the oral commissure, & the larynx (thyroid notch). A bite block may depress the tongue away from palate. Shoulders may be pulled down with straps. Immobilize with a thermoplastic head (± shoulder) mask
- With EBRT, a 3D or IMRT plan should be used for any but simple appositional or opposed-lateral fields in order to spare normal tissues
- Computed dosimetry should be used in all cases

Lip
- Lip lesions may be treated with EBRT (100–250 keV orthovoltage or 6–12 MeV electrons), or with brachytherapy, or in combination
- With EBRT, an appositional field is used & borders are determined clinically with a 1–1.5 cm margin for orthovoltage or a 2–2.5 cm margin for electrons. A lead cut-out is made to outline the treatment volume. Lead shields are placed behind the lip to minimize dose to the mandible & oral cavity
- The neck is treated for T1/2 tumors with commissure involvement, & T3/4, N+, or poorly differentiated tumors

- T3/4 tumors are conventionally treated with opposed lateral 4–6 MV fields. The tumor is treated with 1–1.5 cm margin. The inferior border is at the thyroid notch, & the posterior border is at the posterior aspect of the spinous processes
- When N+, a low-neck field is matched to the inferior border of the opposed lateral fields. If the posterior chain requires RT, the portals are reduced off-cord at 42–45 Gy and the area is boosted with electrons
- With conventional 3-field techniques, the spinal cord is shielded on the AP field at the matchline. A small midline larynx block on the AP field may also be used
- 3DCRT or IMRT techniques are generally recommended, however, for more advanced lesions and in order to spare adjacent normal structures
- Wedges &/or compensating filters may be required
- Afterloading implants use temporary Ir-192 seeds in angiocaths (or wires in Europe) spaced 1 cm apart. A gauze roll is placed between the lip & the gingiva
- EBRT dose: T1-2N0 = 2/50 Gy → boost to 56–60 Gy. (T1 lesions may also be treated with 3/45 Gy.) T3N0 = 2/50 Gy → boost to 60–70 Gy & levels I/II are treated. T4 or N+ = 2/50 Gy → boost to 66–70 Gy & levels I–IV are treated
- When used alone for T1-2, brachytherapy dose is 60–70 Gy at 0.8–1 Gy/hr
- If used 2–4 wks after EBRT (50–54 Gy), LDR brachytherapy boost is 15–30 Gy
- Afterloading Ir-192 HDR brachytherapy may be used instead of LDR

Floor of mouth

- The floor of mouth has lower RT tolerance due to increased risk of soft tissue injury & osteoradionecrosis
- For early superficial T1-2 lesions, brachytherapy or intra-oral cone RT is used
  - LDR brachytherapy dose is 60–70 Gy
  - Intraoral cone dose is 3 Gy/fraction to 45 Gy over 3 weeks
- For larger lesions, EBRT is used with brachytherapy boost
- 3DCRT or IMRT techniques are generally recommended for advanced lesions and in order to spare adjacent normal structures. Brachytherapy or intraoral cone may be used for the boost

- With opposed laterals, the superior border is 1–1.5 cm above the dorsum of the tongue (2 cm above tumor). Level I nodes are always treated, & level II is included for depth of invasion >1.5 mm (with posterior border at the posterior aspect of the spinous processes). The inferior border is at the thyroid notch. The lower lip is excluded when possible. When N+, a low-neck field is matched to the inferior border of the opposed lateral fields
- Definitive RT dose for more advanced lesions is 1.8–2 Gy/ fraction to ≥72 Gy without chemo (concomitant boost used)
- With chemo, EBRT dose is 2 Gy/fraction to 70 Gy
- As a boost after EBRT (~45 Gy), interstitial brachytherapy (25–30 Gy) or intraoral cone (15–24 Gy) may be used
- With post-op RT, fields include the primary site & the dissected neck
- Post-op EBRT doses are 1.8–2 Gy/fraction to 50–54 Gy followed by boost to 60–66 Gy to high-risk areas

Oral tongue

- Brachytherapy or intraoral cone may be used as with floor of mouth lesions
- A prosthesis is used to keep the tongue down and to exclude the palate
- 3DCRT or IMRT techniques are generally recommended for advanced lesions and in order to spare adjacent normal structures. Brachytherapy or intraoral cone may be used for the boost
- With opposed laterals, the superior border is 1–1.5 cm above the dorsum of the tongue or 2 cm above tumor. The inferior border is at the thyroid notch. The posterior border is placed at the posterior aspect of the spinous processes. The anterior border is 2 cm anterior to the tumor. When N+, a low-neck field is matched to the inferior border of the opposed lateral fields
- Doses are similar to floor of mouth lesions

Buccal mucosa

- Wire ipsilateral commissure. Place intraoral stent to displace & shield tongue. May insert metal seeds into the periphery of the tumor for localization
- Treatment is usually with an ipsilateral mixed photon/ electron beam (or wedged photon pair) & a boost is given with brachytherapy or intraoral cone if possible

- Field borders are 2 cm anterior & superior to the lesion; the posterior aspect of the spinous processes if nodes are irradiated; inferiorly at the thyroid notch
- The oral commissures & lips are shielded if possible
- Post-op volumes include the tumor bed, scars, & ipsilateral IB & II nodes
- Pts with + nodes receive bilateral neck RT to the upper & lower neck
- Doses are similar to other oral cavity lesions

Gingiva and hard palate

- EBRT, rather than brachytherapy, is used due to the risk of osteoradionecrosis
- For gingival lesions, if PNI is present, the entire hemimandible from mental foramen to the temporomandibular joint is treated
- Fields cover the primary with 2 cm margins & the upper neck nodes
- The low-neck is treated for T3/4 or N+
- Definitive RT dose is 60–66 Gy for T1 lesions, 66–70 Gy for T2, & ≥72 Gy for T3-4 lesions without chemo (concomitant boost used). With chemo, give 2/70 Gy
- Post-op EBRT doses are 1.8–2 Gy/fraction to 50–54 Gy followed by boost to 60–66 Gy to high-risk areas

Retromolar trigone

- An ipsilateral mixed photon/electron beam (or wedged photon pair) is used for lateralized lesions
- Fields cover the primary with 2 cm margins & the upper neck nodes. The superior border includes the pterygoid plates. The low-neck is treated for T3/4 or N+
- Doses are similar to other oral cavity tumors

IMRT

- With IMRT, GTV = clinical &/or radiographic gross disease (primary & nodal). CTV1 = 0.5–2 cm margin on the primary & nodal GTV (with margin size depending on presence or absence of anatomic boundaries to microscopic spread). CTV2 = elective neck. Individualized PTVs are used for the GTV, CTV1, & CTV2
- Definitive IMRT doses (at UCSF): GTV = 2.12/70 Gy; CTV1 = 1.8/59.4 Gy; CTV2 = 1.64/54 Gy in 33 fractions. Alternative is GTV = 2.2/66 Gy; CTV1 = 2/60 Gy; CTV2 = 1.8/54 Gy in 30 fractions

- Post-op IMRT doses (at UCSF): GTV (residual) = 70 Gy; CTV1 = 60–66 Gy; CTV2 = 54 Gy

Dose limitations
- Spinal cord maximum dose ≤45–50 Gy. Brainstem maximum dose ≤54 Gy. Keep 50% of the volume of each parotid ≤20 Gy (if possible). Mandible maximum dose ≤70 Gy

COMPLICATIONS
- Complications of RT include mucositis, dermatitis, xerostomia, dysgeusia, soft tissue fibrosis, hypothyroidism, & rarely soft tissue or osteoradionecrosis (more common with brachytherapy), pharyngocutaneous fistula, or carotid rupture
- Perioperative complications of surgery include bleeding, airway obstruction, infection, & wound complications. Post-op complications include webs, stenosis, chondritis, fistulas, aspiration, as well as functional speech &/or swallowing deficits
- Patients need ≥2000 calories/day to avoid malnutrition. Supplements (e.g., Boost or Ensure) &/or feeding tubes may be used
- Amifostine may decrease xerostomia & mucositis, but it is associated with significant side effects (hypotension, nausea) (Peters, *IJROBP* 1993 & Brizel, *JCO* 2000)

FOLLOW-UP
- H&P every 1–3 mo for year 1, every 2–4 mo for year 2, every 6 mo for years 3–5, then annually. CXR annually. TSH every 6–12 mo if neck irradiated
- If recurrence is suspected but biopsy is negative, follow closely (at least monthly) until resolves

REFERENCES
Adelstein DJ, Li Y, Adams GL, et al. An intergroup phase III comparison of standard radiation therapy and two schedules of concurrent chemoradiotherapy in patients with unresectable squamous cell head and neck cancer. J Clin Oncol 2003;21:92–98.

Ang KK, Trotti A, Brown BW, et al. Randomized trial addressing risk features and time factors of surgery plus radiotherapy in advanced head-and-neck cancer. Int J Radiat Oncol Biol Phys 2001;51: 571–578.

Bernier J, Domenge C, Ozsahin M, et al. Postoperative irradiation with or without concomitant chemotherapy for locally advanced head and neck cancer. N Engl J Med 2004;350:1945–1952.

Brizel DM, Albers ME, Fisher SR, et al. Hyperfractionated irradiation with or without concurrent chemotherapy for locally advanced head and neck cancer. N Engl J Med 1998;338:1798–1804.

Cooper JS, Pajak TF, Forastiere AA, et al. Postoperative concurrent radiotherapy and chemotherapy for high-risk squamous-cell carcinoma of the head and neck. N Engl J Med 2004;350:1937–1944.

Cooper JS. The oral cavity. In: Cox JD, Ang KK, editors. Radiation Oncology: Rationale, Technique, Results. 8th ed. St. Louis: Mosby; 2003. pp. 219–255.

de Visscher JG, Grond AJ, Botke G, et al. Results of radiotherapy for squamous cell carcinoma of the vermilion border of the lower lip. A retrospective analysis of 108 patients. Radiother Oncol 1996;39:9–14.

Emami B. Oral cavity. In: Perez CA, Brady LW, Halperin EC, et al., editors. Principles and Practice of Radiation Oncology. 4th ed. Philadelphia: Lippincott Williams & Wilkins; 2004. pp. 997–1021.

Fu KK, Pajak TF, Trotti A, et al. A Radiation Therapy Oncology Group (RTOG) phase III randomized study to compare hyperfractionation and two variants of accelerated fractionation to standard fractionation radiotherapy for head and neck squamous cell carcinomas: first report of RTOG 9003. Int J Radiat Oncol Biol Phys 2000; 48:7–16.

Fujita M, Hirokawa Y, Kashiwado K, et al. Interstitial brachytherapy for stage I and II squamous cell carcinoma of the oral tongue: factors influencing local control and soft tissue complications. Int J Radiat Oncol Biol Phys 1999;44:767–775.

Greene FL, American Joint Committee on Cancer, American Cancer Society. AJCC Cancer Staging Manual. 6th ed. New York: Springer-Verlag; 2002.

Lee N, Phillips TL. Cancer of the oral cavity. In: Leibel SA, Phillips TL, editors. Textbook of Radiation Oncology. 2nd ed. Philadelphia: Saunders; 2004. pp. 631–656.

McLaughlin MP, Mendenhall WM, Million RR, et al. Oral cavity cancers. In: Gunderson LL, Tepper JE, editors. Clinical Radiation Oncology. 1st ed. Philadelphia: Churchill Livingstone; 2000. pp. 428–453.

National Cancer Institute. Lip and Oral Cavity Cancer (PDQ): Treatment. Available at: http://cancer.gov/cancertopics/pdq/treatment/lip-and-oral-cavity/healthprofessional/. Accessed on January 19, 2005.

National Comprehensive Cancer Network. Clinical Practice Guidelines in Oncology: Head and Neck Cancers. Available at: http://www.nccn.org/professionals/physician_gls/PDF/head-and-neck.pdf. Accessed on January 19, 2005.

NOTES

Chapter 9
Cancer of the Larynx and Hypopharynx

Eric K. Hansen and Naomi R. Schechter

PEARLS

- Larynx cancer is the most common cancer of the head & neck
- Risk factors include tobacco, alcohol, betel and areca nuts, & deficiencies of iron, vitamin B12, & vitamin C
- Larynx subsites:
  - Supraglottis = suprahyoid & infrahyoid epiglottis, aryepiglottic folds, arytenoids, & false cords
  - Glottis = true vocal cords including the anterior & posterior commissures
  - Subglottis = extends from the lower boundary of the glottis to the inferior aspect of the cricoid cartilage
- True vocal cords attach to the thyroid cartilage at the center of the "figure of 8" on a lateral X-ray
- LN drainage is common from the supraglottis (to levels II–V) & subglottis [to pretracheal (Delphian), paratracheal, & inferior jugular nodes]. Glottic tumors rarely spread to LN when ≤T1-2 (<3%) but more commonly spread to LN when T3-4 (~20–30%)
- Superior laryngeal nerve innervates the cricothyroid muscles that produce tension and elongation of the vocal cords. All other laryngeal muscles are innervated by the recurrent laryngeal nerve
- Hypopharynx is the portion of the pharynx extending from the plane of the superior border of the hyoid bone to the inferior border of the cricoid cartilage
- Hypopharynx subsites:
  - Pyriform sinuses
  - Posterior & lateral hypopharyngeal walls
  - Postcricoid area

- LN drainage from the hypopharynx is to levels II–V, the retropharyngeal LN, & to paratracheal & paraesophageal LN (when tumor involves the lowest portion of the hypopharynx and the postcricoid area)
- 95% of tumors of the larynx & hypopharynx are SCC
- External auditory canal pain may be referred via the superior laryngeal nerve though the auricular nerve of Arnold (branch of CN X)
- A "hot potato" voice may be due to involvement of the base of tongue

WORKUP

- H&P. EUA with laryngoscopy. Esophagoscopy for hypopharnx tumors or if clinically indicated for laryngeal tumors. Bronchoscopy if clinically indicated
- Biopsy tumor &/or lymph node(s)
- Labs include CBC, chemistries, BUN/Cr, LFTs
- Imaging includes CT &/or MRI of the head & neck & a CXR. PET scans may be informative for stage III–IV
- Preventive dental care & extractions should occur 10–14 days before RT

STAGING

Primary tumor (both Larynx & Hypopharnx)

TX: Primary tumor cannot be assessed
T0: No evidence of primary tumor
Tis: Carcinoma in situ

Primary tumor (Supraglottis)

T1: Tumor limited to 1 subsite of supraglottis with normal vocal cord mobility
T2: Tumor invades mucosa of more than one adjacent subsite of supraglottis or glottis or region outside the supraglottis (e.g., mucosa of base of tongue, vallecula, medial wall of pyriform sinus), without fixation of the larynx
T3: Tumor limited to larynx with vocal cord fixation and/or invades any of the following: postcricoid area, preepiglottic tissues, paraglottic space, and/or minor thyroid cartilage erosion (e.g., inner cortex)
T4a: Tumor invades through the thyroid cartilage, and/or invades tissues beyond the larynx (e.g., trachea, soft tissues of the neck including deep extrinsic muscle of the tongue, strap muscles, thyroid, or esophagus)
T4b: Tumor invades prevertebral space, encases carotid artery, or invades mediastinal structures

Primary tumor (Glottis)

T1:   Tumor limited to the vocal cord(s) (may involve anterior or posterior commissure) with normal mobility
      T1a: Tumor limited to one vocal cord
      T1b: Tumor involves both vocal cords
T2:   Tumor extends to supraglottis and/or subglottis, and/or with impaired vocal cord mobility
T3:   Tumor limited to larynx with vocal cord fixation &/or invades paraglottic space, and/or minor thyroid cartilage erosion (e.g., inner cortex)
T4a: Tumor invades through the thyroid cartilage, and/or invades tissues beyond the larynx (e.g., trachea, soft tissues of the neck including deep extrinsic muscle of the tongue, strap muscles, thyroid, or esophagus)
T4b: Tumor invades prevertebral space, encases carotid artery, or invades mediastinal structures

Primary tumor (Subglottis)

T1:   Tumor limited to subglottis
T2:   Tumor extends to vocal cord(s) with normal or impaired mobility
T3:   Tumor limited to larynx with vocal cord fixation
T4a: Tumor invades cricoid or thyroid cartilage, and/or invades tissues beyond the larynx (e.g., trachea, soft tissues of the neck including deep extrinsic muscle of the tongue, strap muscles, thyroid, or esophagus)
T4b: Tumor invades prevertebral space, encases carotid artery, or invades mediastinal structures

Primary tumor (Hypopharynx)

T1:   Tumor limited to one subsite of hypopharynx and 2 cm or less in greatest dimension
T2:   Tumor invades more than one subsite of hypopharynx or an adjacent site, or measures more than 2 cm but not more than 4 cm in greatest diameter, without fixation of hemilarynx
T3:   Tumor more than 4 cm in greatest dimension or with fixation of hemilarynx
T4a: Tumor invades thyroid/cricoid cartilage, hyoid bone, thyroid gland, esophagus, or central compartment soft tissues (including prelaryngeal strap muscles and subcutaneous fat)
T4b: Tumor invades prevertebral fascia, encases carotid artery, or involves mediastinal structures

Regional lymph nodes (both Larynx & Hypopharynx)

NX: Regional lymph nodes cannot be assessed
N0:   No regional lymph node metastasis
N1:   Metastasis in a single ipsilateral lymph node, 3 cm or less in greatest dimension

N2a: Metastasis in a single ipsilateral lymph node, more than 3 cm but not more than 6 cm in greatest dimension
N2b: Metastasis in multiple ipsilateral lymph nodes, none more than 6 cm in greatest dimension
N2c: Metastasis in bilateral or contralateral lymph nodes, none more than 6 cm in greatest dimension
N3: Metastasis in a lymph node more than 6 cm in greatest dimension

Distant Metastases (both Larynx & Hypopharynx)
MX: Distant metastasis cannot be assessed
M0: No distant metastasis
M1: Distant metastasis

Stage Grouping		~2/5 year OS	
		Larynx	Hypopharynx
0:	TisN0M0		
I:	T1N0M0	I: 90/70%	65/35%
II:	T2N0M0	II: 80/60%	60/30%
III:	T3N0M0, T1-3N1M0	III: 70/50%	50/30%
IVA:	T4aN0-1M0, T1-4aN2M0	IV: 60/35%	35/15%
IVB:	T4b any N M0,		
	Any T N3 M0		
IVC:	Any T, any N, M1		

Used with the permission of the American Joint Committee on Cancer (AJCC), Chicago, Illinois. The original source for this material is the AJCC Cancer Staging Manual, Sixth Edition (2002) published by Springer-Verlag New York, www.springeronline.com.

TREATMENT RECOMMENDATIONS
Surgical options
- Limited surgery (stripping or laser)
- Cordectomy
- Vertical partial laryngectomy (removes 1 cord & up to 1/3 of other cord)
- Total laryngectomy (removes hyoid, thyroid, & cricoid cartilages, epiglottis, strap muscles, & patient left with a permanent tracheostoma & reconstruction of the pharynx)

Stage	Larynx
Tis	Endoscopic removal (stripping/ laser) or definitive RT
T1-2N0 glottic	Definitive RT. Or, cordectomy or partial laryngectomy ± selective neck dissection. Post-op chemo-RT for + margin; post-op RT for close margin, PNI, LVSI
T1-2N0 supraglottic	Definitive RT. Or, partial supraglottic laryngectomy ± selective neck dissection. Post-op chemo-RT for + margin; post-op RT for close margin, PNI, LVSI
Resectable T1-2N+, T3N0/+ requiring total laryngectomy	Concurrent chemo-RT as in RTOG 91-11 (preferred). If < complete response, salvage surgery & neck dissection may be performed. If residual neck mass or initial N2-3, post-RT neck dissection considered. Alternative is total laryngectomy, & ipsilateral or bilateral neck dissection (N0-1) or bilateral comprehensive neck dissection (N2-3). Post-op chemo-RT for + margin or nodal ECE; post-op RT or chemo-RT for close margin, PNI, LVSI, multiple + LN, ≥1 cm subglottic extension, T3-4 tumors, &/or cartilage invasion
Resectable T4N0/+	Total laryngectomy & ipsilateral or bilateral neck dissection (N0-1) or bilateral comprehensive neck dissection (N2-3). Post-op chemo-RT for + margin or nodal ECE; post-op RT or chemo-RT for close margin, PNI, LVSI, multiple + LN, ≥1 cm subglottic extension, T3-4 tumors, &/or cartilage invasion

Stage	Larynx
	Alternative is definitive concurrent chemo-RT as in RTOG 91-11
Unresectable T3-4 or N+	Concurrent chemo-RT. If unable to tolerate chemo, definitive RT with concomitant boost

Stage	Hypopharynx
Early T1-2 not requiring total laryngectomy (T1N0-1, small T2N0, T1N2)	Definitive RT. If < complete response, salvage surgery & neck dissection as indicated. If complete response, neck dissection considered for N2-3. Alternatively, partial laryngopharyngectomy & ipsilateral or bilateral selective neck dissection (N0) or comprehensive neck dissection (N+). Post-op chemo-RT for + margin or nodal ECE; post-op RT or chemo-RT for close margin, PNI, LVSI, multiple + LN
T2-4N0/+ requiring total laryngectomy	Induction chemo ×2c (with a 3rd cycle if PR) → RT (≥70 Gy). Non-responders to chemo should undergo surgery → post-op RT or chemo-RT as indicated. If residual neck mass after definitive RT or initial N2-3, post-RT neck dissection considered. Or, laryngopharyngectomy & selective (N0) or comprehensive neck dissection (N+ or T4). Post-op chemo-RT for + margin or nodal ECE; post-op RT or chemo-RT for close margin, PNI, LVSI, multiple + LN cartilage invasion. Definitive concurrent chemo-RT may be considered (as for larynx & oropharynx)

Stage	Hypopharynx
Unresectable T3-4 or N+	Concurrent chemo-RT. If unable to tolerate chemo, definitive RT with concomitant boost

STUDIES
RT dose fractionation

- Le (*IJROBP* 1997). reviewed 398 pts with T1-2 glottic cancer treated with RT alone. On multivariate analysis, overall treatment time ≤43 days, fraction size ≥2.25 Gy, & total dose ≥65 Gy improved LC for T2 lesions. Anterior commissure involvement decreased T1 LC, & impaired cord mobility & subglottic extension decreased T2 LC

- Garden (*IJROBP* 2003). reviewed 230 pts treated with RT alone for T2 glottic cancer. Treatment with ≤2 Gy/fraction had decreased 5 yr LC (68%) compared to >2 Gy/fraction (82%) or bid RT (79%)

- RTOG 95-12 (closed) randomized pts with T2 glottic cancer to 70 Gy/2 Gy qd or 79.2 Gy/1.2 Gy bid

Chemo-RT and altered fractionation

- RTOG 91-11 (Forastierre, *NEJM* 2003). 547 pts with stage III/IV larynx randomized to one of three arms: RT alone, chemo → RT, or concurrent chemo-RT. RT was 2/70 Gy in all arms. Induction chemo was cisplatin/5-FU ×2c → reassessment. If progression or <PR, treated with laryngectomy & post-op RT. If PR/CR → 3rd cycle chemo → RT. Concurrent chemo was cisplatin ×3c. All pts with cN2 had neck dissection within 8 weeks after RT. Concurrent chemo-RT increased the portion of pts with an intact larynx (88% vs C→RT 75%, RT 70%) & LRC (78% vs C→RT 61%, RT 56%). Chemo suppressed DM & improved DFS. There was no difference in 2/5 yr OS (74–76/54–56%). Concurrent chemo increased mucosal toxicity

- VA larynx trial (*NEJM* 1991). 332 pts with III/IV larynx (T1N1 excluded), randomized to surgery & post-op RT (50–74 Gy) vs induction cisplatin/5-FU ×2c (with a 3rd cycle if PR/CR) → RT (66–76 Gy). No routine neck dissection for N+ pts. Chemo allowed 64% larynx preservation at 2 years. There was no difference in 2 yr OS (68%). Chemo-RT decreased distant recurrences but had higher LF (12% vs 2%). Organ preservation improved quality of life

- EORTC (Lefebvre, *J Natl Cancer Inst* 1996). 202 pts with operable pyriform sinus tumors randomized to surgery → post-op RT (50–70 Gy) vs induction cisplatin/5-FU ×2c (with a 3rd cycle if PR/CR) → RT (70 Gy). Non-responders to chemo underwent surgery → RT. 51–54% of pts had a CR after chemo. There was no difference in LRF, and chemo decreased DM (36→25%). The 3/5 year functional intact larynx rates were 42/35% with chemo

- RTOG 90-03 (Fu, *IJROBP* 2000). 268 pts with locally-advanced cancer of the oral cavity, oropharynx, supra-glottic larynx, or hypopharynx randomized to 2/70 Gy vs 1.2 bid/81.6 Gy vs split-course 1.6 bid/67.2 Gy (with 2 wk break) vs concomitant boost RT to 72 Gy (1.8 Gy/fraction with a 1.5 Gy boost on the last 12 treatment days). Concomitant boost & continuous bid RT improved the 2 year LRC (54%), DFS (38–39%), & OS (51–54%) vs standard or split-course bid RT. Altered fractionation increased the acute side effects

- Adelstein (*JCO* 2003). 295 pts with unresectable cancer of the oral cavity, oropharynx, larynx, or hypopharynx randomized to RT (2/70 Gy) vs chemo-RT (2/70 Gy & cisplatin ×3c) vs split-course chemo-RT (2/30 Gy → 2/30–40 Gy with cisplatin/5-FU ×3c). Continuous chemo-RT with cisplatin improved 3 yr OS (37% vs RT 23% vs split C-RT 27%) & DFS (51% vs RT 33% vs split C-RT 41%), but increased grade 3-4 toxicity (89% vs RT 52% vs split C-RT 77%)

- Brizel (*NEJM* 1998). 116 pts with T3-T4N0/+ or T2N0 (base of tongue) cancers of the oral cavity, oropharynx, hypo-pharynx, larynx, nasopharynx, & paranasal sinus randomized to RT (1.25 bid/75 Gy) vs concurrent chemo-RT (1.25 bid/70 Gy with 1 wk break at 40 Gy with cisplatin/5-FU weeks 1 & 6). Most pts received 2 cycles of adjuvant cisplatin/5-FU. Chemo-RT improved 3 yr LC (44→70%), DFS (41→61%), & OS (34→55%) but did not significantly increase toxicity

- Bonner (*NEJM* 2006). 424 pts with locoregionally advanced resectable or unresectable stage III–IV SCC of orophar-ynx, larynx, or hypopharynx randomized to RT or RT + cetuximab given 1wk before RT & weekly during RT. RT options included 2/70 Gy, 1.2 bid/72–76.8 Gy, or concomi-tant boost 72 Gy. Cetuximab increased 3 yr LRC (34 → 47%) & OS (45 → 55%). With the exception of acneiform rash & infusion reactions with cetuximab, toxicity was similar

Post-op RT and post-op chemo-RT

- Ang (*IJROBP* 2001). 213 pts with locally-advanced oral cavity, oropharynx, larynx, & hypopharynx cancers treated with surgery randomized by risk factors to post-op RT. Risk factors included >1 node group, ≥2 nodes, nodes >3 cm, microscopic +margins, PNI, oral cavity site, & nodal extracapsular extension. Low-risk = no risk factors → no RT. Intermediate risk = 1 risk factor (but not ECE) → 1.8/57.6 Gy. High-risk = ECE or ≥2 risk factors → 1.8/63 Gy in 7 weeks or in 5 weeks with a concomitant boost. The 5 yr LRC/OS for low-risk was 90/83%, for intermediate risk 94/66%, & for high-risk 68/42%. Overall treatment time <11 weeks increased LRC, and concomitant boost had a trend for improved OS
- EORTC 22931 (Bernier, *NEJM* 2004). 334 pts with operable stage III/IV oral cavity, oropharynx, larynx, & hypopharnx cancer randomized to post-op RT (2/66 Gy) vs post-op chemo-RT (2/66 Gy & cisplatin 100 mg/m^2 on days 1, 22, 43). All patients received 54 Gy to the low risk neck. Eligible stages included pT3-4N0/+, T1-2N2-3, & T1-2N0-1 with ECE, +margin, or PNI. Chemo-RT improved 3/5 yr DFS (41/36→59/47%), 3/5 yr OS (49/40→65/53%), & 5 yr LRC (69→82%), but increased grade 3-4 toxicity (21→41%)
- RTOG 95–01 (Cooper, *NEJM* 2004). 459 pts with operable cancer of the oral cavity, oropharynx, larynx, or hypopharynx who had ≥2 involved lymph nodes, nodal extracapsular extension, or a + margin randomized to post-op RT (2/60–66 Gy) vs post-op chemo-RT (2/60–66 Gy & cisplatin ×3c as in EORTC 22931). Chemo-RT improved 2 yr DFS (43→54%), LRC (72→82%), & had a trend for improved OS (57→63%), but increased grade 3-4 toxicity (34→77%)

RADIATION TECHNIQUES

Simulation and field design

- Simulate the patient supine with the head hyperextended. Wire neck scars & the tracheostoma (if present). Shoulders may be pulled down with straps. Immobilize with a thermoplastic head & shoulder mask. Bolus may be needed for anterior commissure tumors & over the tracheostoma (if present)
- A 3D or IMRT plan should be used for any but simple opposed-lateral fields in order to spare normal tissues
- Computed dosimetry should be used in all cases

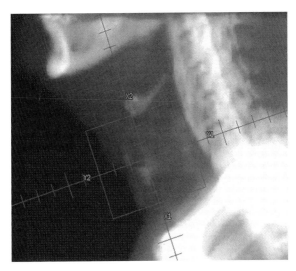

FIGURE 9.1. Lateral DRR of a field used to treat a T1 glottic carcinoma.

- Glottic larynx: For T1N0, use a 5 × 5 cm field with the superior border at the top of the thyroid cartilage, the inferior border at the bottom of the cricoid, a 1 cm skin flash anteriorly, and a 2 cm margin posteriorly (or the anterior edge of the vertebral body). For glottic T2N0, the field size is increased to 6 × 6 cm with the inferior border 1 tracheal ring below the cricoid. For T3-4N0, extend the superior border to 2 cm above the angle of the mandible, the posterior border behind the spinous processes, and the inferior border to include 1.5–2 cm margin on the subglottic extent of the tumor. Match the lateral fields to the low neck AP field. Treat the lateral fields to 42–45 Gy with a small cord block, then move the posterior border off-cord and use an electron boost to treat the elective posterior neck to 50 Gy. Boost the primary with a 1.5 cm margin to 70 Gy with chemo or to 72 Gy with a concomitant boost if chemo not used
- Supraglottic larynx: For T1N0 treat the primary & levels II–III. For T2-3, also treat with a matched low-neck AP field because of increased risk of microscopic nodal disease. For advanced cases, treat as described above

- Hypopharynx: Treat primary & levels II–V & retropharyngeal nodes in all cases. The superior border is the skull base & mastoid. The inferior border is 1 cm below the inferior extent of disease (or 1 cm below cricoid) on the laterals & matched to the AP low neck field. With posterior pharyngeal wall tumors, the anterior border does not need to flash the skin. A clothespin may be used to spare the skin anteriorly
- Post-op: Use 3-field technique with stoma in low-neck AP field. Lateral fields cover neopharynx, adenopathy, & 1.5–2 cm margin on preoperative extent of disease
- With conventional 3-field techniques, the spinal cord is shielded on the lateral fields at the matchline if no gross disease is present. If gross disease is present at the matchline, angling the lateral fields to match the divergence of the AP field may help. A small midline block on the AP field may be necessary
- Wedges &/or compensating filters may be required
- IMRT: GTV = clinical &/or radiographic gross disease. CTV1 = 0.5–2 cm margin on primary &/or nodal GTV (depending on presence or absence of anatomic boundaries to microscopic spread). CTV2 = elective neck. Individualized planning target volumes are used for the GTV, CTV1, & CTV2.
- IMRT not recommended for T1-2N0 glottic cancers

Dose prescriptions

- Larynx: Use >2 Gy/fraction for Tis & T1-2N0 glottic tumors. UCSF uses 2.25 Gy/fraction to 56.25–58.5 Gy for Tis, 63 Gy for T1N0, & 65.25 Gy for T2N0. Alternatively, 60 Gy may be used for T1 tumors after all visible tumor has been removed (e.g., with stripping). For all other cases, if chemo-RT is used, the dose is 2/70 Gy. If the patient is unable to tolerate chemo, altered fractionation to ≥72 Gy may be used
- Hypopharynx: For early-stage, 1.8–2 Gy/fraction to 50–54 Gy followed by a boost to 70–75 Gy. For advanced cases, if chemo-RT is used, the dose is 2/70 Gy. If the patient is unable to tolerate chemo, concomitant boost to 72 Gy may be used
- Post-op RT: 1.8–2 Gy/fraction to 50–54 Gy followed by boost to 60–66 Gy to high-risk areas and the post-operative bed

- <u>IMRT</u> (UCSF): GTV = 2.12/70 Gy, CTV1 = 1.8/59.4 Gy, CTV2 = 1.64/54 Gy

Dose limitations

- Spinal cord maximum dose ≤45–50 Gy. Brainstem maximum dose ≤54 Gy. Keep 50% of the volume of each parotids ≤20 Gy (if possible). Mandible maximum dose ≤70 Gy
- Tracheostomas are limited to ≤50 Gy unless concerned about involvement, significant subglottic extension, or emergent tracheostomy (then boost to 60–66 Gy)

COMPLICATIONS

- Complications of RT include mucositis, dermatitis, xerostomia, dysgeusia, soft tissue fibrosis, hypothyroidism, & rarely radionecrosis, pharyngocutaneous fistula, or carotid rupture
- Perioperative complications of surgery include bleeding, airway obstruction, infection, & wound complications. Post-op complications include webs, stenosis, chondritis, fistulas, & aspiration
- Patients need ≥2000 calories/day to avoid malnutrition. Supplements (e.g., Boost or Ensure) &/or feeding tubes may be used
- Amifostine may decrease xerostomia & mucositis, but it is associated with significant side effects (hypotension, nausea) (Peters, *IJROBP* 1993 & Brizel, *JCO* 2000)

FOLLOW-UP

- H&P every 1–3 mo for year 1, every 2–4 mo for year 2, every 6 mo for years 3–5, then annually. CXR annually. TSH every 6–12 mo if neck irradiated
- If recurrence is suspected but biopsy is negative, follow closely (at least monthly) until resolves

REFERENCES

Adelstein DJ, Li Y, Adams GL, et al. An intergroup phase III comparison of standard radiation therapy and two schedules of concurrent chemoradiotherapy in patients with unresectable squamous cell head and neck cancer. J Clin Oncol 2003;21:92–98.

Ang KK, Trotti A, Brown BW, et al. Randomized trial addressing risk features and time factors of surgery plus radiotherapy in advanced head-and-neck cancer. Int J Radiat Oncol Biol Phys 2001;51: 571–578.

Bernier J, Domenge C, Ozsahin M, et al. Postoperative irradiation with or without concomitant chemotherapy for locally advanced head and neck cancer. N Engl J Med 2004;350:1945–1952.

Bonner JA, Harari PM, Giralt J, et al. Radiotherapy plus cetuximab for squamous-cell carcinoma of the head and neck. N Engl J Med 2006;354:567–578.

Brizel DM, Albers ME, Fisher SR, et al. Hyperfractionated irradiation with or without concurrent chemotherapy for locally advanced head and neck cancer. N Engl J Med 1998;338:1798–1804.

Cooper JS, Pajak TF, Forastiere AA, et al. Postoperative concurrent radiotherapy and chemotherapy for high-risk squamous-cell carcinoma of the head and neck. N Engl J Med 2004;350:1937–1944.

Emami B, Schmidt-Ullrich RK. Hypopharynx. In: Perez CA, Brady LW, Halperin EC, et al., editors. Principles and Practice of Radiation Oncology. 4th ed. Philadelphia: Lippincott Williams & Wilkins; 2004. pp. 1071–1093.

Forastiere AA, Goepfert H, Maor M, et al. Concurrent chemotherapy and radiotherapy for organ preservation in advanced laryngeal cancer. N Engl J Med 2003;349:2091–2098.

Fu KK, Pajak TF, Trotti A, et al. A Radiation Therapy Oncology Group (RTOG) phase III randomized study to compare hyperfractionation and two variants of accelerated fractionation to standard fractionation radiotherapy for head and neck squamous cell carcinomas: first report of RTOG 9003. Int J Radiat Oncol Biol Phys 2000; 48:7–16.

Garden AS, Forster K, Wong PF, et al. Results of radiotherapy for T2N0 glottic carcinoma: does the "2" stand for twice-daily treatment? Int J Radiat Oncol Biol Phys 2003;55:322–328.

Garden AS, Morrison WH, Ang KK. Laryngeal and hypopharyngeal cancer. In: Gunderson LL, Tepper JE, editors. Clinical Radiation Oncology. 1st ed. Philadelphia: Churchill Livingstone; 2000. pp. 485–503.

Garden AS. The larynx and hypopharynx. In: Cox JD, Ang KK, editors. Radiation Oncology: Rationale, Technique, Results. 8th ed. St. Louis: Mosby; 2003. pp. 255–281.

Greene FL, American Joint Committee on Cancer, American Cancer Society. AJCC Cancer Staging Manual. 6th ed. New York: Springer-Verlag; 2002.

The Department of Veterans Affairs Laryngeal Cancer Study Group. Induction chemotherapy plus radiation compared with surgery plus radiation in patients with advanced laryngeal cancer. N Engl J Med 1991;324:1685–1690.

Le QT, Fu KK, Kroll S, et al. Influence of fraction size, total dose, and overall time on local control of T1-T2 glottic carcinoma. Int J Radiat Oncol Biol Phys 1997;39:115–126.

Lee N, Phillips TL. Cancer of the larynx. In: Leibel SA, Phillips TL, editors. Textbook of Radiation Oncology. 2nd ed. Philadelphia: Saunders; 2004. pp. 679–698.

Lefebvre JL, Chevalier D, Luboinski B, et al. Larynx preservation in pyriform sinus cancer: preliminary results of a European Organization for Research and Treatment of Cancer phase III trial. EORTC Head and Neck Cancer Cooperative Group. J Natl Cancer Inst 1996;88:890–899.

Mendenhall WM, Hinerman RW, Amdur RJ, et al. Larynx. In: Perez CA, Brady LW, Halperin EC, et al., editors. Principles and Practice of Radiation Oncology. 4th ed. Philadelphia: Lippincott Williams & Wilkins; 2004. pp. 1094–1116.

National Cancer Institute. Hypopharyngeal Cancer (PDQ): Treatment. Available at: http://cancer.gov/cancertopics/pdq/treatment/hypopharyngeal/healthprofessional/. Accessed on January 19, 2005.

National Comprehensive Cancer Network. Clinical Practice Guidelines in Oncology: Head and Neck Cancers. Available at: http://www.nccn.org/professionals/physician_gls/PDF/head-and-neck.pdf. Accessed on January 19, 2005.

Zelefsky MJ. Cancer of the hypopharynx. In: Leibel SA, Phillips TL, editors. Textbook of Radiation Oncology. 2nd ed. Philadelphia: Saunders; 2004. pp. 657–678.

Chapter 10
Salivary Gland Tumors

Allen Chen and Naomi R. Schechter

PEARLS

- Salivary gland neoplasms account for ~3–7% of H&N cancers
- Major salivary glands consist of the paired parotid, submandibular, & sublingual glands
- Minor salivary glands located throughout oral cavity, pharynx, and paranasal sinuses
- Parotid glands located lateral to the mandibular ramus and masseter muscle
- Facial nerve divides parotid gland into superficial and deep lobes
- Parotid gland drains into oral cavity through Stensen's duct adjacent to upper second molar
- Lymphatic drainage from parotid gland is to intraparotid and periparotid nodes followed by ipsilateral level I, II, and III nodes
- Submandibular gland is located under the horizontal mandibular ramus
- Submandibular gland is lateral to and abuts lingual (V3) and hypoglossal nerves, & is medial to mandibular and cervical branches of CN VII
- Submandibular glands drain into oral cavity through Wharton's duct
- Submandibular lymphatic drainage is to levels I, II, III
- Drainage from parotid and submandibular glands to contralateral nodes is rare
- Sublingual gland located superior to mylohyoid muscle & deep to mucous membrane
- Sublingual glands drain into oral cavity through Rivinus ducts or Bartholin's duct
- Majority of salivary gland neoplasms are benign

- Inverse relationship exists between size of parotid gland and ratio of malignant to benign cancer
- For tumors of the parotid gland, 80% are benign and 20% malignant
- Most parotid tumors present as painless swelling
- Pleomorphic adenoma is most common benign salivary gland neoplasm
- Salivary gland cancer is notable for its remarkable histologic diversity
- Most common malignant histology of parotid gland is mucoepidermoid carcinoma
- Most common malignant histology of submandibular & minor salivary glands is adenoid cystic carcinoma
- Acinic cell carcinoma usually occurs only in the parotid gland
- Incidence of LN involvement varies according to histology and site
- Overall risk of lymph node involvement is less common than for SCC
- Adenoid cystic carcinoma has the lowest frequency of cervical node metastasis (5–8%) but the highest propensity for perineural spread
- LN metastases are most common with minor salivary gland tumors followed by submandibular gland tumors followed by parotid tumors
- Prognostic variables include grade, post-surgical residual disease, & LN status
- Larger tumor size and cranial nerve involvement associated with poor prognosis
- Patterns of failure generally dominated by high rates of distant metastases
- Most likely sites for DM is lung, followed by bone and liver
- Adenoid cystic, ductal, & undifferentiated carcinoma have highest rates of DM
- Loss of salivary function is permanent and complete after 35 Gy with standard fx
- Despite high DM rate, there is generally no role for chemotherapy

WORKUP

- H&P with bimanual palpation. Carefully examine cranial nerves & for trismus

- CT &/or MRI of head and neck. PET scan is still investigational for salivary gland cancers
- Fine-needle aspiration biopsy
- Chest X-ray
- Dental evaluation prior to the start of RT

STAGING (MAJOR SALIVARY GLANDS ONLY)

Primary Tumor

TX: Primary tumor cannot be assessed

T0:   No evidence of primary tumor

T1:   Tumor 2 cm or less in greatest dimension without extraparenchymal extension

T2:   Tumor more than 2 cm but not more than 4 cm in greatest dimension without extraparenchymal extension

T3:   Tumor more than 4 cm and/or having extraparenchymal extension

T4a: Tumor invades skin, mandible, ear canal, and/or facial nerve

T4b: Tumor invades skull base and/or pterygoid plates and/or encases carotid artery

Note: Extraparenchymal extension is clinical or macroscopic evidence of invasion of soft tissues. Microscopic evidence alone does not constitute extraparenchymal extension for classification purposes.

Regional lymph nodes

NX: Regional lymph nodes cannot be assessed

N0:   No regional lymph nodes metastasis

N1:   Metastasis in a single ipsilateral lymph node, 3 cm or less in greatest dimension

N2:   Metastasis in a single ipsilateral lymph node, more than 3 cm but not more than 6 cm in greatest dimension, or in multiple ipsilateral lymph nodes, none more than 6 cm in greatest dimension, or in bilateral or contralateral lymph nodes, none more than 6 cm in greatest dimension

N2a: Metastasis in single ipsilateral lymph node, more than 3 cm but not more than 6 cm in greatest dimension

N2b: Metastasis in multiple ipsilateral lymph nodes, none more than 6 cm in greatest dimension

N2c: Metastasis in bilateral or contralateral lymph nodes, none more than 6 cm in greatest dimension

N3:   Metastasis in a lymph node, more than 6 cm in greatest dimension

Distant Metastasis

MX: Distant metastasis cannot be assessed

M0:   No distant metastasis

M1:   Distant metastasis present

Stage Grouping		~2/5 yr OS	
I:	T1N0M0	I:	88/75%
II:	T2N0M0	II:	77/59%
III:	T3N0M0, T1-3N1M0	III:	68/47%
IVA:	T4aN0-2M0, T1-3N2M0	IV:	47/28%
IVB:	T4b any NM0, any TN3M0		
IVC:	Any T, any N, M1		

Used with the permission of the American Joint Committee on Cancer (AJCC), Chicago, Illinois. The original source for this material is the AJCC Cancer Staging Manual, Sixth Edition (2002) published by Springer-Verlag New York, www.springeronline.com.

- Note that minor salivary gland cancer is staged according to systems for the anatomic site of involvement

TREATMENT RECOMMENDATIONS

Stage	Recommended Treatment
0–II	Surgical excision +/– RT
III–IV	Surgical excision + RT

General points

- Surgery forms the mainstay of definitive treatment for salivary gland malignancies
- Complications of surgery include facial nerve dysfunction and Frey's syndrome
- Frey's syndrome consists of gustatory flushing, sweating, auriculotemporal syndrome
- Superficial parotidectomy can generally be performed for low-grade parotid tumors
- Facial nerve-sparing approaches can often be performed to preserve function, cosmesis
- Neck dissection recommended for clinically + LN or high-grade histology
- Indications for post-op RT are currently controversial as there is no randomized data analyzing the role of post-op RT
- Consider post-op RT for PNI, close/+ margins, high-grade tumors, and T3-4 tumors
- Pts with pathological LN involvement should receive post-op RT
- RT alone is indicated for medically inoperable and unresectable tumors. LC rates with RT alone range from 20% to 80%

- Neutron therapy may achieve better LC for unresectable or inoperable tumors
- Brachytherapy or intraoperative RT can be considered for recurrent tumors
- IMRT reduces mean doses to normal structures and allows dose-escalation to tumor
- Chemotherapy is considered investigational

STUDIES

- Fu (*Cancer* 1977). Retrospective analysis of 100 cases of major and minor salivary gland cancer treated with surgery or surgery + RT. The addition of post-op RT significantly improved LC for pts with adenoid cystic carcinoma, locally advanced (stage III/IV) disease, and + margins
- Garden (*IJROBP* 1997). Retrospective analysis of 166 pts with parotid gland malignancies treated with surgery + RT. On multivariate analysis, facial nerve sacrifice and pathologic cervical nodal disease was associated with LF. The actuarial 5-, 10-, and 15-yr LC rates were 92%, 90%, and 90%, respectively
- Garden (*IJROBP* 1995). Retrospective analysis of 198 pts with adenoid cystic carcinoma of the H&N treated with surgery + RT. 5- and 10-yr LC was 95% and 86%, respectively. Pts with positive margins and major (named) nerve involvement were at significantly increased risk of LR
- Armstrong (*Arch Otolaryngol Head Neck Surg* 1990). Matched-pair analysis of 92 pts treated with surgery vs surgery & post-op RT. The addition of post-op RT improved outcome for pts with stage III/IV disease and for pts with pathological + LN
- Armstrong (*Cancer* 1992). Retrospective review of 474 previously untreated pts with major salivary gland cancers in an attempt to define indications for elective treatment of the neck. Overall, clinically occult, pathologically + LN occurred in only 12% of pts. On multivariate analysis, only primary tumor size and grade were significant risk factors
- North (*IJROBP* 1990). Retrospective analysis of 87 pts with major salivary gland cancer treated with surgery or surgery + post-op RT. The addition of post-op RT significantly improved 5 yr OS (59→75%) LF (26→4%)

- Storey (*IJROBP* 2001). Retrospective analysis of 83 pts treated with surgery and postoperative RT for submandibular gland malignancies. Actuarial 10 yr LRC was 88%, 10 yr DFS was 53%, & OS was 55%

- Terhaard (*IJROBP* 2005). Retrospective analysis of 538 pts treated for major salivary gland tumors. Post-op RT improved 10 yr LC compared with surgery alone for pts with T3-4 tumors (18→84%), close (55→95%) & incomplete resection (44→82%), bone invasion (54→86%), & PNI (60→88%).

- Spiro (*Cancer* 1993). Retrospective analysis of 62 pts with parotid gland malignancies treated with surgery and post-op RT. Actuarial 5/10 yr LC was 95/84%. Pts with larger tumors, recurrent disease, or facial nerve involvement had lower DFS.

- Boahene (*Arch Otolaryngol Head Neck Surg* 2004). Retrospective analysis of 89 pts with mucoepidermoid carcinoma of parotid gland treated predominantly with surgery alone. DFS at 5, 15, & 25 yrs were 99%, 97%, and 97%, respectively

- Garden (*IJROBP* 1994). Retrospective analysis of 160 pts treated with surgery and post-op RT for minor salivary gland cancer. 15 yr LC, DFS, & OS was 78%, 54%, and 43%, respectively. On multivariate analysis, paranasal primary site associated with increased risk of LF

- RTOG/MRC (Laramore, *IJROBP* 1993). Randomized trial of 32 pts with inoperable primary or recurrent salivary gland cancer compared fast neutron RT vs conventional RT with photons and/or electrons. Trial was stopped early due to advantage with neutrons [improved 10 yr LRC, but not OS (15–25%)]. Distant metastases accounted for most failures

- Wang (*IJROBP* 1991). Retrospective analysis of 24 pts treated with RT alone for salivary gland malignancies. All lesions were irradiated by accelerated hyperfractionated photons (bid) with 1.6 Gy per fraction, intermixed with various boost techniques including electron beam, intraoral cone, interstitial implant, and/or submental photons for a total of 65–70 Gy. 5 yr LC for parotid gland lesions was 100% with 65% OS. For minor salivary gland tumors, the 5 yr LC was 78% and OS was 93%

- Mendenhall (*Head and Neck* 2004). Retrospective analysis of 101 pts treated with RT for adenoid cystic carcinoma of the H&N. 10 yr LC was 43% for pts treated with RT alone compared to 91% for pts treated with surgery and post-op RT. On multivariate analysis, T-stage and clinical nerve invasion influenced CSS

RADIATION TECHNIQUES
Simulation and field design
- Simulate supine with customized immobilization devices
- Head secured in holder with face mask and neck hyperextended
- All incisional scars and masses are wired for visualization
- Bite block used to facilitate immobilization and reduce amount of normal tissue in field
- Shoulder pull board can be employed to maximally depress shoulders
- CT-planning allows for more accurate dose distribution
- Various techniques have been described for salivary gland radiation
- Post-op tumor volume includes operative bed with at least 2 cm margin
- Mixed photon/electron beam can be used en face to cover target volume with margin. Weighting is generally 50% to 80% weighting towards electrons. Electron energy depends on distance from skin of ipsilateral cheek to oral mucosa. Typically 12 to 16 MeV electrons are used in combination with 4- to 6-MV photons
- Wedge pair technique with photons can also be used with anterior/posterior obliques. To avoid exit dose through contralateral eye, slightly angle beams inferiorly. Include entire surgical bed in irradiated tumor volume with bolus over the scar
- Consider neutron therapy for unresectable or medically inoperable tumors
- IMRT may be used to spare normal tissues & dose-escalate
- Elective RT to the neck depends on histology, primary site, and presentation
- Treatment of contralateral lymph nodes is unnecessary since failure there is rare
- Using photons, AP/PA or direct AP fields can be used
- Neck field is angled obliquely to keep off spinal cord
- With neck RT, attention to geometric match with primary field is essential

- Half-beam block is used for the cranial edge of the neck field to eliminate divergence
- For adenoid cystic carcinoma, irradiate pathways of cranial nerves to base of skull

Dose prescriptions
- Post-op RT, negative margins: 60–63 Gy at 1.8–2 Gy/fx
- Post-op RT, + margins 66 Gy at 1.8–2 Gy/fx
- RT alone or post-op RT for gross residual disease: 70 at 1.8–2 Gy/fx
- Elective neck RT: 50–54 Gy at 1.8–2 Gy/fx

Dose limitations
- Spinal cord ≤45 Gy, brainstem ≤54 Gy, optic chiasm and nerves ≤54 Gy, cochlea ≤50 Gy, mandible ≤60–70 Gy, temporal brain ≤60 Gy, uninvolved salivary glands ≤24 Gy

COMPLICATIONS
- Xerostomia, trismus, otitis media, hair loss, skin erythema and desquamation, dental problems, taste loss, hypothyroidism, mucositis, oral candidiasis, esophagitis, CN palsy, second malignancy

FOLLOW-UP
- H&P every 1–3 mo for 1 yr, every 2–4 mo for 2nd yr, every 4–6 mo for yrs 3–5, & annually thereafter. Regular head imaging with MRI & CXR as indicated. TSH every 6–12 mo if neck irradiated

REFERENCES

Armstrong JG, Harrison LB, Thaler HT, et al. The indications for elective treatment of the neck in cancer of the major salivary glands. Cancer 992;69:615–619.

Armstrong JG, Harrison LB, Spiro RH, et al. Malignant tumors of major salivary gland origin. A matched-pair analysis of the role of combined surgery and postoperative radiotherapy. Arch Otolaryngol head Neck Surg 1990;116:290–293.

Boahene DK, Olsen KD, Lewis, JE, et al. Mucoepidermoid carcinoma of the parotid gland. Arch Otolaryngol Hed Neck Surg 2004;130:849–856.

Bragg CM, Conway J, Robinson MH. The role of intensity-modulated radiotherapy in the treatment of parotid tumors. Int J Radiat Oncol Biol Phys 2002;52:729–738.

Douglas JG, Koh WJ, Austin-Seymour M, et al. Treatment of salivary gland neoplasms with fast neutron radiotherapy. Arch Otolaryngol Head Neck Surg 2003;129:944–948.

Fu KK, Leibel SA, Levine ML, et al. Carcinoma of the major and minor salivary glands. Cancer 1977;40:2882–2890.

Garden AS, El-Naggar AK, Morrison WH, et al. Postoperative radiotherapy for malignant tumors of the parotid gland. Int J Radiat Oncol Biol Phys 1997;37:79–85.

Garden AS, Weber RS, Ang KK, et al. Postoperative radiation therapy for malignant tumors of minor salivary glands. Cancer 1994;73:2563–2569.

Garden AS, Weber RS, Morrison WH, et al. The influence of positive margins and nerve invasion in adenoid cystic carcinoma of the head and neck treated with surgery and radiation. Int J Radiat Oncol Biol Phys 1995;32:619–626.

Laramore GE, Krall JM, Griffin TW, et al. Neutron versus photon irradiation for unresectable salivary gland tumors: final report of an RTOG-MRC randomized clinical trial. Radiation Therapy Oncology Group. Medical Research Council. Int J Radiat Oncol Biol Phys 1993;27:235–240.

Mendenhall WM, Morris CG, Amdur RJ, et al. Radiotherapy alone or combined with surgery for adenoid cystic carcinoma of the head and neck. Head Neck 2004;26:154–162.

North CA, Lee DJ, Piantadosi S, et al. Carcinoma of the major salivary glands treated by surgery or surgery plus postoperative radiotherapy. Int J Radiat Oncol Biol Phys 1990;18:1319–1326.

Spiro IJ, Wang CC, Montgomery WW. Carcinoma of the parotid gland. Analysis of treatment results and patterns of failure after combined surgery and radiation therapy. Cancer 1993;71:2699–2705.

Storey MR, Garden AS, Morrison WH, et al. Postoperative radiotherapy for malignant tumors of the submandibular gland. Int J Radiat Oncol Biol Phys 2001;51:952–958.

Terhaard CH, Lubsen H, Rasch CR, et al. The role of radiotherapy in the treatment of malignant salivary gland tumors. Int J Radiat Oncol Biol Phys 2005;61:103–111.

Wang CC, Goodman M. Photon irradiation of unresectable carcinomas of salivary glands. Int J Radiat Oncol Biol Phys 1991;21:569–576.

NOTES

Chapter 11
Thyroid Cancer

Joy Coleman and Jeanne Marie Quivey

PEARLS

- Thyroid cancer is rare – 1% of malignancies & 0.2% of cancer deaths in the U.S. Incidence increasing which may in part be related to increased detection of subclinical disease by extensive use of ultrasound & FNA. Female : male ratio of 3 : 1. Incidence begins increasing in teenage yrs, peaking in the 5th decade

- Prior RT exposure is the main environmental factor linked to development. It can result in benign (goiter, nodular disease) & malignant thyroid disease. RT-induced tumors are usually well-differentiated and behave similar to spontaneous thyroid cancer. Periodic clinical and bio-chemical testing (serum thyroglobulin) is prudent for those who have undergone prior thyroid irradiation (including incidental irradiation during mantle or head and neck radiation)

- Pathology – listed in order of declining prognosis:
  - Papillary thyroid carcinoma (several variants; all arise from follicular cells)
    - Solid papillary thyroid carcinoma – good prognosis
    - Follicular variant, formerly called mixed papillary-follicular, but not to be confused with follicular carcinoma (demonstrates biologic and prognostic characteristics of papillary carcinoma). Good prognosis
    - Diffuse sclerosing, tall cell, columnar cell – all have poor prognosis
  - Follicular thyroid carcinoma (arises from follicular cells)
    - No cytologic features distinguish minimally inva-sive carcinomas from benign follicular adenomas. Therefore cannot diagnose on FNA.

- Hurthle Cell (oncocytic carcinoma).
    - Cell of origin unclear: historically thought to be a follicular variant, but molecular studies suggest it may be more similar to papillary.
    - Can be benign or malignant – if they do not demonstrate evidence of microscopic invasion they behave like adenomas. If they have histologic evidence of malignancy they are usually more aggressive than ordinary follicular/papillary carcinomas (10 yr survival 76% vs 85%).
- Medullary thyroid cancer
    - Arises from the parafollicular/C-cells that produce calcitonin
    - 20–30% familial
    - MEN 2 is autosomal dominant; it involves the RET proto-oncogene on chromosome 10. MEN 2A – Pheochromocytoma, parathyroid tumors, medullary thyroid cancer. MEN 2B – Marfanoid habitus, ganglioneuromas of the mucosa and GI tract, pheochromocytomas, mucosal neuromas of tongue and lips, medullary thyroid cancer. Lifetime risk for carriers ~90%. It is codon dependent & age dependent. Prophylactic total thyroidectomy produces cure rate >90%
- Anaplastic thyroid carcinoma
    - Rare; aggressive
    - Must be distinguished from poorly differentiated medullary carcinoma, lymphoma, and poorly differentiated follicular carcinoma (all have different treatment and better prognosis)
- Lymphatic drainage initially to the central compartment, nodes in the tracheo-esophageal groove, and the nodes anterior to the larynx just above the isthmus (Delphian nodes). Drainage proceeds to the cervical nodes then to the anterior mediastinum and occasionally the supraclavicular nodes. All of these sites must be included in treatment planning
- Age is the most important prognostic factor determining survival. Larger tumor size, higher histologic grade, postoperative macroscopic residual disease, male sex, and presence of distant metastases are also poor prognostic factors

WORKUP

- Many present with asymptomatic palpable nodules. Advanced cases can present with hoarseness caused by recurrent laryngeal nerve paralysis or invasion into the larynx, pharynx, or esophagus. Can also present in a thyroglossal duct cyst (rare) or with cervical nodal mets. Occasionally can present with DM in lung or skeleton
- FNA is the most important diagnostic tool. Sensitivity 98%, specificity 99%, accuracy 98%. Results can be benign, suspicious, malignant, or unsatisfactory/indeterminant. A negative FNA still requires careful consideration of all clinical factors before a decision to perform repeat FNA or advance to an excisional bx/lobectomy can be made. A suspicious or indeterminate finding on FNA does not exclude follicular carcinoma
- Radionuclide scintigraphy and thyroid ultrasound are complementary tests that can help provide additional information. Should be performed after FNA (if FNA is positive they are superfluous and not cost effective for evaluating the thyroid gland.)
- US of the neck or MRI are useful to detect adenopathy. Do not perform a contrast CT scan as this will interfere with the ability to treat with I-131 for up to 6 months.
- Blood tests: T3, T4, TSH, thyroglobulin
- If FNA indicates medullary carcinoma, check serum calcitonin, CEA, and calcium as well as urine and serum catecholamines (to screen for pheochromocytoma). If positive for pheochromocytoma, this should be treated first. With more advanced disease, medullary carcinoma can present with diarrhea from calcitonin production. This carries a poor prognosis. Medullary carcioma can be a finding in MEN 2 pts, and families must be screened for the RET proto-oncogene. If a RET proto-oncogene germline mutation is detected, other family members should undergo codon oriented prophylactic surgery (COPS). The specific codon involved will dictate the appropriate timing of surgery for other family members

STAGING

Primary tumor
Note: All categories may be subdivided: (a) solitary tumor, (b) multifocal tumor (the largest determines the classification)

TX: Primary tumor cannot be assessed

T0:   No evidence of primary tumor
T1:   Tumor 2 cm or less in greatest dimension limited to the thyroid
T2:   Tumor more than 2 cm but not more than 4 cm in greatest dimension limited to thyroid
T3:   Tumor more than 4 cm in greatest dimension limited to thyroid or any tumor with minimal extrathyroid extension (e.g., extension to sternothyroid muscle or perithyroid soft tissues)
T4a: Tumor of any size extending beyond the thyroid capsule to invade subcutaneous soft tissues, larynx, trachea, esophagus, or recurrent laryngeal nerve
T4b: Tumor invades prevertebral fascia or encases carotid artery or mediastinal vessels

All anaplastic carcinomas are considered T4 with T4a being surgically resectable and T4b being surgically unresectable

- T4a: Intrathyoidal anaplastic carcinoma – surgically resectable
- T4b: Extrathyroidal anaplastic carcinoma – surgically unresectable

Regional lymph nodes
Regional lymph nodes are the central compartment, lateral cervical, and upper mediastinal lymph nodes

NX: Regional lymph nodes cannot be assessed.
N0:   No regional lymph node metastasis
N1:   Regional lymph node metastasis
N1a: Metastasis to Level VI LN (pretracheal, paratracheal, and prelaryngeal/Delphian lymph nodes)
N1b: Metastasis to unilateral, bilateral, or contralateral cervical or superior mediastinal lymph nodes

Distant Metastases
MX: Distant metastasis cannot be assessed
M0:   No distant metastasis
M1:   Distant metastases

Stage Grouping	Survival
Separate stage grouping are recommended for papillary or follicular, medullary, and anaplastic (undifferentiated) carcinoma.	
Papillary or Follicular: *Under age 45*	Follicular & papillary: 95–97% DSS at 20 yrs (follicular and papillary respectively)
I: Any T any N M0 II: Any T any N M1	Tumor size >1.5 cm, male, and age >45 have increased mortality

Papillary or Follicular: *Age 45 years and older or Medullary Carcinoma*			Medullary: 60–80% DSS at 10 yrs
I:	T1	N0	M0	
II:	T2	N0	M0	
III:	T3	N0	M0	
	T1–3	N1a	M0	
IVA:	T4a	N0-1b	M0	
	T1–3	N1b	M0	
IVB	T4b	any N	M0	
IVC	Any T	any N	M1	
Anaplastic Carcinomas			Anaplastic: 25% 1 yr DSS
IVA	T4a	any N	M0	
IVB	T4b	any N	M0	
IVC	Any T	any N	M1	

Used with the permission of the American Joint Committee on Cancer (AJCC), Chicago, Illinois. The original source for this material is the AJCC Cancer Staging Manual, Sixth Edition (2002) published by Springer-Verlag New York, www.springeronline.com.

TREATMENT RECOMMENDATIONS

Papillary/Follicular/Hurthle Cell	Recommended Treatment
Low risk disease Well differentiated, age 15–45 yrs, no prior RT, no LN or DM, no extrathyroidal extension, no FH of thyroid cancer, & tumor <4 cm in diameter	Total thyroidectomy. At 4–6 weeks post op, THS, thyroglobulin, and antithyroglobulin antibodies measured along with total body RAI scan → RAI treatment if indicated. Common indications include elevated thyroglobulin >1 ng/ml or a positive RAI scan. Lobectomy + isthmusectomy with no RAI is an option for low risk pts but not considered standard because it makes follow-up with THS, thyroglobulin, and RAI difficult/impossible.
High risk disease Age <15 yr or >45 yrs, RT history, known regional or DM, multifocal tumor, ECE, tumor >4 cm, or +FH	Thyroidectomy with LN dissection followed by RAI scan and tx. If LN+, then post op RAI ± EBRT

Papillary/Follicular/Hurthle Cell	Recommended Treatment
Local/Regional Recurrence	LN recurrence: neck dissection followed by RAI. Small volume disease in the superior mediastinum: RAI alone. Large volume mediastinal disease: superior mediastinal dissection followed by RAI. EBRT used for persistent/ recurrent disease after surgery and RAI. Other indications include pts with unresectable disease or pts with no uptake on RAI.
Metastatic Disease	Can have long survival so treat aggressively with RAI & EBRT depending on site of metastasis. Survival times longest for patients with diffuse, small lung metastases that concentrate RAI. Chemo not very effective. Most effective is single agent doxorubicin. Total thyroidectomy important even in the face of DM to allow for treatment with RAI

Medullary Carcinoma	Recommended Treatment
Local/Regional Disease	Total thyroidectomy with central level 6 LN dissection. Consider ipsilateral cervical level 2–5. Contralateral cervical LN dissection only if ipsilateral nodes are positive. EBRT for pts with gross/ microscopic residual disease after surgery, extensive regional LN involvement, T4a disease, or unresectable disease. Check serum calcitonin & CEA post-op to help determine if residual/ metastatic disease is present. No role for chemo or RAI

Medullary Carcinoma	Recommended Treatment
Metastatic disease	Palliative chemo (doxorubicin ± cisplatin), hormonal therapy (octreotide), and/or local RT. Consider a clinical trial: EGFR receptors being tested in phase II clinical trials.

Medullary Carcinoma	Recommended Treatment
Anaplastic	Complete surgical resection gives only chance of cure. If GTR not possible, then radical surgery is not indicated but airway management is needed. EBRT used for LC and to palliate symptoms. Altered fractionation & concurrent chemo-RT is under investigationdue to poor LC with EBRT alone. Clinical trials preferred. No role for RAI. No role for RAI

TRIALS

- No major prospective, randomized trials have been successful in enrolling adequate patient numbers. However, large international groups are studying the incidence, biology, and treatment of thyroid cancers, such as EUROMEN and the International RET Mutation Consortium for MTC
- EBRT in the management of differentiated thyroid cancer (*Clin Oncol* (*R Coll Radiol*), 2003). Retrospective review of 41 pts treated with EBRT with curative intent from 1988–2001. Doses ranged from 37.5–66 Gy over 3–6.5 weeks. 5 yr LR/OS were: papillary 26%/67%; follicular 43%/48%; well differentiated 21%/67%; focus of poor differentiation/ Hurthle cell variants 69%/32%; complete excision 25%/61%; residual disease 37%/59%; EBRT total dose < 50 Gy 63%/42%; 50–54 Gy 15%/72%; >54 Gy 18%/68%
- Value of EBRT for locally advanced papillary thyroid cancer (*IJROBP* 2003). 91 pts with T4 or N1 papillary thyroid cancer treated with surgical resection between 1981 and 1997. After surgery, 23 pts received post-op EBRT ± ablative radioiodine therapy. 68 pts were treated with ablative radioiodine therapy alone. 7 yr OS was not significantly different (no EBRT 98.1% vs EBRT 90%; p =

0.506), whereas 5 yr LRC was improved with EBRT (no EBRT 67.5% vs EBRT 95.2%; p = 0.0408)

- Is there a role for RT in the management of Hurthle cell carcinoma? (*IJROBP* 2003). Retrospective review of 18 pts receiving RT for Hurthle cell carcinoma of the thyroid gland between 1943 and 1995. Five pts received adjuvant RT, 7 received salvage RT for unresectable recurrent disease, and 6 received palliative RT for DM. 5-yr OS and CSS rates were 66.7% and 71.8%. Adjuvant & salvage RT prevented recurrence in 4/5 and 3/5 patients, respectively. Salvage RT was successful in 3 of 5 pts treated with EBRT
- Anaplastic thyroid carcinoma. Treatment outcome and prognostic factors. (*Cancer* 2005). 516 pts diagnosed between 1973 and 2000 drawn from the SEER database. 64% of patients underwent resection of their tumor, and 63% received EBRT. The overall CSS was 68.4% at 6 months and 80.7% at 12 months. On multivariate analysis, only age <60 yrs, an intrathyroidal tumor, and the combined use of surgery and EBRT were independent predictors of lower cause-specific mortality

RADIATION TECHNIQUES
Simulation & field design
- Must decide when to treat thyroid bed alone (for differentiated thyroid carcinoma without extensive extrathyroidal disease) vs thyroid, neck, and superior mediastinum (essentially all other definitive treatment)
- When treating the thyroid alone treat from the hyoid superiorly to just below the suprasternal notch. CT treatment planning is encouraged to ensure adequate coverage of substernal thyroid. Can use an anterior electron beam vs anterolateral wedged pair
- For large volume treatment there are many different treatment possibilities, but 3DCRT or IMRT is essential due to the target volume's size, shape, and proximity to other critical structures (including the spinal cord, larynx, and lungs). Target must include the tumor bed, the B cervical nodes, and the superior mediastinal nodes from the mastoid tip to the carina.
- Simulate patient supine with neck extended using an aquaplast mask to immobilize head and shoulders. Boost gross residual disease or any areas of extrathryoidal extension to doses listed below

Nuclear medicine

- The details of treatment with RAI are beyond the scope of this book. Readers are referred to nuclear medicine literature for details about the procedure

- Treatment with ^{131}I requires preparation with thyroxine withdrawal and a low iodine diet. Synthroid (T4) is stopped for 6 wks and cytomel (T3) given for the 1st three weeks prior to scanning & treatment. For the last two to three weeks, pts are given no replacement at all and started on a low iodine diet

- Recombinant TSH (thyrogen) allows scanning without thyroxine withdrawal, which does not require induced hypothyroidism and thus is better tolerated by patients, but its use is relatively new and it is still gaining acceptance. The patient still needs to be on the low iodine diet

- RAI scan is performed 1st to determine if treatment is appropriate and to determine the appropriate therapeutic dose. Treat with 100–200 mCi within 5 days of the diagnostic scan. Some physicians skip the diagnostic scan for fears of blunting uptake at the time of treatment and prescribe a fixed dose of 100 mCi. Others standardly prescribe 30 mCi as this is easier to deal with from a nuclear regulatory commission perspective, but this lower dose is much less effective. Rescan 7–10 d after treatment to identify additional foci of uptake undetected on the diagnostic scan and to document sites of disease treated.

- Repeat diagnostic RAI scan ~4–6 mo later if the first scan is positive. If repeat scan is positive can retreat or rescan in 6 mo. Continue rescanning & retreating until all detectable tumor has disappeared by I-131 scan. Once scan is negative, repeat in 1–2 yrs. If this is negative then follow clinically

- Never use iodinated contrast in a patient who will need RAI within 3–6 months

Dose prescriptions

- Papillary/Follicular/Medullary: Treat CTV to 45–50 Gy, microscopic disease to 55–60 Gy, and macroscopic disease to ≥65 Gy

- Anaplastic: Conventional fractionation to ≥65 Gy. Due to poor response with standard fractionation some use 1.5 Gy BID to 60 Gy ± chemo. For patients with poor KPS or known metastasis a palliative approach can be used

Dose limitations
- From EBRT: Esophagus <50–60 Gy. Salivary gland <24 Gy mean dose (consider RAI already affects salivary function). Cord ≤45–50 Gy. Brachial plexus <60 Gy. Lung $^2/_3$ <20 Gy
- From RAI: Total dose to bone marrow is 2 Gy

COMPLICATIONS

- From EBRT: Acute – skin breakdown, esophagitis, mucositis, changes in taste, xerostomia, laryngitis. Late – skin changes, fibrosis, lymphedema under chin, xerostomia, dental carries, esophageal stenosis.
- From RAI: Acute – sialadenitis xerostomia, cystitis (encourage good hydration), radiation gastritis (nausea, vomiting), diarrhea, pain (from localized tumor picking-up RAI very well), transient leucopenia/thrombocytopenia. Transient oligospermia in males. Rarely, thyrotoxicosis during the 1st 1–2 weeks of tumor lysis must be managed with propranolol. Acute acute radiation pneumonitis if extensive pulmonary metastases are present. Chronic side effects include increased risk of leukemia with cumulative doses >800 mCi, increased risk of breast & bladder cancer with doses >1000 mCi; late pulmonary fibrosis in pts with diffuse pulmonary metastases. No increased incidence of infertility, miscarriages, stillbirth, prematurity, and congenital anomalies, although most advise that patients wait 6 mo before attempting pregnancy

FOLLOW-UP

- H&P, labs (thyrotropin, free T3, thyroglobulin, TSH), US of the neck every 6 mo. MRI neck increasing in use. Frequency of RAI scans controversial. Disadvantage is the requirement for thyroxine withdrawl and resultant hypothyroidism, but use of recombinant TSH (thyrogen) may allow scanning without thyroxine withdrawl. PET/CT scans are sometimes useful in pts with elevation of thyroglobulin but no uptake with RAI. Serum calcitonin useful for following medullary thyroid carcinoma

REFERENCES
Biermann M, Pixberg MK, Schuck A, Heinecke A, Kopcke W, Schmid KW, Dralle H, Willich N, Schober O. Multicenter study differentiated thyroid carcinoma (MSDS). Diminished acceptance of adjuvant external beam radiotherapy. Nuklearmedizin. 2003 Dec;42(6): 244–250.

Foote RL, Brown PD, Garces YI, et al. Is there a role for radiation therapy in the management of Hurthle cell carcinoma? Int J Radiat Oncol Biol Phys 2003 Jul 15;56(4):1067–1072.

Ford D, Giridharan S, McConkey C, et al. External beam radiotherapy in the management of differentiated thyroid cancer. Clin Oncol (R Coll Radiol) 2003 Sep;15(6):337–341.

Fraker DL, Skarulis M, Livolsi V. Thyroid Tumors. In: Davita VT, Hellman S, and Rosenberg SA, editors. 6th ed. Philadelphia: Lippincptt Williams & Wilkins. Pp. 1740–1763.

Kebebew E, Greenspan FS, Clark OH, et al. Anaplastic thyroid carcinoma. Treatment outcome and prognostic factors. Cancer 2005 Apr 1;103(7):1330–1335.

Kim TH, Yang DS, Jung KY, et al. Value of external irradiation for locally advanced papillary thyroid cancer. Int J Radiat Oncol Biol Phys 2003 Mar 15;55(4):1006–1012.

Leenhardt L, Grosclaude P, Cherie-Challine L; Thyroid Cancer Committee. Increased incidence of thyroid carcinoma in france: a true epidemic or thyroid nodule management effects? Report from the French Thyroid Cancer Committee. Thyroid 2004 Dec; 14(12):1056–1060.

Machens A, Ukkat J, Brauckhoff M, et al. Advances in the management of hereditary medullary thyroid cancer. J Intern Med 2005 Jan;257(1):50–59.

Nahas Z, Goldenberg D, Fakhry C, et al. The role of positron emission tomography/computed tomography in the management of recurrent papillary thyroid carcinoma. Laryngoscope 2005 Feb;115(2): 237–243.

NCCN Physician Guidelines. http://www.nccn.org/professionals/physician_gls/PDF/thyroid.pdf. Accessed May 8, 2006.

Posner MD, Quivey JM, Akazawa PF, et al. Dose optimization for the treatment of anaplastic thyroid carcinoma: a comparison of treatment planning techniques. Int J Radiat Oncol Biol Phys 2000 Sep.

Reynolds RM, Weir J, Stockton DL, Brewster DH, et al. Changing trends in incidence and mortality of thyroid cancer in Scotland. Clin Endocrinol (Oxf) 2005 Feb;62(2):156–162.

Swift PS, Larson S, Price DC. Cancer of the Thyroid. In: Leibel SA, Phillips TL, editors. Textbook of radiation oncology. 2nd ed. Philadelphia: Saunders; 2004. pp. 757–778.

Tsang RW, Brierly JD. The Thyroid. In: Cox JD, Ang KK, editors. 8th ed. St. Louis: Mosby; 2003. pp. 310–330.

Tubiana M. Role of radioiodine in the treatment of local thyroid cancer. Int J Radiat Oncol Biol Phys 1996 Aug 1;36(1):263–265.

Wilson PC, Millar BM, Brierley JD. The management of advanced thyroid cancer. Clin Oncol (R Coll Radiol) 2004 Dec;16(8):561–568.

Yutan E, Clark OH. Hurthle cell carcinoma. Curr Treat Options Oncol 2001 Aug;2(4):331–335.

Chapter 12
Unusual Neoplasms of the Head and Neck

Eric K. Hansen and M. Kara Bucci

PEARLS

- **Chloromas** are solid extramedullary tumors consisting of early myeloid precursors associated with AML. Its name derives from the green color of affected tissues. It is more frequent with AML M4 & M5 subtypes & is associated with t(8;21). It may herald AML relapse after remission. It presents in the CNS with increased intracerebral pressure, or in the orbit with exophthalmos

- **Chordomas** originate from the primitive notochord. 50% occur in the sacrococcygeal area, 35% in the base of skull, and 15% in cervical vertebrae. Most common age is 50s to 60s. They are more common in men (2–3:1). They are locally invasive with slow growth. Metastases occur in up to 25% of patients, but lymph node spread is uncommon. Gross total resection is accomplished in only 10–20% of patients. Protons offer improved local control

- **Esthesioneuroblastomas** arise in the olfactory receptors of the nasal mucosa or cribiform plate. They present most commonly at ages 11–20 or 40–60 yrs, & the most common symptoms are epistaxis & nasal blockage. LN spread is ≤10% for early-stage disease, but is as high as 50% for Kadish stage C disease

- **Glomus tumors** are also called <u>paragangliomas</u>, <u>chemodectomas</u> (when non-chromaffin producing), or <u>carotid body tumors</u> (when chromaffin producing). They arise from the carotid body, jugular bulb, or middle ear from the tympanic nerve (of Jacobson) or auricular nerve (of Arnold). They rarely spread to nodes or metastasize (<5%). The mean age is 40s. They are more common in women (3:1). They present with ear pain, pulsations, tinnitus, cranial nerve palsies, or a painless mass. Biopsies may cause severe bleeding

- **Hemangioblastomas** are benign vascular tumors. The most common age is in the 20s to 30s. Most are found in the cerebellum. It is the most common cerebellar tumor in adults. It is associated with von Hippel-Lindau disease (cerebellar & retinal hemangioblastomas, pancreatic & renal cysts, renal cell carcinoma)
- **Hemangiopericytomas** are sarcomatous lesions arising from the smooth muscle around vessels. They most commonly present in the base of skull. They grow slowly and are locally invasive & hypervascular. They may be confused for meningioma. In the nose, they present with epistaxis. In the orbit, they present as painless proptosis. Meningeal hemangiopericytomas have >80% LR. Late metastases occur in 50–80% of pts
- **Juvenile nasopharyngeal angiofibromas** arise most frequently in pubertal boys, but age ranges from 9 to 30 yrs. They present with nasal obstruction or epistaxis. They have a pronounced tendency for hemorrhage, so biopsy is contraindicated. They often contain androgen receptors and may regress with estrogen therapy. Less than 4% of pts are female
- **Nasal NK/T cell lymphoma** (lethal midline granuloma or midline polymorphic reticulosis) presents with progressive ulceration & necrosis of midline facial tissues and is associated with EBV. The differential diagnosis includes Wegener's granulomatosis, polymorphic reticulosis, cocaine abuse, sarcoidosis, & infections. Pathology reveals non-specific acute & chronic inflammation with necrosis. The cause is idiopathic. It is more common in men and presents most commonly in the nasal cavity & paranasal sinuses. The most common age is in the 50s. Must rule-out Wegener's because it responds to steroids

WORKUP

- H&P, CT, MRI, angiogram (optional), CBC, chemistries, audiogram (to establish baseline hearing), visual testing (optional)

STAGING

- Esthesioneuroblastoma is staged according to the Kadish system (A = confined to nasal cavity; B = extends to ≥1 of the paranasal sinuses; C = extends beyond nasal cavity or paranasal sinuses; D = distant metastasis)

- Glomus tumors are staged according to the Glassock-Jackson classification or the McCabe-Fletcher classification based on anatomic location, extension, and tumor volume
- Nasopharyngeal angiofibromas are staged according to one of two systems: Chandler (I = confined to nasopharynx; II = extends to nasal cavity or sphenoid sinus; III = extends to antrum, ethmoid, pterygomaxillary and infratemporal fossa, orbit, and/or cheek; IV = intracranial extension) or Sessions (Ia = limited to nasopharynx & posterior nares; Ib = extends to paranasal sinuses; IIa/b/c = extends to other extracranial locations; III = intracranial extension)
- The other listed tumor types do not have commonly used staging systems

TREATMENT RECOMMENDATIONS

Stage	Recommended Treatment	Results
Chloroma	Definitive RT (1.5/30 Gy) with 2–3 cm margin	>80–90% LC
Chordoma	Maximal safe resection. If gross total resection, post-op RT (50–54 Gy). If subtotal resection, post-op RT (60 Gy). For small tumors, may use SRS. Protons beneficial if available	LC ~40%. DFS 10–20% (some long-term survivors)
Esthesioneuro-blastoma	Surgery or RT alone (65–70 Gy) for small, low-grade tumors confined to ethmoids. Otherwise, combine surgery, with pre-op RT (45 Gy) or post-op RT (50–60 Gy), &chemo	LC: Stage A 70%, Stage B 50–65%, Stage C 30–50%
Glomus tumor	Pre-op embolization → maximal safe resection → post-op RT (50 Gy). Alternative SRS	LC >90%
Hemangio-blastoma	Maximal safe resection. Alternative is SRS	
Hemangio-pericytoma	Pre-op embolization → maximal safe resection + post-op RT (60–65 Gy) with wide margins up to 5 cm. Need long-term follow-up because of DM. SRS may be used (12–20 Gy)	LC ~70–90%

Stage	Recommended Treatment	Results
Nasopharyngeal angiofibroma	If extracranial & resectable, surgery ± embolization. Residual disease may be observed, or treated with RT if symptoms develop. If intracranial extension, treat with RT (30–50 Gy in 2–3 Gy fractions)	RT LC ~80% but tumors regress slowly (up to 2 yrs)
NK/T cell lymphoma	Definitive RT (45–54 Gy) with 2–3 cm margin & treat adjacent structures (e.g., paranasal sinuses for nasal) & ± doxorubicin-based chemotherapy	OS 50–60%

RADIATION TECHNIQUES

- Depend on histology & location. Refer to primary literature for details

COMPLICATIONS

- Depend on the location, and they are in common with other head & neck sites described in this handbook

FOLLOW-UP

- Regular H&P, and follow-up imaging. Long-term follow-up may be needed due to late recurrences

REFERENCES

Carew JF, Singh B, Kraus DH. Hemangiopericytoma of the head and neck. Laryngoscope 1999;109:1409–1411.

Chao KS, Kaplan C, Simpson JR, et al. Esthesioneuroblastoma: the impact of treatment modality. Head Neck 2001;23:749–757.

Chen HH, Fong L, Su IJ, et al. Experience of radiotherapy in lethal midline granuloma with special emphasis on centrofacial T-cell lymphoma: a retrospective analysis covering a 34-year period. Radiother Oncol 1996;38:1–6.

Hinerman RW, Mendenhall WM, Amdur RJ. Definitive radiotherapy in the management of chemodectomas arising in the temporal bone, carotid body, and glomus vagale. Head Neck 2001;23:363–371.

Khairi S, Ewend MG. Chordoma. Curr Treat Options Neurol 2002;4:167–173.

Lee JT, Chen P, Safa A, et al. The role of radiation in the treatment of advanced juvenile angiofibroma. Laryngoscope 2002;112:1213–1220.

Pellitteri PK, Rinaldo A, Myssiorek D, et al. Paragangliomas of the head and neck. Oral Oncol 2004;40:563–575.

Perez CA, Chao KSC. Unusual neonepithelial tumors of the head and neck. In: Perez CA, Brady LW, Halperin EC, et al., editors. Principles and Practice of Radiation Oncology. 4th ed. Philadelphia: Lippincott Williams & Wilkins; 2004. pp. 1117–1157.

Tsao MN, Wara WM, Larson DA. Radiation therapy for benign central nervous system disease. Semin Radiat Oncol 1999;9:120–133.

NOTES

CHAPTER 13
Small Cell Lung Cancer

Brian Missett and Daphne A. Haas-Kogan

PEARLS

- SCLC accounts for ~20–25% of lung cancer cases
- Associated with paraneoplastic syndromes: SIADH, ectopic ACTH production, & Eaton-Lambert syndrome
- ~65–75% of cases present with extensive stage disease & the remaining with limited stage disease
- ~10–15% of pts have brain metastases at presentation, & the CNS is a common site of relapse after chemo-RT
- Pathologic subtypes (classic, variant, mixed) carry the same prognosis
- Most important prognostic factors = stage, performance status, & wt loss

WORKUP

- H&P
- Labs: CBC, chemistries, BUN, Cr, LFTs, LDH
- Imaging: CT chest & abdomen, bone scan, & MRI of brain (preferred) or CT brain. PET optional
- Pathology review. If LDH elevated, consider bone marrow aspirate or biopsy
- Recommend smoking cessation intervention

STAGING

Limited stage: Disease confined to one hemithorax and regional nodes (occasionally defined as being able to fit into one RT treatment portal)

Extensive stage: Any disease not fitting the above limited stage criteria

TREATMENT RECOMMENDATIONS

Stage	Recommended Treatment
Limited	Concurrent cisplatin + etoposide (every 3 wks ×4c) with RT (45 Gy/1.5 Gy bid). If CR, prophylactic cranial RT (25 Gy/2.5 Gy fx). Consider resection and chemo for T1N0
Extensive	Combination chemo ± palliative RT

STUDIES

- <u>Turrisi</u> (*NEJM* 1999). 417 pts with limited stage SCLC randomized to concurrent cisplatin, etoposide with 45 Gy at 1.8 Gy QD vs concurrent cisplatin, etoposide with 45 Gy at 1.5 Gy bid. The bid arm increased 5 yr OS (26%) compared to the QD arm (16%)
- <u>Auperin</u> (*NEJM* 1999). Meta-analysis of 7 trials that included pts with SCLC in CR comparing prophylactic cranial irradiation (PCI) vs no PCI. The PCI arm demonstrated an increased 3 yr OS (20.7%) compared to the no PCI arm (15.3%)

RADIATION TECHNIQUES
Simulation and field design

- High dose volume to 1.5 cm margin on GTV. Include ipsilateral hilum, and bilateral mediastinum from thoracic inlet to subcarinal region (5 cm below carina or adequate margin on subcarinal disease). Do not include contralateral hilum or SCV unless involved

Dose prescriptions

- 45 Gy bid fractionation (1.5 Gy bid) or 50–70 Gy with qd fractionation
- PCI if CR to lung irradiation (30 Gy/15 fx or 36 Gy/18 fx or 24 Gy/8 fx or 25 Gy/10 fx)

Dose limitations

- Spinal cord: limit maximum dose to ≤46 Gy at 1.8–2 Gy/fx qd or ≤36 Gy with bid RT
- Lung: Attempt to limit volume receiving ≥20 Gy (V20) to <20–30%. Pneumonitis rates increase rapidly with V20 >25–30%

- Esophagus: limit 1/3 to 60 Gy, 2/3 to 58 Gy, entire esophagus to 55 Gy
- Heart: limit 50% of volume of heart <25–40 Gy
- Brachial plexus: limit maximum dose to <60 Gy

COMPLICATIONS

- Acute: esophagitis. Late: radiation pneumonitis, rib fracture, esophageal stricture or perforation, coronary artery disease

FOLLOW-UP

- Clinic visits every 2–3 mo initially (H&P, chest imaging, and blood work at each visit), then can decrease frequency to every 3–6 mo then annually

REFERENCES

Auperin A, Arriagada R, Pignon JP, et al. Prophylactic cranial irradiation for patients with small-cell lung cancer in complete remission. Prophylactic Cranial Irradiation Overview Collaborative Group. N Engl J Med 1999;341:476–484.

Bradley J, Govindan R, Komaki R. Lung. In: Perez CA, Brady LW, Halperin EC, et al., editors. Principles and Practice of Radiation Oncology. 4th ed. Philadelphia: Lippincott Williams & Wilkins; 2004. pp. 1201–1243.

Komaki R, Travis EL, Cox JD. The Lung and Thymus. In: Cox JD, Ang KK, editors. Radiation Oncology: Rationale, Technique, Results. 8th ed. St. Louis: Mosby; 2003. pp. 399–427.

National Comprehensive Cancer Network. Clinical Practice Guidelines in Oncology: Small Cell Lung Cancer. Available at: http://www.nccn. org/professionals/physician_gls/PDF/sclc.pdf. Accessed on January 19, 2005.

National Cancer Institute. Small Cell Lung Cancer (PDQ): Treatment. Available at: http://cancer.gov/cancertopics/pdq/treatment/small-cell-lung/healthprofessional/. Accessed on January 19, 2005.

Rosenzweig KE, Krug LM. Tumors of the lung, pleura, and mediastinum. In: Leibel SA, Phillips TL, editors. Textbook of Radiation Oncology. 2nd ed. Philadelphia: Saunders; 2004. pp. 779–810.

Turrisi AT, 3rd, Kim K, Blum R, et al. Twice-daily compared with once-daily thoracic radiotherapy in limited small-cell lung cancer treated concurrently with cisplatin and etoposide. N Engl J Med 1999;340:265–271.

NOTES

Chapter 14
Non-Small Cell Lung Cancer

Eric K. Hansen and Daphne A. Haas-Kogan

PEARLS

- Most common non-cutaneous cancer in the world
- 2nd most common cancer in the U.S., behind prostate in men & breast in women
- #1 cause of cancer death in the U.S. & worldwide
- >90% of cases are associated with smoking or involuntary smoking
- The surgical lymph node levels 1–9 correspond to N2 nodes, and levels 10–14 correspond to N1 nodes
  - 1 = high mediastinal, 2 = upper paratracheal, 3 = pre- & retrotracheal, 4 = lower paratracheal, 5 = AP window, 6 = para-aortic, 7 = subcarinal, 8 = paraesophageal below carina, 9 = pulmonary ligament, 10 = hilar, 11 = interlobar, 12 = lobar, 13 = segmental, 14 = subsegmental
- Adenocarcinoma comprises 40–50% of cases. It tends to be peripherally located; it has a high propensity to metastasize (frequently to the brain)
- Bronchioalveolar carcinoma is a subtype of adenocarcinoma that is not associated with smoking. It is associated with prior lung disease
- Squamous cell carcinoma tends to be centrally located
- Large cell carcinoma tends to be peripherally located. It has a high propensity to metastasize
- Carcinoid tumors are rare, and they tend to be endobronchial. They rarely metastasize

WORKUP

- H&P, including performance status & weight loss
  - Superior sulcus (Pancoast) tumor triad = shoulder pain, brachial plexus palsy, & Horner's syndrome (ptosis, meiosis, & ipsilateral anhidrosis)
- Labs: CBC, BUN, Cr, LFTs, alkaline phosphatase, LDH

- Imaging: CXR. CT chest & abdomen (to rule-out adrenal or liver mets). PET scan. MRI of brain for stage ≥IIB or for neurologic symptoms. MRI of the thoracic inlet for superior sulcus tumors
- PFTs for pre-surgical eval. Desire FEV1 >75% predicted & DLCO >60%
- Pathology: thoracentesis for pleural effusions. For central lesions, perform bronchoscopy because sputum cytology has only ~65–80% sensitivity. For peripheral lesions, perform CT-guided biopsy
- Mediastinoscopy or bronchoscopic biopsy should be performed to confirm any CT+ or PET+ nodes, and for all superior sulcus tumors. If T3 or central T1-2, perform mediastinoscopy to evaluate superior mediastinal nodes (95% accurate). Cervical mediastinoscopy assesses nodal levels 1–4 and Chamberlain procedure assesses levels 5 and 6

STAGING

Primary tumor	
TX:	Primary tumor cannot be assessed, or tumor proven by the presence of malignant cells in sputum or bronchial washings but not visualized by imaging or bronchoscopy
T0:	No evidence of primary tumor
Tis:	Carcinoma in situ
T1:	Tumor 3 cm or less in greatest dimension, surrounded by lung or visceral pleura, without bronchoscopic evidence of invasion more proximal than the lobar bronchus (i.e., not in the main bronchus)
T2:	Tumor with any of the following features of size or extent: more than 3 cm in greatest dimension; involves main bronchus, 2 cm or more distal to the carina; invades visceral pleura; associated with atelectasis or obstructive pneumonitis that extends to the hilar region but does not involve the entire lung
T3:	Tumor of any size that directly invades any of the following: chest wall (including superior sulcus tumors), diaphragm, mediastinal pleura, parietal pericardium; or tumor in the main bronchus less than 2 cm distal to the carina, but without involvement of the carina; or associated atelectasis or obstructive pneumonitis of the entire lung
T4:	Tumor of any size that invades any of the following: mediastinum, heart, great vessels, trachea, esophagus, vertebral body, carina; or separate tumor nodules in the same lobe; or tumor with malignant pleural effusion;

Note: The uncommon superficial tumor of any size with its invasive component limited to the bronchial wall, which may extend proximal to the main bronchus, is classified T1

Regional lymph nodes
NX: Regional lymph nodes cannot be assessed
N0:   No regional lymph node metastasis
N1:   Metastasis to ipsilateral peribronchial and/or ipsilateral hilar nodes, and intrapulmonary nodes including involvement by direct extension of the primary tumor
N2:   Metastasis to ipsilateral mediastinal and/or subcarinal lymph node(s)
N3:   Metastasis to ontralateral mediastinal, contralateral hilar, ipsilateral or contralateral scale or supraclavicular or lymph node(s)

Distant Metastases
MX: Distant metastasis cannot be assessed
M0:   No distant metastasis
M1:   Distant metastasis present. Note: M1 includes separate tumor nodule(s) in a different lobe (ipsilateral or contralateral)

Stage Grouping	~1 yr/5 yr Survival
Occult: TXN0M0	IA: 90–95%/60–80%
0: TisN0M0	IB: 80–90%/50–70%
IA: T1N0M0	IIA: 70–90%/40–70%
IB: T2N0M0	IIB: 60–80%/30–50%
IIA: T1N1M0	IIIA: 40–70%/20–30%
IIB: T2N1M0, T3N0M0	IIIB: 10–40%/< 5–10%
IIIA: T3N1M0, T1-3N2M0	IV: MS 3–6 mo with best
IIIB: Any T, N3, M0 or T4, any N, M0	supportive care, 8–10 mo with chemo
IV: Any T, any N, M1	

Used with the permission of the American Joint Committee on Cancer (AJCC), Chicago, Illinois. The original source for this material is the AJCC Cancer Staging Manual, Sixth Edition (2002) published by Springer-Verlag New York, www.springeronline.com.

TREATMENT RECOMMENDATIONS

Stage	Recommended Treatment
Operable I–II	Lobectomy preferred over pneumonectomy if anatomically feasible. Wedge resection only if physiologically compromised (& is not a cancer operation)

Stage	Recommended Treatment
	■ For completely resected T2N0 & T1-2N1, give adjuvant chemo [CALGB, NCIC BR.10] ■ For completely resected T3N0, give adjuvant chemo [IALT] ■ For +margins or nodal ECE, re-resect or give post-op RT → chemo
I–II marginally operable	Pre-op chemo → surgery → chemo [DePierre] ■ For close/+margin or nodal ECE, give post-op RT
I–II inoperable	Definitive RT to primary ± involved nodes ■ 1.8–2 Gy/fraction to ≥65 Gy [Dosoretz, Sibley] ■ If peripheral tumor or poor PS, may hypofractionate with 4 Gy/fraction to 48 Gy to primary tumor only [Slotman] ■ Dose escalation >70 Gy & radiosurgical techniques are under investigation & appear to provide improved LC ■ If pt can tolerate it, give chemo (induction, concurrent, &/or consolidation)
IIIA operable or marginally operable	Chemo alone → restage* → if no progression → surgery → chemo ± post-op RT for close + margin, nodal ECE, or N2 disease [DePierre, Roth, Rosell] Alternatively, concurrent chemo-RT (45 Gy) → restage* → if no progression → surgery → chemo [Int 0139] * If unresectable after restaging → complete definitive concurrent chemo-RT (63 Gy)
IIIA inoperable	Concurrent chemo-RT (63 Gy) → adjuvant chemo [LAMP, RTOG 9410] (preferred), or induction chemo →

Stage	Recommended Treatment
	concurrent chemo-RT [CALGB 39801]
IIIB (no pleural effusion)	Concurrent chemo-RT (63 Gy) → adjuvant chemo [SWOG 9504, LAMP, RTOG 9410] (preferred), or induction chemo → concurrent chemo-RT [CALGB 39801] If T4N0-1, may treat with surgery → chemo ± RT, or chemo ± RT → surgery → chemo
IIIB (pleural effusion)	Local treatment as necessary (e.g., pleurodesis) & treat as stage IV
IV	ECOG PS 0–2: chemo ± palliative RT. First-line chemo uses 2 agents for 3–4 cycles. Addition of bevacizumab to carboplatin-paclitaxel improves survival (Sandler, ASCO abstract #4, 2005) ECOG PS 3–4: best supportive care
Superior sulcus	If operable, concurrent chemo-RT (45 Gy) → surgery → chemo (preferred). Or, surgery → post-op chemo + RT (60–66 Gy) for close or +margins, nodal ECE If marginally resectable, concurrent chemo-RT (45 Gy) → restage → if no progression → surgery → chemo [INT 0160] If unresectable (initially or after restaging), complete definitive concurrent chemo-RT (63–66 Gy)

STUDIES
Surgery
- <u>LCSG 821</u> (Ginsberg, *Ann Thorac Surg* 1995). 247 pts with peripheral T1N0 randomized to lobectomy vs wedge resection with a 2 cm margin of normal lung. Wedge resection tripled LRF (6→18%)

RT alone
- <u>Dosoretz</u> (*Semin Radiat Oncol* 1996). Review of T1-3N0 medically inoperable pts treated with RT alone. RT >64 Gy improved PFS and increasing field size did not improve outcomes
- <u>Sibley</u> (*Cancer* 1998). Review of 10 studies of medically inoperable T1-2N0 pts treated with RT alone 60–66 Gy. 5 yr OS was ~15%. ~50% of failures were local only vs ~5% regional-only failure. ~30% of pts died of DM, ~30% of pts died after LF, & ~25% died of intercurrent disease
- <u>Slotman</u> (*Radiother Oncol* 1996). Review of 31 pts with T1-2N0 treated with 4 Gy/fraction to the tumor +1.5 cm margin to 40 Gy → conedown to tumor +0.5 cm margin to 48 Gy. 3 yr OS 40%, DFS 76%. Only 6% regional failure
- <u>RTOG 73-01</u> (Perez, *Cancer* 1980). 375 pts with IIIA/IIIB treated with RT alone randomized to 2/40 Gy vs 2/50 Gy vs 2/60 Gy vs 4/40 Gy (split-course). Clinical LC was improved with dose escalation. However, 75–80% of patients developed DM in all arms and 2 yr OS was only 14–18% in continuous RT arms
- <u>RTOG 93-11</u> (Bradley, *IJROBP* 2005). 179 pts with medically inoperable or unresectable I–III disease stratified into RT dose escalation levels of 70.9, 77.4, 83.8, or 90.3 Gy at 2.15 Gy/fx depending on V20. Concurrent chemo not allowed. 25 pts received neoadjuvant chemo. The PTV included the GTV (primary & involved LN) + 1 cm margin. RT was generally well tolerated except in 90.3 Gy group (with 2 dose-related deaths). LRC ranged from 50% to 78%

Induction chemo
- <u>DePierre</u> (*JCO* 2002). 355 pts with resectable clinical stage IB-IIIA randomized to pre-op chemo ×3c → surgery → chemo ×2c vs no pre-op chemo. Chemo was mitomycin C, ifosfamide, cisplatin. Pts with pT3 or pN2 received 60 Gy RT. Pre-op chemo increased DFS (13→27 mo, p = 0.03). On

subset analysis, benefit only for N0-1 pts & not for N2 pts

- Rosell (*NEJM* 1994). 60 pts with IIIA randomized to pre-op chemo ×3c → surgery → 50 Gy to mediastinum vs no pre-op chemo. Pre-op chemo (MMC, ifosfamide, cisplatin) improved MS (8 mo→26 mo) & 2 yr OS (0→30%)
- Roth (*J Natl Cancer Inst* 1994). 60 pts with IIIA randomized to pre-op chemo ×3c → surgery → chemo ×3c vs surgery alone. RT given for unresectable or residual disease. Chemo (cytoxan, etoposide, cisplatin) improved MS (11→64 mo) & 3 yr OS (15→56%)
- S9900 (Pisters, ASCO abstr, 2005). 335 pts with T2N0, T1-2N1, & T3N0-1 randomized to carboplatin-paclitaxel ×3c → surgery vs surgery alone. pCR to chemo was 10%. No difference in median PFS (31 mo vs 20 mo, p = 0.14) or OS (47 mo vs 40 mo, p = 0.32)

Pre-op RT

- There is no improvement in survival with pre-op RT alone (without chemo) as noted in 2 collaborative studies from 1970s (VA & NCI)

Pre-op chemo-RT

- Intergroup/RTOG 0139 (ASCO 2005 abstr.). 396 eligible pts with T1-3pN2 treated with concurrent chemo ×2c + 45 Gy → restaging → randomized to surgery (if no progression) → chemo ×2c vs concurrent chemo-RT to 61 Gy (no surgery) → chemo ×2c. Chemo was cisplatinum & etoposide. With median 81 mo f/u, pCR to induction chemo-RT was 18%. Surgery improved 5 yr PFS (11→22%). OS curves overlapped for 2 yrs, then trended in favor of surgery at 5 yrs (27% vs 20%, p = 0.10). Increased treatment-related deaths with surgery, particularly when pneumonectomy required
- Ruebe (ASTRO 2004 abstr). 525 pts with IIIA/IIIB treated with neoadjuvant cisplatin/etoposide ×3c then randomized to pre-op hyperfractionated chemo-RT vs immediate surgery → post-op RT. Pre-op chemo-RT was 1.5 bid/45 Gy with carboplatin/vindesin ×3c → surgery if possible → RT boost (1.5 bid/24 Gy) if inoperable or R1/R2 resection. Post-op RT was 1.8/54 Gy or 1.8/68.4 Gy if inoperable or R1/R2 resection. There was no difference in 3 yr OS (25–26%) or PFS (18–20%). Hyperfractionated RT

increased esophagitis & hematotoxicity, but reduced pneumonitis

Post-op chemo

- <u>NCIC BR.10</u> (Winton, *NEJM* 2005). 482 pts with completely resected pIB-II were randomized to observation vs cisplatin/vinorelibine ×4c. 45% were IB, 15% IIA, & 40% IIB. Chemo improved 5y OS (54→69%) and RFS (49→61%)
- <u>CALGB 9633</u> (Strauss, ASCO 2004 abstr.). 344 pts with completely resected T2N0 randomized to observation vs carbo/taxol ×4c. Chemo improved 4y OS (59→71%) & decreased lung CA mortality (26→15%)
- <u>Kato</u> (*NEJM* 2004). 980 pts with pT1-2N0 (adenocarcinoma only) randomized to observation vs daily uracil-tegafur (UFT) for 2 yrs. UFT improved 5yr OS (85→88%), due to improvements for T2 (74→85%) but not T1 (89→90%)
- <u>IALT</u> (*NEJM* 2004). 1867 pts with pI (36%), pII (25%), & pIII (39%) randomized to 3-4c adjuvant cisplatinum-based chemo. Most pts received platinum/etoposide. Post-op RT (60 Gy) to the mediastinum was given to 1/3 of N1 pts & 2/3 of N2 pts. Chemo improved 2/5 yr OS (67/40→70/45%) & DFS (55/34→61/39%). However, 0.8% of pts died due to chemo toxicity

Post-op RT, Post-op chemo-RT

- <u>LCSG 773</u> (*NEJM* 1986). 210 pts with pII-IIIA (squamous cell carcinoma only) randomized to observation vs post-op RT to the mediastinum (50 Gy). RT decreased LR overall (41→3%) & for N2 pts, but there were no differences in OS
- <u>MRC</u> (Stephens, *Br J Cancer* 1996). 308 pts with pII-IIIA randomized to observation vs post-op RT (2.67/40 Gy). Subgroup analysis demonstrated a 1 month survival advantage & improved LRC for N2 (but not N1) pts
- <u>Sawyer</u> (*Ann Thorac Surg* 1997). Regression tree analysis of pN2 pts treated with & without post-op RT. RT improved LRC & OS for pts with ≥ two N2 nodes or T3-4 tumors with one N2 node
- <u>PORT meta-analysis</u> (*Lancet* 1998). 9 trials of surgery ± post-op RT. For N0-1 pts, RT produced a 7% absolute OS decrement, but there was no OS difference for N2 patients. Analysis criticized because 25% of pts were N0, many pts

were treated with Co-60, older studies used inadequate staging, and unpublished data was included

- Van Houtte (*IJROBP* 1980). pI-II randomized to observation vs post-op 60 Gy to mediastinum. RT improved local-regional control but 5 yr OS was worse (24% RT vs 43% with observation) due to increased pneumonitis. Study criticized because used Co-60 machines, large field size, & no CT planning
- INT 0115/ECOG 3590 (Keller, *NEJM* 2000). 488 pts with completely resected pII–IIIA randomized to RT (1.8/ 50.4 Gy) +/– concurrent cisplatin/etoposide chemo ×4c. RT boost given for ECE (10.8 Gy). Addition of chemo did not change MS (38–39 mo) or LF (12–13%)

Sequencing and timing of chemo and RT

- LAMP (Belani, *JCO* 2005). Phase II study of 276 pts with unresected stage IIIA/IIIB randomized to sequential chemo ×2c → 63 Gy (arm 1) vs induction chemo ×2c → concurrent 63 Gy + chemo (arm 2) vs upfront concurrent 63 Gy + chemo → consolidation chemo ×2c (arm 3). Chemo was carboplatin & paclitaxel. Up-front concurrent chemo-RT had trend for improved MS (arm 1 = 13 mo, arm 2 = 12.7 mo, arm 3 = 16.3 mo) but was associated with increased acute toxicity
- CALGB 39801 (Vokes, ASCO 2004 abstr.). 366 pts with unresectable IIIA/IIIB randomized to concurrent chemo (weekly) + RT (66 Gy) vs induction chemo ×2c → the same concurrent chemo-RT. Chemo was carboplatin & paclitaxel. No difference in MS (11.4–13.7 mo) or OS. Induction chemo increased toxicity
- RTOG 9410 (Curran, ASCO 2003 abstr.). 610 pts with unresectable or medically inoperable II–III randomized to chemo → 1.8/63 Gy (seq) vs concurrent 1.8/63 Gy + chemo (con-qd) vs concurrent 1.2 bid/69.6 Gy + chemo (con-bid). Chemo was cisplatin/vinblastine, but cisplatin/etoposide for bid arm. Concurrent chemo improved MS (seq = 14.6 mo, con-qd = 17 mo, con-bid = 15.2 mo) & 4 yr OS, but increased toxicity, especially with bid RT
- French NPC 95-01 (Fournel, *JCO* 2005). Randomized 205 pts with unresectable stage III to sequential cisplatin/ vinorelbine → RT (2/66 Gy) vs concurrent cisplatin/etoposide ×2c + RT (2/66 Gy) → consolidation cisplatin/vinorelbine. Although not statistically significant, concurrent chemoRT had improved MS (14.5→16.3 mo) & 2–4 yr OS

(by 7–13%). Esophageal toxicity was more frequent with concurrent

- <u>SWOG 9504</u> (Gandara, *JCO* 2003). Phase II trial of 83 pts with IIIB treated with concurrent chemo (platinum-etoposide) + RT (61 Gy) → consolidation docetaxel. Excellent results (MS 26 mo, 1/3 yr OS 76/37%)
- <u>CALGB 8433</u> (Dillman, *NEJM* 1990). 155 pts with T3 or N2 randomized to RT alone (2/60 Gy) vs sequential cisplatin/vinblastine → RT (60 Gy). Induction chemo improved MS (10→14 mo) & 2/5 yr OS (13/7→26/19%)
- <u>RTOG 8808</u> (Sause, *Chest* 2000). 458 pts with cII, IIIA, IIIB randomized to RT alone (2/60 Gy) vs sequential cisplatin/vinblastine → 2/60 Gy vs bid RT alone (1.2/69.6 Gy). Induction chemo improved MS (13.2 mo) vs RT alone, and there was no difference for qd RT (11.4 mo) vs bid RT (12 mo)

Superior sulcus

- <u>Int 0160</u> (Rusch, *J Thorac Cardiovasc Surg* 2001). Phase II trial of 111 pts with T3-4N0-1 superior sulcus tumors treated with concurrent chemo-RT (45 Gy) → restaging → surgery (if no progression) → chemo ×2c. Chemo was platinum/etoposide. 86% of pts had surgery. 65% had pCR or minimal microscopic residual disease. The 2 yr OS was 55% (70% for pts with pCR). The LR rate was only 23% & the most common site of relapse was in the brain

Prophylactic cranial RT (PCI)

- 3 randomized trials have investigated PCI in advanced NSCLC. PCI delayed and reduced the incidence of brain failure, but had no impact on OS. Extracranial disease was the cause of death for most pts, and may be a source of CNS re-seeding after PCI

RADIATION TECHNIQUES
Simulation and field design

- Simulate pt supine with arms up so that arms do not block the tattoos on the sides of the patient
- Immobilize with a wingboard or with an alpha cradle (with arms behind head)
- Use a 3D conformal or IMRT plan throughout treatment so that beams passing through normal tissues have lower doses per fraction throughout treatment

- Wedges and/or compensating filters may be needed
- GTV: gross primary and nodal disease including LN(s) ≥1 cm or hypermetabolic on PET scan or harboring tumor cells per mediastinoscopy
- CTV: typically includes the GTV plus 1–1.5 cm margin
- PTV: Add 0.5–1.5 cm margin on CTV to account for setup uncertainties and respiratory motion
- The rationale against elective nodal RT for early-stage disease is that there are high rates of local recurrence with current doses and techniques. If gross disease cannot be controlled, then why enlarge the volume & increase complications by including areas that might harbor microscopic disease that will frequently be addressed by chemo
- Only treat the supraclavicular fossa if an upper lobe primary or gross upper mediastinal disease because it is the 1st site of failure in only ~3% of patients
- Contralateral hilar or supraclavicular treatment is discouraged unless involved

Dose prescriptions
- Treat initial volume with 1.8–2 Gy per fraction to 45–50 Gy. Boost to 60–63 Gy for close/+margins or to 66 Gy for gross disease
- For peripheral lesions, may use 4 Gy/fraction to tumor +1.5 cm margin to 40 Gy followed by conedown to tumor +0.5 cm to 48 Gy
- Dose escalation >70 Gy at 1.8–2.15 Gy/fx & radiosurgical techniques are under investigation (especially with concurrent chemotherapy)

Dose limitations
- Spinal cord: limit maximum dose to ≤46 Gy at 1.8–2 Gy/fx qd or ≤36 Gy with bid RT
- Lung: attempt to limit volume receiving ≥20 Gy (V20) to <20–30%. Pneumonitis rates increase rapidly with V_{20} >25–30%
- Esophagus: limit $^1/_3$ to 60 Gy, $^2/_3$ to 55 Gy, entire esophagus to 45 Gy
- Heart: limit 50% of volume <25–40 Gy
- Brachial plexus: limit maximum dose to <60 Gy

COMPLICATIONS

- Acute RT complications include esophagitis, dermatitis, &/or cough
- Subacute and late complications include pneumonitis, pulmonary fibrosis, pericarditis, brachial plexopathy, and Lhermitte's syndrome
- Radiation pneumonitis occurs ~6 weeks after RT. It presents with cough, dyspnea, hypoxia, and fever. Treat radiation pneumonitis with prednisone (1 mg/kg/d) & trimethoprim/sulfamethoxazole for PCP prophylaxis
- Lhermitte's syndrome (sudden electric-like shocks extending down the spine with head flexion) usually resolves spontaneously
- Amifostine may decrease esophageal and pulmonary toxicity (Komaki, *IJROBP* 2004), but hypotension may be problematic

FOLLOW-UP

- H&P & CXR every 3–4 months for 2 years, then every 6 months for 3 years, then annually. CT chest annually. PET scans optional

REFERENCES

Albain KS, Scott CB, Rusch VR, et al. Phase III comparison of concurrent chemotherapy plus radiotherapy (CT/RT) and CT/RT followed by surgical resection for stage IIIA(pN2) non-small cell lung cancer (NSCLC): Initial results from intergroup trial 0139 (RTOG 93-09). Proc Am Soc Clin Oncol 2003 (abstr. 2497);22:621.

Albain KS, Swann RS, Rusch VR, et al. Phase III study of concurrent chemotherapy and radiotherapy (CT/RT) vs CT/RT followed by surgical resection for stage IIIA(pN2) non-small cell lung cancer (NSCLC): Outcomes update of North American Intergroupl 0139 (RTOG 9309). J Clin Oncol, 2005 ASCO Annual Meeting Proceedings, 2005;23;16S (June 1 Supplement): 624S.

Arriagada R, Bergman B, Dunant A, et al. Cisplatin-based adjuvant chemotherapy in patients with completely resected non-small-cell lung cancer. N Engl J Med 2004;350:351–360.

Belani C, Choy H, Bonomi P, et al. Combined chemoradiotherapy regimens of paclitaxel and carboplatin for locally advanced non-small-cell lung cancer: a randomized phase II locally advanced multi-modality protocol. J Clin Oncol 2005;23:5883–5891.

Bradley J, Govindan R, Komaki R. Lung. In: Perez CA, Brady LW, Halperin EC, et al., editors. Principles and Practice of Radiation Oncology. 4th ed. Philadelphia: Lippincott Williams & Wilkins; 2004. pp. 1201–1243.

Bradley J, Graham MV, Winter K. Toxicity and outcome results of RTOG 9311: A phase I–II dose escalation study using three-dimensional conformal radiation therapy in patients with inoperable non-small cell lung carcinoma. Int J Radiat Oncol Biol Phys 2005;61: 318–328.

Choy H, Jr. WJC, Scott CB, et al. Preliminary report of locally advanced multimodality protocol (LAMP): ACR 427: a randomized phase II study of three chemo-radiation regimens with paclitaxel, carboplatin, and thoracic radiation (TRT) for patients with locally advanced non small cell lung cancer (LA-NSCLC). Presented at American Society of Clinical Oncology, 2002.

Crowley R, Ginsberg P, Ellis B, et al. S9900: A phase III trial of surgery alone or surgery plus preoperative (preop) paclitaxel/carboplatin (PC) chemotherapy in early stage non-small cell lung cancer (NSCLC): Preliminary results. J Clin Oncol, 2005 ASCO Annual Meeting Proceedings, 2005;23;16S (June 1 Supplement): 624S.

Curran WJ, Scott CB, Langer CJ, et al. Long-term benefit is observed in a phase III comparison of sequential vs concurrent chemo-radiation for patients with unresected stage III nsclc: RTOG 9410. Proc Am Soc Clin Oncol 2003 (abstr 2499);22:621.

Depierre A, Milleron B, Moro-Sibilot D, et al. Preoperative chemotherapy followed by surgery compared with primary surgery in resectable stage I (except T1N0), II, and IIIa non-small-cell lung cancer. J Clin Oncol 2002;20:247–253.

Dillman RO, Seagren SL, Propert KJ, et al. A randomized trial of induction chemotherapy plus high-dose radiation versus radiation alone in stage III non-small-cell lung cancer. N Engl J Med 1990;323: 940–945.

Dosoretz DE, Katin MJ, Blitzer PH, et al. Medically inoperable lung carcinoma: the role of radiation therapy. Semin Radiat Oncol 1996;6:98–104.

Effects of postoperative mediastinal radiation on completely resected stage II and stage III epidermoid cancer of the lung. The Lung Cancer Study Group. N Engl J Med 1986;315:1377–1381.

Fournel P, Robinet G, Thomas P, et al. Randomized phase III trial of sequential chemoradiotherapy compared with concurrent chemoradiotherapy in locally advanced non-small-cell lung cancer: Groupe Lyon-Saint-Etienne d'Oncologie Thoracique-Groupe Françç5ais de Pneumo-Cancérologie NPC 95-01 Study. J Clin Oncol 2005;23: 5910–5917.

Gandara DR, Chansky K, Albain KS, et al. Consolidation docetaxel after concurrent chemoradiotherapy in stage IIIB non-small-cell lung cancer: phase II Southwest Oncology Group Study S9504. J Clin Oncol 2003;21:2004–2010.

Ginsberg RJ, Rubinstein LV. Randomized trial of lobectomy versus limited resection for T1 N0 non-small cell lung cancer. Lung Cancer Study Group. Ann Thorac Surg 1995;60:615–622; discussion 622–613.

Greene FL, American Joint Committee on Cancer, American Cancer Society. AJCC Cancer Staging Manual. 6th ed. New York: Springer-Verlag; 2002.

Kato H, Ichinose Y, Ohta M, et al. A randomized trial of adjuvant chemotherapy with uracil-tegafur for adenocarcinoma of the lung. N Engl J Med 2004;350:1713–1721.

Keller SM, Adak S, Wagner H, et al. A randomized trial of postoperative adjuvant therapy in patients with completely resected stage II or IIIA non-small-cell lung cancer. Eastern Cooperative Oncology Group. N Engl J Med 2000;343:1217–1222.

Komaki R, Lee JS, Milas L, et al. Effects of amifostine on acute toxicity from concurrent chemotherapy and radiotherapy for inoperable non-small cell lung cancer: report of a randomized comparative trial. Int J Radiat Oncol Biol Phys 2004;58:1369–1377.

Komaki R, Travis EL, Cox JD. The lung and thymus. In: Cox JD, Ang KK, editors. Radiation Oncology: Rationale, Technique, Results. 8th ed. St. Louis: Mosby; 2003. pp. 399–427.

Langer C, Rosenzweig KE. Lung Cancer Part I: Non-Small Cell (#204). Presented at American Society of Therapeutic Radiology and Oncology Annual Meeting, Atlanta, GA, 2004.

National Cancer Institute. Non-Small Cell Lung Cancer (PDQ): Treatment. Available at: http://cancer.gov/cancertopics/pdq/treatment/non-small-cell-lung/healthprofessional/. Accessed on January 19, 2005.

National Comprehensive Cancer Network. Clinical Practice Guidelines in Oncology: Non-Small Cell Lung Cancer. Available at: http://www.nccn.org/professionals/physician_gls/PDF/nscl.pdf. Accessed on January 19, 2005.

Perez CA, Stanley K, Rubin P, et al. A prospective randomized study of various irradiation doses and fractionation schedules in the treatment of inoperable non-oat-cell carcinoma of the lung. Preliminary report by the Radiation Therapy Oncology Group. Cancer 1980;45:2744–2753.

Postoperative radiotherapy in non-small-cell lung cancer: systematic review and meta-analysis of individual patient data from nine randomised controlled trials. PORT Meta-analysis Trialists Group. Lancet 1998;352:257–263.

Rosell R, Gomez-Codina J, Camps C, et al. A randomized trial comparing preoperative chemotherapy plus surgery with surgery alone in patients with non-small-cell lung cancer. N Engl J Med 1994;330:153–158.

Rosenzweig KE, Krug LM. Tumors of the lung, pleura, and mediastinum. In: Leibel SA, Phillips TL, editors. Textbook of Radiation Oncology. 2nd ed. Philadelphia: Saunders; 2004. pp. 779–810.

Roth JA, Fossella F, Komaki R, et al. A randomized trial comparing perioperative chemotherapy and surgery with surgery alone in resectable stage IIIA non-small-cell lung cancer. J Natl Cancer Inst 1994;86:673–680.

Ruebe C, Riesenbeck D, Semik M, et al. Neoadjuvant chemotherapy followed by preoperative radiochemotherapy (hfRTCT) plus surgery or surgery plus postoperative radiotherapy in stage III non-small cell lung cancer: results of a randomized phase III trial of the German Lung Cancer Cooperative Group. Presented at American Society of Therapeutic Radiology and Oncology 46th Annual Meeting, Atlanta, GA, 2004.

Rusch VW, Giroux DJ, Kraut MJ, et al. Induction chemoradiation and surgical resection for non-small cell lung carcinomas of the superior sulcus: Initial results of Southwest Oncology Group Trial 9416 (Intergroup Trial 0160). J Thorac Cardiovasc Surg 2001;121: 472–483.

Sandler AB, Gray R, Brahmer J, et al. Randomized phase II/III trial of paclitaxel (P) plus carboplatin (C) with or without bevacizumab (NSC#704865) in patients with advanced non-squamous non-small cell lung cancer (NSCLC): An Eastern Cooperative Oncology Group (ECOG) Trial – E4599. J Clin Oncol, 2005 ASCO Annual Meeting Proceedings, 2005;23;16S (June 1 Supplement): 2S.

Sause W, Kolesar P, Taylor SI, et al. Final results of phase III trial in regionally advanced unresectable non-small cell lung cancer: Radiation Therapy Oncology Group, Eastern Cooperative Oncology Group, and Southwest Oncology Group. Chest 2000;117: 358–364.

Sawyer TE, Bonner JA, Gould PM, et al. Effectiveness of postoperative irradiation in stage IIIA non-small cell lung cancer according to regression tree analyses of recurrence risks. Ann Thorac Surg 1997;64:1402–1407; discussion 1407–1408.

Sibley GS. Radiotherapy for patients with medically inoperable Stage I nonsmall cell lung carcinoma: smaller volumes and higher doses – a review. Cancer 1998;82:433–438.

Slotman BJ, Antonisse IE, Njo KH. Limited field irradiation in early stage (T1-2N0) non-small cell lung cancer. Radiother Oncol 1996;41:41–44.

Stephens RJ, Girling DJ, Bleehen NM, et al. The role of post-operative radiotherapy in non-small-cell lung cancer: a multicentre randomised trial in patients with pathologically staged T1-2, N1-2, M0 disease. Medical Research Council Lung Cancer Working Party. Br J Cancer 1996;74:632–639.

Strauss GM, Herndon J, Maddaus MA, et al. Randomized clinical trial of adjuvant chemotherapy with paclitaxel and carboplatin following resection in Stage IB non-small cell lung cancer (NSCLC): Report of Cancer and Leukemia Group B (CALGB) Protocol 9633. J Clin Oncol, 2004 ASCO Annual Meeting Proceedings (Post-Meeting Edition) 2004;22; 14S (July 15 Supplement): 7019.

Turrisi III AT. Updates and Issues in Lung Cancer. Presented at American Society of Therapeutic Radiology and Oncology Spring Refresher Course, Chicago, IL, 2004.

Van Houtte P, Rocmans P, Smets P, et al. Postoperative radiation therapy in lung caner: a controlled trial after resection of curative design. Int J Radiat Oncol Biol Phys 1980;6:983–986.

van Meerbeeck JP, Kramer G, van Schil PE, et al. A randomized trial of radical surgery (S) versus thoracic radiotherapy (TRT) in patients (pts) with stage IIIA-N2 non-small cell lung cancer (NSCLC) after response to induction chemotherapy (ICT) (EORTC 08941). J Clin Oncol, 2005 ASCO Annual Meeting Proceedings, 2005;23;16S (June 1 Supplement): 624S.

Vokes EE, Herndon JE, Kelley MJ, et al. Induction chemotherapy followed by concomitant chemoradiotherapy (CT/XRT) versus CT/XRT alone for regionally advanced unresectable non-small cell lung cancer (NSCLC): Initial analysis of a randomized phase III trial. J Clin Oncol, 2004 ASCO Annual Meeting Proceedings (Post-Meeting Edition) 2004;22;14S (July 15 Supplement):7005.

Wagner H. Non-small cell lung cancer. In: Gunderson LL, Tepper JE, editors. Clinical Radiation Oncology. 1st ed. Philadelphia: Churchill Livingstone; 2000. pp. 600–628.

Winton TL, Livingston R, Johnson D, et al. Vinorelbine plus cisplatin vs. observation in resected non-small-cell lung cancer. N Engl J Med 2005;352:2589–2597.

NOTES

Chapter 15
Mesothelioma and Thymoma

Brian Lee and Joycelyn L. Speight

MESOTHELIOMA

PEARLS

- Rare: only 2000–3000 cases per year in U.S.
- 80% cases involve asbestos exposure
- Affects both visceral and parietal pleura
- May mimic adenocarcinoma on pathologic examination

WORKUP

- H&P, CXR, CT/MRI chest, PET
- On CT, look for pleural thickening, effusions, contraction of ipsilateral hemithorax
- Differential diagnosis = adenocarcinoma or benign causes (i.e., empyema, infection, fibrothorax, nonmalignant exudates)
- Circumferential pleural thickening, mediastinal/chest wall/diaphragm involvement, &/or irregular pleural contour are most likely malignant. Pleural calcifications are usually benign

STAGING

Primary tumor	
TX:	Primary tumor cannot be assessed
T0:	No evidence of primary tumor
T1:	Tumor involves ipsilateral parietal pleura, with or without focal involvement of visceral pleura
T1a:	Tumor involves ipsilateral parietal (mediastinal, diaphragmatic) pleura. No involvement of the visceral pleura
T1b:	Tumor involves ipsilateral parietal (mediastinal, diaphragmatic) pleura, with focal involvement of the visceral pleura
T2:	Tumor involves any of the ipsilateral pleural surfaces with at least one of the following:

- confluent visceral pleural tumor (including fissure)
- invasion of diaphragmatic muscle
- invasion of lung parenchyma

T3:   Locally advanced but potentially resectable tumor. Tumor involves any of the ipsilateral
pleural surfaces, with at least one of the following:
  - invasion of the endothoracic fascia
  - invasion into mediastinal fat
  - solitary focus of tumor invading the soft tissues of the chest wall
  - non-transmural involvement of the pericardium

T4:   Locally advanced, technically unresectable tumor. Tumor involves any of the ipsilateral pleural surfaces, with at least one of the following:
  - diffuse or multifocal invasion of soft tissues of the chest wall
  - any involvement of rib
  - invasion through thte diaphragm to the peritoneum
  - invasion of any mediastinal organ(s)
  - direct extension to the contralateral pleura
  - invasion into the spine
  - extension to the internal surface of the pericardium
  - pericardial effusion with positive cytology
  - invasion of the myocardium
  - invasion of the brachial plexus

Regional lymph nodes

NX: Regional lymph nodes cannot be assessed

N0:   No regional lymph node metastases

N1:   Metastases in the ipsilateral bronchopulmonary and/or hilar lymph nodes

N2:   Metastases in the subcarinal and/or ipsilateral internal mammary or mediastinal node(s)

N3:   Metastases in the contralateral mediastinal, internal mammary, or hilar lymph nodes(s) and/or the ipsilateral or contralateral supraclavicular or scalene lymph nodes(s)

Metastases

MX: Distant metastases cannot be assessed

M0:   No distant metastasis

M1:   Distant metastasis

Stage Grouping	Median Survival
Stage I: T1N0M0	I ~35 mo, II ~16 mo,
Stage Ia: T1aN0M0	III ~12 mo, IV ~6 mo
Stage Ib: T1bN0M0	
Stage II: T2N0M0	Resectable Stg I,II: 34 mo

Stage III:	T1/T2	N1	M0	Resectable Adv Stg: 10 mo
	T1/T2	N2	M0	
	T3	N0-2	M0	
Stage IV:	T4	Any N	M0	
	Any T	N3	M0	
	Any T	Any N	M1	

Used with the permission of the American Joint Committee on Cancer (AJCC), Chicago, Illinois. The original source for this material is the AJCC Cancer Staging Manual, Sixth Edition (2002) published by Springer-Verlag New York, www.springeronline.com.

TREATMENT RECOMMENDATIONS

Stage	Recommended Treatment
I–II	If resectable/N0, extrapleural pneumonectomy → 3–6 wk break → RT 1.8/54 Gy. If inoperable → chemo.
III–IV	If resectable, treat as early stage, or with pemetrexed + cisplatin or with cisplatin & gemcitabine

STUDIES

- Rusch (*IJROBP* 2003). Phase II trial of 88 pts treated with extrapleural pneumonectomy & adjuvant hemithoracic RT (54 Gy). MS 34 mo for stage I–II & 10 mo for late stage. Toxicity included fatigue and esophagitis
- Van Meerbeeck/EORTC (*Cancer* 1999). Phase II study of gemcitabine (1000 mg/m^2 on d 1, 8, 15) + cisplatin (100 mg/m^2 day 1) for 21 advanced-stage pts. No CR, but 48% of pts had PR. No treatment-related deaths
- Vogelzang (*JCO* 2003). Phase III single-blinded study of pemetrexed + cisplatin vs cisplatin alone in chemo naïve pts with malignant pleural mesothelioma. Addition of pemetrexed improved response rate (17→41%) and MS (9→12 mo)

RADIATION TECHNIQUES
Simulation and field design

- Hemithoracic RT 3–6 wks after extrapleural pneumonectomy
- Simulate & CT pt supine, arms overhead

- Conventional AP/PA borders: superior = top of T1; inferior = bottom L2; medial = contralateral edge of vertebral body (if mediastinum negative) or 1.5 cm beyond contralateral edge of vertebral body (if mediastinum involved), lateral = flash
- Blocks: liver & stomach (covers diaphragm/abdomen interface), humerus, heart (after 20 Gy), spinal cord (after 41.4 Gy, shift medial border to ipsilateral edge of vertebral body)
- Scar: include in field, bolus or boost to scar may be needed
- Electron boost to areas of chest wall blocked for abdominal or cardiac protection

Dose prescriptions
- 1.8 Gy/fx to 54 Gy (off cord after 41.4 Gy)
- Electrons: give concurrent with photon treatment, 1.53 Gy/fx (15% scatter under blocks from photon fields). Choose energy so that chest wall is covered by 90% IDL

Dose limitations
- Spinal cord <45 Gy, heart <20–40 Gy

COMPLICATIONS
- Fatigue, esophagitis
- Rare esophageal fistula

THYMOMA

PEARLS
- Presents most commonly at age 40–60 yrs. Rare in children
- Most common presentation = anterior mediastinal mass on CXR performed for other reasons. 30–40% are asymptomatic
- Symptoms include ocular muscle weakness, ptosis, dysphagia, or fatigue. Impingement on mediastinal structures may cause chest pain, cough, dyspnea, hoarseness, &/or superior vena cava syndrome
- 35–50% cases associated with myasthenia gravis (MG); 15% of MG pts have thymoma
- Predominant pattern of spread = direct invasion
- Importance of histology controversial. Of the 3 subtypes (cortical, medullary, mixed), cortical has a low but increased risk of late relapse even with minimal invasion.
- Prognosis is related to stage & completeness of resection

WORKUP

- H&P, CXR, & CT chest (MRI does not offer additional info)
- Be careful to note entire pre-op tumor volume including extension to posterior sternum or anterior chest wall
- Serum studies to rule-out germ cell tumor (β-HCG, LDH, AFP, ACH receptor assay)
- Anterior mediastinoscopy with biopsy

STAGING

Stage grouping (Masaoka system)		~5 yr survival	
I:	Macroscopically completely encapsulated and microscopically no capsular invasion	I:	93%
II:	1. Macroscopic invasion into surrounding fatty tissue or mediastinal pleura, or 2. Microscopic invasion into capsule	II:	86%
III:	Macroscopic invasion into neighboring organ, i.e., pericardium, great vessels, or lung	III:	70%
IVA:	Pleural or pericardial dissemination	IV:	50%
IVB:	Lymphatic or hematogenous metastases		

From: Masaoka A, Monden Y, Nakahara K, et al. Follow-up study of thymomas with special reference to their clinical stages. Cancer 1981;48:2485, with permission

TREATMENT RECOMMENDATIONS

Stage	Recommended Treatment
I	Complete resection only
II	Complete resection → post-op RT
III	Complete resection (if possible) → post-op RT. If initially unresectable, pre-op RT +/− chemo (doxorubicin or cisplatin based). Otherwise, definitive RT
IV	Induction combination chemo → RT &/or surgery

STUDIES

- Multiple retrospective reviews demonstrate that RT reduces recurrence rates
- Curran (*JCO* 1988). Retrospective study of 103 pts with stage II/III thymoma. 5 yr actuarial mediastinal relapse after GTR was reduced with adjuvant RT from 53% to 0%
- Mornex (*IJROBP* 1995). Retrospective review of 90 pts treated with surgery + RT (30–70 Gy) +/– chemo (cisplatin based). 5/10 yr OS was 51/39%. Extent of surgery impacted 10 yr OS (43% for partial resection vs 31% for biopsy only). Stage, histology, & chemo were not prognostic
- Monden (*Ann Thorac Surg* 1985). 127 pts treated with surgery +/– RT. RT reduced recurrence from 30% to 15%

RADIATION TECHNIQUES
Simulation and field design
- Simulate pt supine with wing board
- 3DCRT should be used if available to minimize dose to normal structures
- Include mediastinum 5 cm below carina, tumor extensions (e.g., into lung parenchyma) +1–2 cm margin for CTV
- No need for SCV field(s) unless involved

Dose prescriptions
- Pre-op RT: 1.8–2 Gy/fx to 45 Gy
- Stage II post-op: 1.8 Gy/fx to 45 Gy
- Stage III post-op: 1.8 Gy/fx to 50–54 Gy
- Gross residual disease: 1.8 Gy/fx to 54–60 Gy
- Poor LC with total dose <40 Gy

Dose limitations
- Spinal cord <45 Gy, lung 70% <20 Gy, heart 70% <25–40 Gy, esophagus <60 Gy

COMPLICATIONS
- Acute: fatigue, dysphagia, cough, chest tightness, mild skin reaction
- Late: Pericarditis, radiation myelitis, radiation pneumonitis/fibrosis

FOLLOW-UP

- Late recurrences reported in up to 12% pts. Can be as late as 32 yrs post-op, so follow pts for life. Most recurrences remain indolent & confined to thorax

REFERENCES

Batata M. Thymomas: clinicopathologic features, therapy, and prognosis. Cancer 1974;34:389–396.

Ciernik IF, Meier U, Lutolf UM. Prognostic factors and outcome of incompletely resected invasive thymoma following radiation therapy. J Clin Oncol 1994;12:1484–1490.

Curran WJ, Jr., Kornstein MJ, Brooks JJ, et al. Invasive thymoma: the role of mediastinal irradiation following complete or incomplete surgical resection. J Clin Oncol 1988;6:1722–1727.

Eng TY ST, Thomas CR. Mediastinum and trachea. In: Perez CA, Brady LW, Halperin ED, Schmidt-Ullrich RK, editors. Principles and Practice of Radiation Oncology. 4th ed. Philadelphia: Lippincott Williams & Wilkins; 2004. pp. 1244–1281.

Komaki R, Travis EL, Cox JD. The lung and thymus. In: Cox JD, Ang KK, editors. Radiation Oncology: Rationale, Technique, Results. 8th ed. St. Louis: Mosby; 2003. pp. 399–427.

Monden Y, Nakahara K, Iioka S, et al. Recurrence of thymoma: clinicopathological features, therapy, and prognosis. Ann Thorac Surg 1985;39:165–169.

Mornex F. Radiotherapy and chemotherapy for invasive thymomas: a multicentric retrospective review of 90 cases. Int J Radiat Oncol Biol Phys 1995;2:651–659.

Ohara K, Okumura T, Sugahara S, et al. The role of preoperative radiotherapy for invasive thymoma. Acta Oncol 1990;29:425–429.

Rosenzweig KE KL. Tumors of the Lung, Pleura, and Mediastinum. In Leibel SA, Phillips TL, editors. Textbook of Radiation Oncology. 2nd ed. Philadelphia: Saunders; 2004. pp. 779–810.

Rusch VW, Rosenzweig K, Venkatraman E, et al. A phase II trial of surgical resection and adjuvant high-dose hemithoracic radiation for malignant pleural mesothelioma. J Thorac Cardiovasc Surg 2001;122:788–795.

Urgesi A, Monetti U, Rossi G, et al. Role of radiation therapy in locally advanced thymoma. Radiother Oncol 1990;19:273–280.

van Meerbeeck JP, Baas P, Debruyne C, et al. A phase II study of gemcitabine in patients with malignant pleural mesothelioma. European Organization for Research and Treatment of Cancer Lung Cancer Cooperative Group. Cancer 1999;85:2577–2582.

Vogelzang NJ, Rusthoven JJ, Symanowski J, et al. Phase III study of pemetrexed in combination with cisplatin versus cisplatin alone in patients with malignant pleural mesothelioma. J Clin Oncol 2003; 21:2636–2644.

NOTES

Chapter 16
Breast Cancer

Allen Chen, Catherine Park, Alison Bevan, and Lawrence W. Margolis

PEARLS

- Most common cancer among women in the United States (excluding skin)
- Second leading cause of cancer deaths in women
- Most important risk factor for breast cancer development is age
- Risk affected by age at menarche, first pregnancy, menopause, & family history
- Use of exogenous estrogen increases risk for breast cancer
- Approximately 10% of breast cancer cases are associated with germline mutation
- Carriers of BRCA1 have 36–56% probability of developing breast cancer in lifetime
- Medial & lateral borders of breast tissue typically the sternum and mid-axillary line
- Cranial & caudal borders typically the 2nd anterior rib & 6th anterior rib
- Primary lymphatic drainage is to axillary, internal mammary, & SCV nodes
- Axillary lymph nodes divided into 3 levels by relation to pectoralis minor muscle
- Level I (low axillary) = nodes inferior/lateral to pectoralis minor muscle
- Level II (mid-axillary) = nodes directly beneath the pectoralis minor muscle. Rotter's (interpectoral) nodes considered level II
- Level III (apical or infraclavicular) = nodes superior/medial to pectoralis minor muscle
- Pathological status of axillary lymph nodes is the most important prognostic variable
- Internal mammary LN located in 1st to 3rd intercostal spaces, 3–3.5 cm from midline

- Ductal carcinoma *in situ* (DCIS) comprises 15–20% of all breast cancer
- DCIS represents confinement of malignant cells within basement membrane
- Prognostic variables for DCIS include tumor size, margins, nuclear grade, necrosis, and age
- Lobular carcinoma *in situ* (LCIS) is marker for bilateral breast cancer
- Invasive (infiltrating) ductal carcinoma is the most common type of breast cancer
- Invasive lobular carcinoma has prognosis similar to that of ductal carcinoma
- Lobular carcinoma associated with increased risk of bilateral, multifocal breast cancer
- Tubular, medullary, & mucinous carcinomas generally have better prognosis
- Paget's disease is nipple involvement by tumor, usually from an underlying carcinoma
- Multicentricity is disease in multiple quadrants and is contraindication to breast conserving therapy (BCT)
- Multifocality is multiple foci within same quadrant & is not contraindication to BCT
- Extensive intraductal component (EIC) is when 25% or more of primary tumor is DCIS that is located within & adjacent to the invasive component
- EIC is not an independent risk factor for recurrence when margins are considered
- Younger pts are generally felt to be at higher risk for LR
- Positive margins & lymphatic invasion associated with increased LR
- High grade associated with increased LR in some, but not all studies
- Post-lumpectomy mammogram should be routinely obtained to rule-out residual microcalcifications

Locally advanced

- Incidence of locally advanced breast cancer is decreasing with mammography
- Locally advanced = stage III & subset of stage IIB (T3N0)
- Locally advanced can be divided into operable & inoperable disease
- Signs of inoperability: arm edema, satellites, inflammatory, & SCV disease

- Haagensen's grave signs: skin edema, ulceration, chest fixation, fixed/matted nodes
- Metastatic workup is important because high percentage develop distant disease
- SCV involvement no longer considered stage IV but stage IIIC (N3)
- Internal mammary LN involvement more likely with medial tumors, axillary nodes
- Prognostic variables include tumor size & extent of lymph node involvement
- Inflammatory carcinoma is a clinical diagnosis confirmed by pathological findings
- Inflammatory carcinoma presents with rapid onset of erythema, warmth, and edema
- Underlying mass often cannot be appreciated for inflammatory carcinoma
- Characteristic pathology for inflammatory disease is invasion of dermal lymphatics
- Most common site of LRF is the chest wall

WORKUP

- Breast cancer specific history including risk factors, gynecologic history, menopausal status, & general physical exam
- Breast exam (tumor size, satellites, skin/chest wall, nipple changes, symmetry)
- Lymph node exam (axillary, supraclavicular/infraclavicular)
- Bilateral diagnostic mammography, ultrasound
- Biopsy with estrogen & progesterone receptor studies; Her-2-neu status
- CBC, blood chemistries
- CXR
- Bone scan, head imaging, CT abdomen (when clinically indicated & for locally-advanced disease)
- Careful histologic assessment of breast specimens

STAGING

Primary tumor	
TX:	Primary tumor cannot be assessed
T0:	No evidence of primary tumor
Tis:	Carcinoma in situ
	Tis (DCIS): Ductal carcinoma in situ
	Tis (LCIS): Ductal carcinoma in situ
	Tis (Paget's): Paget's disease of the nipple with no tumor
T1:	Tumor 2 cm or less in greatest dimension

T1mic:	Microinvasion 0.1 cm or less in greatest dimension
T1a:	Tumor more than 0.1 cm but not more than 0.5 cm in greatest dimension
T1b:	Tumor more than 0.5 cm but not more than 1 cm in greatest dimension
T1c:	Tumor more than 1 cm but not more than 2 cm in greatest dimension

T2:	Tumor more than 2 cm but not more than 5 cm in greatest dimension
T3:	Tumor more than 5 cm in greatest dimension
T4:	Tumor of any size with direct extension to (a) chest wall or (b) skin
T4a:	Extension to chest wall, not including pectoralis muscle
T4b:	Edema (including peau d'orange) or ulceration of the skin of the breast, or satellite skin nodules confined to the same breast
T4c:	Both T4a and T4b
T4d:	Inflammatory carcinoma

Regional lymph nodes
Clinical

NX:	Regional lymph nodes cannot be assessed (e.g., previously removed)
N0:	No regional lymph node metastasis
N1:	Metastasis to moveable ipsilateral axillary lymph node(s)
N2:	Metastases in ipsilateral axillary lymph nodes fixed or matted, or in clinically apparent ipsilateral internal mammary nodes in the absence of clinically evident axillary lymph node metastasis
N2a:	Metastasis in ipsilateral axillary lymph nodes fixed to one another (matted) or to other structures
N2b:	Metastasis in clinically apparent ipsilateral internal mammary nodes and in the absence of clinically evident axillary lymph node metastasis
N3:	Metastasis in ipsilateral infraclavicular lymph node(s) with or without axillary lymph node involvement, or in clinically apparent ipsilateral internal mammary lymph node(s) and in the presence of clinically evident axillary lymph node metastasis; or metastasis in ipsilateral supraclavicular lymph node(s) with or without axillary or internal mammary lymph node involvement
N3a:	Metastasis in ipsilateral infraclavicular lymph node(s)
N3b:	Metastasis in ipsilateral internal mammary lymph node(s) and axillary lymph node(s)
N3c:	Metastasis in ipsilateral supraclavicular lymph node(s)

*Clinically apparent is defined as detected by imaging studies (excluding lymphoscintigraphy) or by clinical examination or grossly visible pathologically

Pathologic (pN)

pNX:	Regional lymph nodes cannot be assessed (e.g., previously removed, or not removed for pathologic study)
pN0:	No regional lymph node metastasis histologically, no additional examination for isolated tumor cells (ITC)
pN0(i–):	No regional lymph node metastasis histologically, negative IHC
pN0(i+):	No regional lymph node metastasis histologically, positive IHC, no IHC cluster greater than 0.2 mm
pN0(mol–):	No regional lymph node metastasis histologically, negative molecular findings (RT-PCR)
pN0(mol+):	No regional lymph node metastasis histologically, positive molecular findings (RT-PCR)
pN1:	Metastasis in 1–3 axillary lymph nodes, and/or in internal mammary nodes with microscopic disease detected by sentinel lymph node dissection but not clinically apparent
pN1mi:	Micrometastasis (greater than 0.2 mm, none greater than 2.0 mm)
pN1a:	Metastasis in 1–3 axillary lymph nodes
pN1b:	Metastasis in internal mammary nodes with microscopic disease detected by sentinel lymph node dissection but not clinically apparent

pN1c: Metastasis in 1–3 axillary lymph nodes and in internal mammary nodes with microscopic disease detected by sentinel lymph node dissection but not clinically apparent. (If associated with greater than 3 positive axillary lymph nodes, the internal mammary nodes are classified as pN3b to reflect increased tumor burden)

pN2:   Metastasis in 4–9 axillary lymph nodes, or in clinically apparent internal mammary lymph nodes in the absence of axillary lymph node metastasis

        pN2a: Metastasis in 4–9 axillary lymph nodes (at least one tumor deposit greater than 2.0 mm)

        pN2b: Metastasis in clinically apparent internal mammary lymph nodes in the absence of axillary lymph node metastasis

pN3:   Metastasis in 10 or more axillary lymph nodes, or in infraclavicular lymph nodes, or in clinically apparent ipsilateral internal mammary lymph nodes in the presence of 1 or more positive axillary lymph nodes; or in more than 3 axillary lymph nodes with clinically negative microscopic metastasis in internal mammary lymph nodes; or in ipsilateral supraclavicular lymph nodes

        pN3a: Metastasis in 10 or more axillary lymph nodes (at least one tumor deposit greater than 2.0 mm), or metastasis to the infraclavicular lymph nodes

        pN3b: Metastasis in clinically apparent ipsilateral internal mammary lymph nodes in the presence of 1 or more positive axillary lymph nodes; or in more than 3 axillary lymph nodes and in internal mammary lymph nodes with microscopic disease detected by sentinel lymph node dissection but not clinically apparent

        pN3c: Metastasis in ipsilateral supraclavicular lymph nodes

Note: Isolated tumor cells (ITC) are defined as single tumor cells or small cell clusters not greater than 0.2 mm, usually detected only by immunohistochemical (IHC) or molecular methods but which may be verified on H&E stains. ITCs do not usually show evidence of malignant activity e.g., proliferation or stromal reaction

Classification is based on axillary lymph node dissection with or without sentinel lymph node dissection. Classification solely based on sentinel lymph node dissection without subsequent axillary lymph node dissection is designated (sn) for "sentinel node," e.g., pN0(i+) (sn).

Distant Metastasis
MX   Distant metastasis cannot be assessed
M0:   No distant metastasis
M1:   Distant metastasis

*Rules: The pathologic tumor size is a measure of only the invasive component. For multiple ipsilateral primaries, use largest primary to designate T stage. Do not assign separate T stage for smaller tumor. Enter into the record that it is a case of multiple ipsilateral primaries. For bilateral disease, each primary is staged separately. If surgery occurs after neoadjuvant chemotherapy, hormonal therapy, immunotherapy, or radiation therapy, the prefix "y" should be used with the TNM classification, e.g., ypTNM

Stage Grouping		~5-yr Survival
0	TisN0M0	100%
I	T1N0M0	98%
IIA	T2N0M0, T0-1N1M0	88%
IIB	T3N0M0, T2N1M0	76%
IIIA	T3N1M0, T0-3N2M0	56%
IIIB	T4N0-2M0	49%
IIIC	Any T, N3 M0	
IV	Any T, any N, M1	16%

Used with the permission of the American Joint Committee on Cancer (AJCC), Chicago, Illinois. The original source for this material is the AJCC Cancer Staging Manual, Sixth Edition (2002) published by Springer-Verlag New York, www.springeronline.com.

TREATMENT RECOMMENDATIONS (GENERAL POINTS)
DCIS

- DCIS treatment is individualized based on clinical & pathological features, & pt preference
- Both total mastectomy & breast-conserving therapy (BCT) with lumpectomy ±RT reasonable options for DCIS
- For widely excised, small, low-grade DCIS without necrosis, RT is controversial
- Prospective data has failed to identify subsets of DCIS that may not require RT
- Tamoxifen for DCIS reduces local recurrence after lumpectomy + RT, although absolute benefit may be small

Early stage

- Breast-conserving therapy (BCT) is equivalent to mastectomy for early-stage disease
- BCT with lumpectomy + RT is considered standard of care
- Mastectomy reserved for pts ineligible for BCT due to medical/surgical/personal reasons
- Contraindications to BCT include multicentricity, ratio of tumor size to breast, locally-advanced tumors, diffuse microcalcifications, persistently positive margins, previous breast RT, pregnancy, & collagen vascular disease (relative)
- Attempts to define subsets with early-stage disease not requiring RT unsuccessful
- Lymph node involvement not a contraindication to BCT
- Sentinel node dissection indicated for small primaries with clinically negative axilla
- Adjuvant chemotherapy generally recommended for >1 cm tumors or node positive
- Adjuvant chemotherapy reduces LR after lumpectomy + RT
- Adjuvant hormonal therapy generally recommended for ER-positive tumors
- Trastuzumab (Herceptin), a humanized monoclonal antibody for HER2/neu, is also often indicated for pts with HER2 overexpression

Locally advanced

- Multi-modality approach is critical for all patients

- With standard therapy, OS is 50–60% at 5 yrs & 30–40% at 10 yrs
- Traditional approach is to treat upfront with mastectomy
- Modified radical mastectomy: removal of breast to level of pectoralis minor muscle
- Level I/II axillary node dissection performed with modified radical mastectomy
- Total (simple) mastectomy is removal of breast tissue without axillary dissection
- Patients with 4+ involved axillary lymph nodes should have SCV RT
- Indications for SCV RT for 1–3 involved axillary lymph nodes less clear
- Tangential RT usually covers a large percentage of the level I and II axillary nodes
- Early post-mastectomy RT trials limited by selection, technique, no systemic therapy. Survival detriment attributed to RT in early trials due to cardiac/pulmonary toxicity
- Contemporary randomized trials have shown OS benefit for post-mastectomy RT
- Post-mastectomy RT indications: T3/4, + margins, gross ECE, & ≥4+ nodes
- For 1–3 axillary lymph nodes involved, indications for post-mastectomy RT unclear
- Consider tumor size, margins, LVSI, extent of axillary dissection in decision-making
- Post-mastectomy RT needed for gross residual tumor or inadequate node dissection
- Neoadjuvant chemotherapy as initial therapy has gained increasing popularity
- Advantages of neoadjuvant chemotherapy: assessment of response, increased rate of BCT
- Neoadjuvant chemotherapy converts 20–30% of pts initially ineligible for BCT to eligible
- Complete clinical (cCR) & pathological response rates (pCR) depend on initial extent of disease
- For locally advanced disease, 20–40% achieve cCR after neoadjuvant chemotherapy & 10–20% achieve pCR
- Clinical response frequently does not correlate with pathological response
- Approximately 1/3 with a cCR found to have pathological residual disease
- BCT may be possible after neoadjuvant chemotherapy in properly selected patients

- Selection criteria for BCT after neoadjuvant chemotherapy remain to be defined
- MRI to assess treatment response to neoadjuvant chemo appears promising
- Adjuvant chemotherapy recommended for all patients with locally advanced disease
- Adjuvant hormonal therapy generally recommended for ER-positive tumors
- RT can usually begin within 2–4 weeks of surgery
- For patients receiving chemotherapy, RT begins 3–4 weeks after last cycle
- Median time to breast cancer recurrence is 2–5 yrs, but may occur up to 15–20 yrs later

Stage	Recommended Treatment
DCIS	BCT with lumpectomy ± RT. RT generally indicated for all pts to reduce LR, but some pts may choose no RT [e.g., with small (<0.5cm), unicentric, low-grade tumors excised with wide negative margins]. Alternative is total mastectomy (TM) without LN dissection, indicated for diffuse suspicious microcalcifications, multicentric disease, persistently + margins, or pt desire. Consider adjuvant tamoxifen for ER+ tumors
LCIS	Lifelong close observation ± tamoxifen for risk reduction. If young & strong FH or genetic predisposition, consider prophylactic bilateral mastectomy

Stage	Recommended Treatment
I–IIB (T1-2N0-1)	BCT with lumpectomy & surgical axillary staging + RT. Some consider RT optional for T1N0 ER+ pts ≥70yrs of age who receive adjuvant hormone therapy (HT). Alternative: TM with surgical axillary staging + RT as indicated. Adjuvant chemo, HT, &/or trastuzumab as indicated
IIB (T3N0) & IIIA	Neoadjuvant chemo → surgery (mastectomy or BCT) with surgical axillary staging + RT. Alternative: TM with surgical axillary staging + RT. Adjuvant chemo, HT, &/or trastuzumab as indicated
IIIB–IIIC	Neoadjuvant chemo → surgery (mastectomy or BCT) with surgical axillary staging + RT. Adjuvant chemo, HT, &/or trastuzumab as indicated
IV	HT, chemo, &/or trastuzumab as indicated. Consider bisphosphonates for bone metastases. Palliative RT may be needed
Isolated axillary LN(s)	Workup: H&P, bilateral mammography, CT chest, abdomen, & pelvis, US of axilla(e) ± breast(s), & serum tumor markers. Consider MRI of breast(s) Treatment: Neoadjuvant chemo → axillary lymph node dissection (ALND) + RT to breast & axilla ± SCV. Alternative: TM with ALND + RT as indicated. Adjuvant chemo, HT, &/or trastuzumab as indicated

Stage	Recommended Treatment
During pregnancy	1st trimester: Discuss termination. If pregnancy not terminated, mastectomy & ALND → chemo (as indicated) in 2nd trimester ± post-partum RT &/or HT
	2nd /3rd trimester: Surgery (mastectomy or BCT) + ALND → adjuvant chemo (as indicated) ± post-partum RT &/or HT. Alternative: neoadjuvant chemo → surgery (mastectomy or BCT)& ALND post-partum ± RT &/or HT

PREVENTION TRIAL

- NSABP P-1 (*J Natl Cancer Inst* 1998). 13,388 pts at elevated risk for breast cancer (>60 yrs old, 35–59 yrs old with 5 yr predicted risk of at least 1.66% based on Gail model, history of LCIS) randomized to placebo vs tamoxifen ×5 yrs. At 69 mo F/U, tamoxifen reduced relative risk of invasive breast cancer by 49% and noninvasive breast cancer by 50%. However, reductions in absolute risk were only 2% & 0.9%, respectively

DCIS STUDIES

- NSABP B-17 (*JCO* 1998 *Semin Oncol* 2001). 818 pts with DCIS (negative margins) randomized to lumpectomy vs lumpectomy +50 Gy RT. At 12 yrs F/U, addition of RT reduced rates of noninvasive LF from 15% to 8% & invasive LF from 17% to 8% (total LF: 32% to 16%)
- EORTC 10853 (*Lancet* 2000). 1010 pts with DCIS (negative margins) randomized to lumpectomy vs lumpectomy +50 Gy RT. At 4 yrs F/U, addition of RT reduced LF (invasive and noninvasive) rates from 16% to 9%
- NSABP B-24 (*Lancet* 1999 *Semin Oncol* 2001). 1804 pts with DCIS (16% + margins; all unknown ER status) treated with lumpectomy & 50 Gy RT randomized to placebo vs tamoxifen (20 mg daily ×5 yrs). At 7 yrs F/U, addition of tamoxifen reduced incidence of LF (invasive and

noninvasive) from 11% to 8% and contralateral events from 4.9% to 2.3%

- **VNPI** (Silverstein, *Am J Surg* 2003). Retrospective review of 706 pts s/p BCT with or without RT scored based on four parameters: tumor size (≤1.5 cm, 1.6–4.0 cm, ≥4.1 cm); pathology (non-high grade without necrosis, non-high grade with necrosis, high grade); margins (≥1 cm, 0.1–0.9 cm, <0.1 cm); & age (>60 yrs, 40–60 yrs, <40 yrs). For low-risk (score 4, 5, 6), no significant difference in 12 yr local RFS (>90–95%) with or without RT. For intermediate-risk (score 7, 8, 9), addition of RT provided 12–15% 12 yr local RFS benefit. For high-risk (score 10, 11, 12) mastectomy recommended due to high 5 yr LR (~50%) with or without RT

- **Silverstein** (*NEJM* 1999). Retrospective study of 469 pts s/p lumpectomy with or without RT. For the 90 pts with >1 cm lumpectomy alone with median F/U 81 mos (2.2% vs 2.5%)

- **Wong** (*J Clin Oncol* 2006). Phase II trial of 158 women with predominantly grade 1–2 DCIS measuring ≤2.5 cm on mammography with final margins ≥1 cm observed after lumpectomy (no RT or Tamoxifen). 12% LF at 5 yrs

- **UKCCR** (*Lancet* 2003). 1701 pts status post lumpectomy (negative margins) for DCIS randomized to 50 Gy RT; tamoxifen ×5 yrs; neither; or both. At median F/U 53 months, rates of all breast events were 8%, 18%, 22%, and 6%, respectively. When analyzing those randomized to RT vs no RT, RT reduced LF (invasive or noninvasive) in ipsilateral breast from 14% to 6%

EARLY-STAGE BREAST CANCER STUDIES

- **NSABP B-04** (*NEJM* 2002). 1079 pts with clinically negative axillary LN randomized to 1 of 3 arms: radical mastectomy vs total mastectomy without axillary dissection but with post-op RT vs total mastectomy plus axillary dissection if LN pathologically positive. Also 586 pts with clinically + axillary LN randomized to 1 of 2 arms (radical mastectomy vs total mastectomy without axillary dissection but with post-op RT). None received adjuvant systemic therapy. At 25 yrs F/U, no significant differences in LF, DFS, or OS among the 3 groups of pts with clinically negative LN or the 2 groups of pts with clinically + LN

- **NSABP B-06** (*NEJM* 2002). 1851 pts with stage I/II breast ca (<4 cm, negative margins) randomized to total mastectomy vs lumpectomy alone vs lumpectomy + 50 Gy RT. At 20 yrs F/U, no significant differences observed among 3 groups with respect to DFS, OS, or DM-free survival. Addition of RT to lumpectomy reduced LF from 39% to 14%

- EORTC 10801 (*J Natl Cancer Inst* 2000). 902 pts with stage I/II breast ca randomized to modified radical mastectomy vs lumpectomy + 50 Gy RT + boost. At 10 yrs F/U, no difference in OS (66% vs 65%), but there was a difference in rate of LF (12% vs 20%, p = 0.01). However, 48% in lumpectomy group had + margins

- Milan I (*NEJM* 2002). 701 pts with T1N0 breast ca randomized to radical mastectomy vs quadrantectomy +60 Gy RT. At median F/U 20 yrs, no difference in OS (59% vs 58%) or breast ca-specific survival (76% vs 74%). However, LF was 2.3% vs 8.8% (p < 0.001)

- Milan III (*Ann Oncol* 2001). 570 pts with tumors <2.5 cm randomized to surgery alone (quadrantectomy + axillary dissection) versus surgery + 60 Gy RT. At 10 yrs F/U, addition of RT reduced LF (23.5 → 5.8%), but there was no difference in OS. Pts <45 yrs had highest LF but also derived most benefit from RT

- EORTC boost trial (*NEJM* 2001). 5569 pts with stage I/II breast ca s/p lumpectomy (negative margins) randomized to 50 Gy RT vs 50 Gy + 16 Gy boost. Boost decreased LF from 7.3% to 4.3% with largest benefit observed in patients ≤40 yrs

- Lyon boost trial (*JCO* 1997). 1024 pts with early-stage breast ca s/p lumpectomy (<3 cm tumor), axillary LN dissection, and 50 Gy RT randomized to boost (10 Gy) vs no boost. At median F/U 3 yrs, addition of boost reduced LF (3.6% vs 4.5%). No difference in self-assessed cosmetic response between 2 arms

- NSABP B-21 (*JCO* 2002). 1009 pts s/p lumpectomy for tumors ≤1 cm (both ER/PR −/+) randomized to tamoxifen vs RT + placebo vs RT and tamoxifen. At 8 yrs F/U, both tamoxifen and RT independently reduced LF (16.5%, 9.3%, and 2.8%). However, OS and DM-free survival did not differ between the 3 groups

- CALGB C9343/INT trial (*NEJM* 2004). 636 pts (>70 yrs) with T1N0, ER+ breast ca s/p lumpectomy randomized to tamoxifen + RT vs tamoxifen alone. Addition of RT to tamoxifen improved 5 yr LF (1% vs 4%, p < 0.001). No difference in breast ca-specific survival or OS

- <u>PMH/Canada</u> (*NEJM* 2004). 769 pts with stage I/II breast cancer (ER/PR +/–) s/p lumpectomy randomized to tamoxifen + RT vs tamoxifen alone. Addition of RT to tamoxifen reduced 5 yr LR (7.7% vs. 0.6%, p < 0.001) and improved DFS (91% vs. 84%, p = 0.004). For pts with tumors <1 cm and ER+, 5 yr LF was 2.6% vs 0% (p = 0.02). At 8 yrs, with 86 pts at risk, addition of RT reduced LR from 17.6% to 3.5%

- <u>Scottish trial</u> (*Lancet* 1996). 585 pts with stage I/II breast ca s/p lumpectomy (tumors <4 cm, gross margins >1 cm) randomized to lumpectomy vs lumpectomy + 50 Gy RT. All patients received systemic therapy (tamoxifen if ER+ or CMF if ER–). LF was 24.5% with adjuvant systemic therapy alone vs 5.8% with addition of RT (p < 0.01). Thus, systemic therapy does not obviate need for RT

- <u>NSABP B-20</u> (*J Natl Cancer Inst* 1997). 2306 pts s/p surgery with pathologically LN–, ER+ breast ca randomized to tamoxifen alone vs tamoxifen + MF chemotherapy vs tamoxifen + CMF chemotherapy. At 5 yrs F/U, the addition of chemotherapy to tamoxifen resulted in better DFS (85% vs 90%)

- <u>NSABP B-18</u> (*J Natl Cancer Inst Monogr* 2001). 1523 pts with breast ca randomized to AC chemo ×4 pre-op vs AC chemo ×4 post-op. At 9 yrs F/U, no significant difference in DFS, DM-free survival, or OS. Pts assigned to pre-op group underwent more BCT than post-op pts, especially among pts with tumors >5 cm at study entry

- <u>JCRT sequencing</u> (*JCO* 2005). 244 pts with stage I/II breast ca s/p lumpectomy randomized to adjuvant doxorubicin-based chemo followed by RT versus adjuvant RT followed by four cycles of same chemo. With 11 yrs F/U, there are no differences in OS, DM, time to any event, or site of first failure. For close margins, crude LR was 32% with chemo first vs 4% with RT first; for + margins, crude LR was 20–23% in both arms

- <u>NSABP B-14</u> (*NEJM* 1989). 2644 pts s/p surgery for breast ca (pathologically LN–, ER+) randomized to tamoxifen ×5 yrs vs placebo. At 4 yrs F/U, adjuvant tamoxifen reduced LF (3 → 1%) & improved DFS (77 → 83%). No difference in OS

- <u>ATAC Trial</u> (*Lancet* 2002). 9366 postmenopausal patients (both ER–/+) s/p definitive therapy for early-stage breast ca randomized to anastrozole, tamoxifen, or both. Anastrozole alone improved 3-yr DFS compared with tamoxifen (89% vs 87%) or both (87%). Benefit observed only in ER pos pts. Anastrozole better tolerated with respect to side-effects

- Goss (*N Eng L Med* 2003). 5187 postmenopausal patients (98% ER+) s/p definitive therapy and adjuvant tamoxifen ×5 yrs for early-stage breast ca randomized to letrozole (2.5 mg) or placebo daily ×5 yrs. Addition of letrozole improved 4 yr DFS (87 → 93%)
- Vicini (*J Natl Cancer Int* 2003). Phase II trial with 199 pts with early-stage breast ca treated with limited-field RT to region of tumor bed only (LDR 60%, HDR 40%). At median F/U 65 mos, LF was 1% and comparable to matched-pair controls treated with whole-breast RT

LOCALLY-ADVANCED BREAST CANCER STUDIES

- EBCTCG RT (*Lancet* 2005). Meta-analysis of 78 randomized trials including 42,000 women. RT after BCS, & RT after mastectomy with axillary clearance in LN+ disease, produced significant absolute improvements in 5 yr LR (17–19% benefit) & 15 yr breast cancer mortality (5.4% benefit). RT produced similar proportional reductions in LR risk (~70% risk reduction) irrespective of age, grade, tumor size, ER status, or amount of LN involvement. Among pts treated with systemic therapy, the absolute benefits of RT on LR & breast cancer mortality were 20% (at 5 yrs) & 5.9% (at 15 yrs), respectively. Therefore, better local treatment adds to the effect of systemic therapy on LR, which can translate into a moderate breast cancer mortality benefit (4:1 ratio). RT was associated with excess contralateral breast cancer, lung cancer, & mortality from heart disease. Yet, addition of RT improved 15 yr OS by 5.3% after BCS & by 4.4% after mastectomy with axillary clearance for LN+ disease
- EBCTCG chemo/HT (*Lancet* 2005). Meta-analysis of 194 randomized trials with ~150,000 women. ~6 months of anthracycline-based polychemotherapy reduced annual breast cancer death rate by 38% for women < 50 yrs (15 yr absolute gain: 10/15% for LN–/LN+) & by 20% for women 50–69 yrs (15 yr absolute gain: 5/6% for LN–/LN+). Anthracycline regimens were significantly more effective than CMF chemo. Tamoxifen × 5 yrs for ER+ (any age) reduced annual breast cancer death rate by 31% (5 yr absolute gains: without chemo 12%, in addition to chemo 11%,

<50 yrs 10%, ≥50 yrs 12%, LN– 9%, LN+ 16%). 5 yrs tamoxifen significantly better than 1–2 yrs of tamoxifen

- Cuzick (*JCO* 1994). Meta-analysis of 8 randomized trials analyzing post-mastectomy RT. At 10 yrs F/U, post-mastectomy RT improved breast ca-specific survival, although this benefit was offset by increase in cardiac deaths. However, there is still a non-significant OS benefit with addition of RT

- Danish 82b (*New Engl J Med* 1997). 1708 pre-menopausal pts s/p modified radical mastectomy randomized to adjuvant CMF chemo alone vs chemo + RT (37.5 Gy/18 fractions). At median F/U 114 mos, addition of post-mastectomy RT reduced LRF (32% vs 9%). RT also improved 10 yr DFS (34% vs 48%) and OS (45% vs 54%). Improvement in LC and OS observed in all subsets regardless of tumor size or number of involved LN

- Danish 82c (*Lancet* 1999). 1460 postmenopausal pts s/p modified radical mastectomy randomized to adjuvant tamoxifen alone vs tamoxifen + RT (48–50 Gy). At 10 yrs F/U, addition of RT improved LRF (35% vs 8%), DFS (24% vs 36%), and OS (36% vs 45%)

- British-Columbia trial (*J Natl Cancer Inst* 2005). 318 premenopausal pts s/p modified radical mastectomy (LN+) randomized to CMF chemo alone vs chemo + RT. At 20 yrs F/U, addition of post-mastectomy RT reduced LRF (26 → 10%), & improved breast ca-specific survival (38 → 53%), & OS (37 → 47%)

- Whelan (*JCO*, 2000). Meta-analysis of 18 contemporary post-mastectomy trials (6367 pts) demonstrated that the addition of post-mastectomy RT reduced LRF by 75% and improved OS by 17%

- ECOG, Recht (*JCO* 1999). Retrospective review of 2016 pts s/p mastectomy and adjuvant CMF chemo without RT demonstrated that 10 yr LRF was 13% for those with 1–3 LN+ compared to 29% for those with ≥4 LN+

- ECOG, Fowble (*JCO* 1988). Retrospective review of pts treated with mastectomy and CMF. Features predictive of LRF include tumor >5 cm, pectoralis fascia invasion, ER-tumors, and ≥4 LN+

- Katz (*JCO* 2000). Retrospective review of 1031 pts treated with mastectomy and doxorubicin-based chemo without adjuvant RT. 10 yr LRF were 4%, 10%, 21%, and 22% for patients with 0, 1–3, 4–9, or >10 LN involved. T-stage, tumor size and >2 mm ECE predictive for LRF

- Katz (*IJROBP* 2001). Retrospective review of 1031 pts treated with mastectomy and doxorubicin-based chemo without adjuvant RT demonstrated on multivariate analysis that ≥4 LN+, tumor >5 cm, close/+ margins, lymphatic invasion, and gross multicentric disease were independent predictors of LRF

- Kuerer (*JCO* 1999). Retrospective review of 372 patients with locally advanced breast cancer treated with neoadjuvant AC ×4. With median F/U 58 mos, 12% of patients had a pCR in both primary tumor and axillary nodes. 5 yr OS was significantly higher in pts with a pCR vs those with less than pCR (89% vs 64%).

- Chen (*JCO* 2004). Retrospective review of 340 pts treated with neoadjuvant chemo + BCT demonstrated that acceptably low rates of LF (5% at 5 yrs) can be obtained when appropriate selection criteria are used

- Huang (*JCO* 2004). Retrospective review of 679 pts treated with neoadjuvant chemo + mastectomy with or without post-mastectomy RT. At 10 yrs F/U, addition of RT reduced LRF (11% vs 22%) and improved breast ca-specific survival for pts with clinical T3 tumors or stage III disease and for pts with ≥4 LN+

- ASTRO post-mastectomy consensus (*IJROBP* 1999). Practice guidelines issued by multidisciplinary expert panel recommend post-mastectomy RT for pts with ≥4 LN+. Pts with 1–3 LN+ should be enrolled on protocol. Controversy regarding sites requiring RT

- ASCO post-mastectomy consensus (*JCO* 2001). Practice guidelines issued by multidisciplinary expert panel recommended post-mastectomy RT for pts with ≥4 LN+ and with T3 or stage III tumors. Insufficient evidence to make recommendations for pts with 1–3 LN+

- NSABP B-31 & NCCTG N9831 (Romond, *NEJM* 2005). 3351 pts with resected LN+ or high-risk LN−, HER2+ breast cancer randomized to chemo (doxorubicin, cyclophosphamide, & paclitaxel) vs chemo + trastuzumab. Trastuzumab increased 3 yr DFS (75 → 87%) & OS (92 → 94%), but was associated with increased risk of heart failure or cardiac death (3–4%)

- HERA BIG 01–01 (Piccart-Gebhart, *NEJM* 2005). 5090 pts s/p surgery ± RT & neoadjuvant or adjuvant chemo ± HT (if ER/PR+) with HER2 overexpression randomized to observation, 1 yr trastuzumab (q3wk), or 2 yr trastuzumab.

On interim analysis, trastuzumab × 1 yr improved 2 yr DFS (77 → 86%), but no difference in OS (95–96%)

RADIATION TECHNIQUES: EARLY-STAGE
Simulation and field design

- Pts usually treated in supine position with customized immobilization device
- Ipsilateral arm abducted and externally rotated
- Wire all surgical scars
- Target volume is entire breast using tangential fields
- Mark estimated medial, lateral, cranial, and caudal field borders
- Medial border at mid-sternum
- Lateral border placed 2 cm beyond all palpable breast tissue (mid-axillary line)
- Inferior border is 2 cm from inframammary fold
- Superior border is at head of clavicle or second intercostal space
- Deep (intrathoracic) field border must be non-divergent and edges made coplanar
- Isocenter typically placed in center of treatment field
- In general, 1–2 cm of underlying lung in the treatment field is acceptable
- For left-sided lesions, minimize the amount of heart in tangential fields
- CT-planning increasingly common and allows for more accurate dose distribution
- Rarely need to treat completely dissected axilla since axillary failure is uncommon
- High tangent technique can be used to treat greater percentage of axilla
- When using third field, attention to geometric match with tangential fields is essential
- Half-beam block for caudal edge of supraclavicular field to eliminate divergence
- Divergence of tangential fields superiorly can be eliminated with various techniques
- Supraclavicular field is angled obliquely 10–15 degrees laterally to keep off spinal cord
- Inferior border of supraclavicular field placed at inferior aspect of clavicular head
- Superior border of supraclavicular field is above acromioclavicular joint, top of T1/first rib, short of flash

- Medial border of supraclavicular field placed at the pedicles of vertebral bodies
- Lateral border of supraclavicular field is coracoid process or lateral to humeral head
- Monoisocentric technique can also be employed to treat supraclavicular field
- RT to the internal mammary chain is controversial
- Internal mammary RT performed with matched electrons or with wide tangential field
- Boost field is delivered with appositional field using electrons to tumor bed
- Partial breast irradiation is becoming increasingly popular although still investigational

Dose prescriptions

- 45–50 Gy at 1.8–2 Gy/fx to whole breast with tangential fields
- 45–50 Gy at 1.8–2 Gy/fx to supraclavicular fossa (when included)
- Boost irradiation with electrons to bring total tumor bed dose to 60–66 Gy
- Electron energy is selected to allow the 85–90% isodose line to encompass target
- Each field should be treated on a daily basis, Monday through Friday
- Bolus should not be used

RADIATION TECHNIQUES: LOCALLY-ADVANCED
Simulation and field design

- Pt simulated in similar manner to early-stage disease
- Target volume includes chest wall and supraclavicular fossa
- Wire all surgical scars and drain sites
- Entire mastectomy scar, flaps, surgical clips and drain sites included in treatment field
- Attention to geometric match with SCV field to avoid junctional overdose
- Boost field is delivered using electrons in appositional field to chest wall and skin
- BCT after good response to neoadjuvant chemotherapy typically requires 3-field RT
- RT is given to internal mammary nodes if they are clinically or pathologically positive, otherwise internal mammary node irradiation is controversial and at the

discretion of the treating radiation oncologist. CT treatment planning should be utilized in all cases where RT is delivered to the internal mammary lymph nodes

Dose prescriptions

- 45–50 Gy at 1.8–2 Gy/fx to chest wall using tangential fields
- 45–50 Gy at 1.8–2 Gy/fx to supraclavicular fossa
- Consider electron boost to bring total scar dose to 60 Gy in high-risk patients
- Two electron fields often necessary to cover skin and subcutaneous tissue at risk
- Electron energy selected to allow the 85–90% isodose line to encompass target
- Each field should be treated on a daily basis, Monday through Friday
- 5–10 mm bolus typically used every other day until moist desquamation occurs

DOSE LIMITATIONS

- Goal of treatment is to achieve homogeneous distribution throughout target volume
- Careful attention must be paid to amount of lung tissue and heart in treatment field
- Wedging and weighting can achieve better dose distribution
- Field-within-field technique using static IMRT often used to optimize dose distribution

COMPLICATIONS

- Acute skin reaction
- Cosmetic impairment (edema, fibrosis, telangiectasia)
- Upper extremity lymphedema: 1–5% risk with RT alone, 10% risk with axillary LN dissection (ALND), 12% risk with ALND + RT, & 16–20% risk with ALND + SCV/axillary RT
- Uncommon: brachial plexopathy, pneumonitis, cardiac toxicity, rib fracture, secondary malignancies

FOLLOW-UP

- Regular H&P
- Annual mammography
- Cosmetic assessment

■ Follow-up every 3–6 mo, yrs 1–3; every 6 mo, yrs 4–5; annually thereafter

REFERENCES

Arriagada R, Le MG, Mouriesse H, et al. Long-term effect of internal mammary chain treatment. Results of a multivariate analysis of 1195 patients with operable breast cancer and positive axillary nodes. Radiother Oncol 1988;11:213–222.

Bartelink H, Horiot JC, Poortsmans P, et al. Recurrence rates after treatment of breast cancer with standard radiotherapy with or without additional radiation. N Engl J Med 2001;245:1378–1387.

Bellon JR, Come SE, Belman RS, et al. Sequencing of chemotherapy and radiation therapy in early-stage breast cancer: updated results of a prospective randomized trial. J Clin Oncol 2005;23:1934–1940.

Bijker N, Peterse JL, Duchateau L, et al. Risk factors for recurrence and metastases after breast-conserving therapy for ductal carcinoma in-situ: analysis of European organization for research and treatment cancer trial 10853. J Clin Oncol 2001;19:226–2271.

Boice JD, Harvey EB, Blettner M, et al. Cancer in the contralateral breast after radiotherapy for breast cancer. N Engl J Med 1992; 326:781–785.

Bonadonna G, Valagussa P, Moliterni A, et al. Adjuvant cyclophospha-mide, methotrexate, and fluorouracil in node-positive breast cancer: the results of 20 years of follow-up. N Engl J Med 1995;332: 901–906.

Brito RA, Valero V, Buzdar AU, et al. Long-term results of combined-modality therapy for locally advanced breast cancer with ipsilateral supraclavicular metastases: the university of texas M.D. Anderson Cancer Center experience. J Clin Oncol 2001;19:628–633.

Buchholz TA, Tucker SL, Masullo L, et al. Predictors of local-regional recurrence after neoadjuvant chemotherapy and mastectomy without radiation. J Clin Oncol 2001;20:17–23.

Burstein HJ, Polyak K, Wong JS, et al. Ductal carcinoma in situ of the breast. N Engl J Med 2004;350:1430–1441.

Chen AM, Meric-Bernstam F, Hunt KK, et al. Breast conservation after neoadjuvant chemotherapy: the M.D. Anderson Cancer Center experience. J Clin Oncol 2004;22:2303–2312.

Chen AM, Obedian E, Haffty BG. Breast-conserving therapy in the setting of collagen vascular disease. Cancer J 2001;7:480–491.

Cole BF, Gelber RD, Gelber S, et al. Polychemotherapy for early breast cancer: an overview of the randomized clinical trials with quality-adjusted survival analysis. Lancet 2001;358:277–286.

Cuzick J, Stewart H, Rutqvist L, et al. Cause-specific mortality in long-term survivors of breast cancer who participated in trials of radio-therapy. J Clin Oncol 1994;12:447–453.

Early Breast Cancer Trialists' Collaborative Group. Effects of radio-therapy and of differences in the extent of surgery for early breast cancer on local recurrence and 15-year survival: an overview of the randomized trials. Lancet 2005;366:2087–2106.

Early Breast Cancer Trialists' Collaborative Group. Effects of chemotherapy and hormonal therapy for early breast cancer on recurrence and 15-year survival: an overview of the randomized trials. Lancet 2005;365:1687–1717.

Esserman L, Kaplan E, Partridge S, et al. MRI phenotype is associated with response to doxorubicin and cyclophosphamide neoadjuvant chemotherapy in stage III breast cancer. Ann Surg Oncol 2001;8:549–559.

Fisher B, Anderson S, Bryant J, et al. Twenty-year follow-up of a randomized trial comparing total mastectomy, lumpectomy, and lumpectomy plus irradiation for the treatment of invasive breast cancer. N Engl J Med 2002;347:1233–1241.

Fisher B, Bryant J, Dignam JL, et al. Tamoxifen, radiation therapy, or both for prevention of ipsilateral breast tumor recurrence after lumpectomy in women with invasive breast cancers of one centimeter or less. N Engl J Med 2002;20:4141–4149.

Fisher B, Bryant J, Wolmark N, et al. Effect of preoperative chemotherapy on the outcome of women with operable breast cancer. J Clin Oncol 1998;16:2672–2685.

Fisher B, Cosantino J, Redmond C, et al. A randomized clinical trial evaluating tamoxifen in the treatment of patients with node-negative breast cancer who have estrogen-receptor positive tumors. N Engl J Med 1989;320:479–484.

Fisher B, Costantino JP, Wickerham DL, et al. Tamoxifen for prevention of breast cancer: report of the National Surgical Adjuvant Breast and Bowel Project P-1 Study. J Natl Cancer Inst. 1998;16;90: 1371–1388.

Fisher B, Dignam J, Bryant J, et al. Five versus more than five years of tamoxifen for lymph node-negative breast cancer: updated findings from the national surgical adjuvant breast and bowel project B-14 randomized trial. J Natl Cancer Inst 2001;93:684–690.

Fisher B, Dignam J, Wolmark N, et al. Lumpectomy and radiation therapy for the treatment of intraductal breast cancer: findings from the national surgical adjuvant breast and bowel project B-17. J Clin Oncol 1998;16:441–452.

Fisher B, Dignam J, Wolmark N, et al. Tamoxifen and chemotherapy for lymph node-negative, estrogen receptor-positive breast cancer. J Natl Cancer Inst 1997;89:1673–1682.

Fisher B, Dignam J, Wolmark N, et al. Tamoxifen in treatment of intraductal breast cancer: national surgical adjuvant breast and bowel project B-24 randomized controlled trial. Lancet 1999;353: 1993–2000.

Fisher B, Jeong JH, Anderson S, et al. Twenty-five year follow-up of a randomized trial comparing radical mastectomy, total mastectomy, and total mastectomy followed by irradiation. N Engl J Med 2002; 347:567–575.

Fisher B, Land S, Mamounas E, et al. Prevention of invasive breast cancer in women with ductal carcinoma in situ: an update of the national surgical adjuvant breast and bowel project experience. Semin Oncol 2001;28:400–418.

Forrest AP, Stewart HJ, Everington D, et al. Randomized controlled trial of conservation therapy for breast cancer: 6-year analysis of the Scottish trial. Lancet 1996;348:708–713.

Fowble B, Gray R, Gilchrist K, et al. Identification of a subgroup of patients with breast cancer and histologically positive axillary lymph nodes receiving adjuvant chemotherapy who may benefit from postoperative radiotherapy. J Clin Oncol 1988;6:1107–1117.

Fyles AW, McCready DR, Manchul LA, et al. Tamoxifen with or without breast irradiation in women 50 years of age or older with early stage breast cancer. N Engl J Med 2004;351:963–970.

Gage I, Schnitt SJ, Nixon AJ, et al. Pathologic margin involvement and the risk of recurrence in patients treated with breast-conserving therapy. Cancer 1996;78:1921–1928.

Galper S, Recht A, Silver B, et al. Factors associated with regional nodal failure in patients with early stage breast cancer with 0–3 positive axillary lymph nodes following tangential irradiation alone. Int J Radiat Oncol Biol Phys 1999;45:1157–1166.

Goss PE, Ingle JN, Martino S, et al. A randomized trial of letrozole in postmenopausal women after five years of tamoxifen therapy for early stage breast cancer. N Engl J Med 2003;349:1793–1802.

Haffty BG, Fischer D, Rose M, et al. Prognostic factors for local recurrence in the conservatively treated breast cancer patient: a cautious interpretation of the data. J Clin Oncol 1991;9:997–1003.

Harris JR, Halpin-Murphy P, McNeese M, et al. Consensus statement on postmastectomy radiation therapy. Int J Radiat Oncol Biol Phys 1999;44:989–990.

Huang EH, Tucker SL, Strom EA, et al. Postmastectomy radiation improves local-regional control and survival for selected patients with locally advanced breast cancer treated with neoadjuvant chemotherapy and mastectomy. J Clin Oncol 2004; 22:4639–4647.

Hughes KS, Schnaper LA, Berry D, et al. Lumpectomy plus tamoxifen with or without irradiation in women 70 years of age or older with early breast cancer. N Engl J Med 2004;351:971–977.

Jaiyesimi IA, Buzdar AU, Hortobagyi GN, et al. Inflammatory breast cancer: a review. J Clin Oncol 1992;10:1014–1024.

Julien JP, Bijker N, Fentiman IS, et al. Radiotherapy in breast conserving treatment for ductal carcinoma in situ: first results of the EORTC randomized phase III trial 10853. Lancet 2000;353:528–533.

Katz A, Buchholz TA, Strom EA, et al. Recursive partitioning analysis of locoregional recurrence following mastectomy and doxorubicin-based chemotherapy: implications for postoperative irradiation. Int J Radiat Oncol Biol Phys 2001;50:397–403.

Katz A, Strom EA, Buchholz TA, et al. Locoregional recurrence patterns after mastectomy and doxorubicin-based chemotherapy:

implications for postoperative irradiation. J Clin Oncol 2000;18: 2817–2827.

Krag D, Weaver D, Ashikaga A, et al. The sentinel node in breast cancer. N Engl J Med 1998;339:941–946.

Kuerer HM, Newman LA, Smith TL, et al. Clinical course of breast cancer patients with complete pathological primary tumor and axillary lymph node response to doxorubicin-based neoadjuvant chemotherapy. J Clin Oncol 1999;14:460–469.

Meric F, Buchholz TA, Mirza NQ, et al. Long-term complications associated with breast-conservation surgery and radiotherapy. Ann Surg Oncol 2002;9:543–549.

Morrow M, Strom EA, Bassett LW, et al. Standard for breast conservation therapy in the management of breast carcinoma. CA Cancer J Clin 2002;52:277–230.

Olson JE, Neuberg D, Pandya KJ, et al. The role of radiotherapy in the management of operable locally advanced breast carcinoma. Cancer 1997;79:1138–1149.

Overgaard M, Hansen PS, Overgaard J, et al. Postoperative radiotherapy in high-risk premenopausal women with breast cancer who receive adjuvant chemotherapy. N Engl J Med 1997;337:949–955.

Overgaard M, Jensen MB, Overgaard J, et al. Postoperative radiotherapy In high-risk postmenopausal breast cancer patients given adjuvant tamoxifen: Danish Breast Cancer Cooperative Group DBCG 82c randomized trial. Lancet 1999;353:1641–1648.

Park CC, Mitsumori M, Nixon A, et al. Outcome at 8 years after breast-conserving surgery and radiation therapy for invasive breast cancer: influence of margin status and systemic therapy on local recurrence. J Clin Oncol 2000;18:1668–1675.

Piccart-Gebhart MJ, Procter M, Leyland-Jones B, et al. Trastuzumab after adjuvant chemotherapy in HER2-postive breast cancer. N Engl J Med 2005;353:1659–1672.

Ragaz J, Jackson SM, Le N, et al. Adjuvant radiotherapy and chemotherapy in node-positive premenopausal women with breast cancer. N Engl J Med 1997;337:956–962.

Ragaz J, Olivotto I, Spinelli J, et al. Locoregional radiation therapy in patients with high-risk breast cancer receiving adjuvant chemotherapy: 20-year results of the British Columbia randomized trial. J Natl Cancer Inst 2005;97:116–126.

Recht A, Come SE, Henderson IC, et al. The sequencing of chemotherapy and radiation therapy after conservative surgery for early-stage breast cancer. N Engl J Med 1996;334:1356–1361.

Recht A, Edge SB, Solin LJ, et al. Postmastectomy radiotherapy: guidelines of the American society of clinical oncology. J Clin Oncol 2001;19:1539–1569.

Recht A, Gray R, Davidson NE, et al. Locoregional failure 10 years after mastectomy and adjuvant chemotherapy with or without tamoxifen without irradiation: experience of the easten cooperative oncology group. J Clin Oncol 1999;17:1689–1700.

Romestaing P, Lehingue Y, Carrie C, et al. Role of a 10 Gy boost in the conservative treatment of early breast cancer: results of a randomized trial. J Clin Oncol 1997;15:963–968.

Romond EH, Perez EA, Bryant J, et al. Trastuzumab plus adjuvant chemotherapy for operable HER2-positive breast cancer. N Engl J Med 2005;353:1673–1684.

Shapiro CL, Recht A. Side effects of adjuvant treatment of breast cancer. N Engl J Med 2001;344:1997–2008.

Silverstein MJ, Lagios MD, Groshen S, et al. The influence of margin width on local control of ductal carcinoma in situ of the breast. N Engl J Med 1999;340:1455–1461.

Silverstein MJ. The University of Southern California/Van Nuys prognostic index for ductal carcinoma in situ of the breast. Am J Surg 2003;186:337–343.

Singletary SE, McNeese MD, Hortobagyi GN, et al. Feasibility of breast-conservation surgery after induction chemotherapy for locally advanced breast carcinoma. Cancer 1992;69:2849–2852.

Strom EA, McNeese MD. Postmastectomy irradiation: rationale for treatment field selection. Semin Radiat Oncol 1999;9:247–253.

The ATAC (Arimidex, Tamoxifen Alone or in Combination) Trialists Group. Anastrozole alone or in combination with tamoxifen versus tamoxifen alone for adjuvant treatment of postmenopausal women with early breast cancer: first results of the ATAC randomized trial. Lancet 2002;359:2131–2139.

UK Coordinating Committee on Cancer Research. Radiotherapy and tamoxifen in women with completely excised ductal carcinoma in situ of the breast in the UK, Australia, and New Zealand: randomized controlled trial. Lancet 2003;362:95–102.

Van Dongen JA, Voogd AC, Fentiman IS, Legrand C, et al. Long-term results of a randomized trial comparing breast-conserving therapy with mastectomy: European organization for research and treatment of cancer 10801 trial. J Natl Cancer Inst 2000;92:1143–1150.

Veronesi U, Cascinelli N, Mariani L, et al. Twenty-year follow-up of a randomized study comparing breast-conserving surgery with radical mastectomy for early stage breast cancer. N Engl J Med 2002;347:1227–1232.

Veronesi U, Luini A, Del Vecchio M, et al. Radiotherapy after breast-preserving surgery in women with localized cancer of the breast. N Engl J Med 1993;328:1587–1591.

Veronesi U, Marubini E, Marian L, et al. Radiotherapy after breast-conserving surgery in small breast carcinoma: long-term results of a randomized trial. Ann Oncol 2001;12:997–1003.

Veronesi U, Saccozzi R, Del Vecchio M, et al. Comparing radical mastectomy with quadrantectomy, axillary dissection, and radiotherapy in patients with small cancers of the breast. N Engl J Med 1981;305:6–11.

Veronesi U, Salvadori, Luini A, et al. Breast conservation is a safe method in patients with small cancer of the breast: long-term results of three randomized trials on 1973 patients. Eur J Cancer 1995;31:1574–1599.

Veronesi U, Zucali R, Luini A. Local control and survival in early breast cancer: the Milan Trial. Int J Radiat Oncol Bio Phys 1986;12: 717–720.

Vicini FA, Kestin L, Chen P, et al. Limited-field radiation therapy in the management of early stage breast cancer. J Natl Cancer Inst 2003;95:1205–1211.

Whelan TJ, Julian J, Wright J, et al. Does locoregional radiation therapy improve survival in breast cancer? A meta-analysis. J Clin Oncol 2000;18:1220–1229.

Wong JS, Kaelin CM, Troyan SL, et al. Prospective study of wide excision alone for ductal carcinoma in situ of the breast. J Clin Oncol 2006;24:1031–1036.

Wong JS, Recht A, Beard CJ, et al. Treatment outcome after tangential radiation therapy without axillary dissection in patients with early-stage breast cancer and clinically negative axillary lymph nodes. Int J Radiat Oncol Biol Phys 1997;39:915–920.

NOTES

Chapter 17
Esophageal Cancer

Charlotte Y. Dai

PEARLS

- Esophageal cancer accounts for 5% of all GI cancers. There are 13,900 new cases & 13,000 deaths from esophageal cancer each year in the U.S. It is the 6th leading cause of death from cancer worldwide
- Incidence increases with age, peaks at 6th to 7th decade
- Male:female = 2.7:1
- African-American males:white males = 5:1
- Most common in China, Iran, South Africa, and the former Soviet Union
- Risk factors: tobacoo, EtOH, nitrosamines, Tylosis (congenital hyperkeratosis), Plummer Vinson syndrome, achalasia, GERD, and Barrett's esophagus
- Four regions of the esophagus: cervical = cricoid cartilage to thoracic inlet (18 cm from the incisor); upper thoracic = thoracic inlet to tracheal bifurcation (18–24 cm); Mid thoracic = tracheal bifurcation to just above the GE junction (24–32 cm); lower thoracic = includes GE junction (32–40 cm)
- Barrett's esophagus: metaplasia of the esophageal epithelial lining. The squamous epithelium is replaced by columnar epithelium, with 0.5% annual rate of neoplastic transformation
- Adenocarcinoma: rapid rise in incidence. Comprises 60–80% of all new cases compared to 10–15% 10 years ago. Predominately white men. Associated with Barrett's, GERD, & hiatal hernia. Locations: 75% in the distal esophagus & 25% in the upper and mid esophagus

Special acknowledgement: We thank Richard M. Krieg, M.D. for his valuable advice in the preparation of this chapter.

■ Squamous cell carcinoma: Associated with tobacco, alcohol, or prior history of H&N cancers. Locations: 50% mid esophagus, 50% distal esophagus

WORKUP

■ H&P: dysphagia, odynophagia, cough, hoarseness (laryngeal nerve involvement), weight loss, use of EtOH, tobacco, nitrosamines, history of GERD. Examine for cervical or supraclavicular adenopathy
■ Labs: CBC, chemistries, LFTs
■ EGD: allow direct visualization and biopsy
■ EUS: assess the depth of penetration & LN involvement. Limited by the degree of obstruction
■ Barium swallow: can delineate proximal and distal margins
■ CT chest & abdomen: assess adenopathy and metastasis
■ PET scan: can detect up to 15–20% of metatases not seen on CT and EUS
■ Bronchoscopy: rule-out fistula in mid-esophageal lesions
■ Bone scan: recommended if elevated alkaline phosphatase or bone pain
■ Nutritional assessment

STAGING

Primary Tumor (T)
TX: Primary tumor cannot be assessed
T0: No evidence of primary tumor
Tis: Carcinoma *in situ*
T1: Tumor invades lamina propria or submucosa
T2: Tumor invades muscularis propria
T3: Tumor invades adventitia
T4: Tumor invades adjacent structures

Regional Lymph Nodes (N)
NX: Regional lymph node metastasis cannot be assessed
N0: No regional lymph node metastasis
N1: Regional lymph node metastasis

Distant metastasis (M)
MX: Distant metastasis cannot be assessed
M0: No distant metastasis
M1: Distant metastasis

Tumors of the lower thoracic esophagus:
M1a: Metastasis in celiac lymph nodes
M1b: Other distant metastasis

Tumors of the midthoracic esophagus:
M1a: Not applicable
M1b: Nonregional lymph nodes and/or other distant metastasis

Tumors of the upper thoracic esophagus:
M1a: Metastasis in cervical nodes
M1b: Other distant metastasis

Stage Grouping		~3 yr OS by Stage	
0:	TisN0M0	I:	70–100%
I:	T1N0M0	II:	65–100%
IIA:	T2N0M0, T3N0M0	III:	60–90%
IIB:	T1N1M0, T2N1M0	IV:	50–70%
III:	T3N1M0, T4 Any N M0		
IV:	Any T, Any N, M1		
IVA:	Any T, Any N, M1a		
IVB:	Any T, Any N, M1b		

Used with the permission of the American Joint Committee on Cancer (AJCC), Chicago, Illinois. The original source for this material is the AJCC Cancer Staging Manual, Sixth Edition (2002) published by Springer-Verlag New York, www.springeronline.com.

SURGICAL TECHNIQUES

- Transhiatal esophagectomy: for tumors anywhere in esophagus or gastric cardia. No thoracotomy. Blunt dissection of the thoracic esophagus. Left with cervical anastomosis. Limitations are lack of exposure of mid-esophagus & direct visualization and dissection of the subcarinal LN cannot be performed
- Right thoracotomy (Ivor-Lewis procedure): good for exposure of mid to upper esophageal lesions. Left with thoracic or cervical anastomosis
- Left thoracotomy: appropriate for lower third of esophagus and gastric cardia. Left with low to mid-thoracic anastomosis
- Radical (en block) resection: for tumor anywhere in esophagus or gastric cardia. Left with cervical or thoracic anastomosis. Benefit is more extensive lymphadenectomy & potentially better survival, but increased operative risk

TREATMENT RECOMMENDATIONS

Stage I-III Resectable Medically-fit	Surgery (with post-op RT for close/+ margins) Or, pre-op chemo-RT (5-FU+cisplatin, 50 Gy) → surgery [Walsh, Bossett, Urba] Or, definitive chemo-RT (5-FU+cisplatin, 50 Gy) [RTOG 85-01, RTOG 94-05, INT0123]. Chemo-RT is preferred for cervical esophagus lesions
Stage I-III Inoperable	Definitive chemo-RT (5-FU+cisplatin, 50 Gy) [RTOG 85-01, RTOG 94-05, INT0123]
Stage IV Palliative	Concurrent chemo-RT (5-FU+cisplatin, 50 Gy) or RT alone (2.5 Gy ×14 fx) or chemo alone or best supportive care Obstruction: stenting, laser, RT, chemo, or dilatation Pain: medications ± RT Bleeding: endoscopic therapy, surgery, or RT

STUDIES
Surgery alone
- 3 yr OS 6–35% (~20%). See control arms in Kelsen, Medical Research Council, and EORTC trials below

RT alone
- 3 yr OS 0%. See control arm in RTOG 85-01

Pre-op & post-op RT
- 5 randomized trials of pre-op RT vs surgery alone demonstrate no difference in LF and OS
- Phase III data from outside the U.S. demonstrates decreased LF but no difference in OS or DM with post-op RT

Pre-op chemo
- Kelsen (*NEJM* 1998). Phase III. 467 pts with resectable T1-2N×M0 SCC and adenocarcinoma randomized to surgery alone vs pre-op chemo ×3c (cisplatin, 5-FU) → surgery. Pre-op chemo did not improve MS (16 mo vs

15 mo) or OS at 4 yrs (26% vs 23%). 12% cCR and 2.5% pCR. No difference between histologies

- <u>Medical Research Council</u> (*Lancet* 2002). Phase III. 802 pts with resectable SCC and adenocarcinoma randomized to surgery alone vs preop chemo ×2c (5-FU, cisplatin) → surgery. 9% of patients from each arm received pre-op RT. Pre-op chemo improved 2 yr OS (34 → 43%) and complete resection rate (54 → 60%)

Pre-op chemo-RT

- <u>Walsh</u> (*NEJM* 1996). Phase III. 113 pts, adenocarcinoma only, randomized to surgery alone vs pre-op chemo-RT → surgery. RT was 40 Gy/15 fx. Chemo was 5-FU and cisplatin ×2c. Pre-op chemo-RT improved OS at 1 and 3 yrs (52/32% vs 44/6%) & MS (16 mo vs 11 mo). 25% pCR rate in chemo-RT arm. Caveats: small pt #, adenocarcinoma only, poor outcome of surgery alone arm, non-US fractionation, and short f/u (only 11 mo)
- <u>EORTC</u> (Bossett, *NEJM* 1997). Phase III. 282 pts, T1-3N0 & T1-2N1M0, SCC only, randomized to surgery alone vs pre-op chemo-RT → surgery. Chemo was cisplatin ×2c. RT was 37/10 fx in two one-wk courses separated by 2 wks. Surgery was one-stage en bloc esophagectomy and proximal gastrectomy. pCR 26%. No difference in OS and MS (18.6 mo). Pre-op chemo-RT improved DFS (p = 0.003), had a higher rate of curative resection (p = 0.017), a lower rate of death from cancer (p = 0.002), and a higher rate of post-op death (p = 0.012)
- Caveats: split course RT, non-US fractionation, no 5-FU
- <u>Urba</u> (*JCO* 2001). Phase III. 100 pts, localized CA, 75% adenocarcinoma, 25% SCC randomized to pre-op chemo-RT → surgery vs surgery alone. Chemo was cisplatin, vinblastine, and 5-FU. RT was 1.5 Gy bid to 45 Gy. Surgery was transhiatal esophagectomy. Pre-op chemo-RT significantly decreased LR (19 vs 42%). Improved 3 yr OS (30 vs 15%) did not reach statistical significance
- <u>Bates</u> (*JCO* 1996). Phase II. 35 pts, localized CA, 80% SCC, 20% adenocarcinoma treated with pre-op chemo-RT → surgery. Chemo was 5-FU + cisplatin. RT was 1.8/45 Gy. Surgery was Ivor-Lewis esophagectomy. pCR 51%, DFS 32.8 mo, MS 25.8 mo (all pts) with 36.8 mo for pCR & 12.9 mo for no pCR. 41% pts with negative pathology from post-chemo-RT, pre-resection EGD had residual tumor at

surgery indicating that pre-resection EGD not reliable for detecting residual disease

Definitive chemo-RT

▪ RTOG 85-01 (Herskovic, *NEJM* 1992; Al-Sarraf, *JCO* 1997; Cooper, *JAMA* 1999). Phase III. 121 pts, T1-3N0-1M0, adenocarcinoma and SCC, rand omized to RT alone vs chemo-RT. Chemo was 5-FU & cisplatin on wks 1, 5, 8, 11. RT alone arm was 50 Gy + 14 Gy boost at 2 Gy/fx. Concurrent chemo-RT dose was 50 Gy. Interim analysis showed improved OS with chemo-RT. Additional 69 pts were treated according to the chemo-RT protocol and followed prospectively. 5 yr OS for RT alone was 0%, for chemo-RT (randomized) 26%, & for chemo-RT (non-randomized) 14%. No differences in OS based on histology

▪ RTOG 94-05, INT0123 (Minsky, *JCO* 2002). Phase III. 236 pts, T1-4N0-1M0, SCC and adenocarcinoma, rand-omized to chemo-RT to 50 Gy vs chemo-RT to 65 Gy. Chemo was 5-FU + cisplatin ×4c. Trial was stopped after an interim analysis. High-dose arm had higher treatment-related death (10 vs 2%). Of the 11 deaths in high dose arm, 7 occurred at ≤50.4 Gy. No differences in MS (13 vs 18 mo), 2 yr OS (31 vs 40%) or LF (56 vs 52%)

Chemo-RT with and without surgery in high risk pts

▪ Stahl (*JCO* 2005). Phase III. 172 pts, T3-4N0-1M0, SCC, treated with chemo × 3c & then randomized to chemo-RT (2/40 Gy) → surgery (arm 1) vs definitive chemo-RT (64–65 Gy, arm 2). Chemo was 5-FU, leucovorin, etopo-side, & cisplatin when given alone, and cisplatin/etopo-side when given with RT. RT in arm 2 was 2/50 Gy + 1.5 Gy bid/15 Gy boost (total 65 Gy) or 2/60 Gy + 4 Gy HDR boost (total 64 Gy). 66% of pts in arm 1 & 88% of pts in arm 2 completed treatment. pCR was 35% at surgery. No difference in MS (16 mo vs 15 mo) or 3 yr OS (31% vs 24%). Surgery improved 2 yr freedom from local progression (64% vs 41%), but definitive chemo-RT had less treatment-related mortality (13% vs 4%) & preserved the esophagus. Pts with response to induction chemo had improved prognosis regardless of treatment group (3 yr OS ~50%)

Brachytherapy

- <u>RTOG 9207 PhaseI/II</u> (Gaspar, *Cancer* 2000). 49 pts T1-2N0-1M0, 92% SCC, 8% adenocarcinoma treated with concurrent chemo (5-FU, cisplatin) + RT (EBRT 50 Gy/25 fx + HDR 5 Gy ×3 or LDR 20 Gy ×1). 24% Grade 4 toxicity, 12% fistula, 10% treatment related deaths with MS 11 mo. Brachytherapy not recommended due to high toxicity

RTOG trials

- <u>RTOG 0246</u>. Phase II study of resectable locoregionally advanced CA treated with induction chemo (5-FU, cisplatin, paclitaxel) → chemo-RT (50 Gy, 5-FU, cisplatin) → salvage surgery. Trial closed 3/17/2006. Result pending
- <u>RTOG 0113</u>. Randomized phase II study of inoperable local-regional esophageal CA treated with 5-FU based vs non-5-FU based induction chemo → chemo-RT. Trial closed 4/2005. Result pending

RADIATION TECHNIQUES
General principles

- Simulate patient supine with arms up so that lateral fiducials are possible
- Immobilize with wing board or alpha cradle with arms above head
- Use esophatrast to outline the esophagus and barium (2%, ReadiCat) to outline the stomach and small bowel
- Target volume: 5 cm proximal and distal margins beyond primary tumor, 2.5 cm radial margin, and regional nodes

Field design

- AP/PA fields deliver higher dose to the heart & lower dose to the lungs, whereas obliques & laterals deliver higher dose to the lungs & lower dose to the heart
- At UCSF, we consider using a 3DCRT plan throughout treatment so that normal tissues such as the lungs receive a lower total integral dose. We generally weight AP/PA > obliques
- Wedges and/or compensators may be needed
- Tumors above the carina: treat SCV and mediastinal LN
- Two options for field design:
  - SCV and primary tumor treated in one field. Consider AP 6 MV and PA 18 MV with off cord boost to primary

(after cord dose reaches 45 Gy). This technique might not be suitable if tumor volume includes excessive heart
- SCV field matched to primary tumor fields. Isocenter is placed at the matchline. SCV field is AP 6 MV to 50 Gy with half-beam block at clavicle and block placed over spinal cord. Primary tumor fields are beam-split from above and use AP/PA & obliques. AP/PA fields are weighted >> obliques and laterals
- Tumors at or below the carina: treat mediastinal LN, & include celiac LN for lower 1/3 and gastroesophageal junction tumors
  - Use a multi-field technique including AP/PA and obliques or laterals. Weigh AP/PA >> obliques and laterals

Dose prescriptions
- 1.8 Gy/fx to 50.4 Gy
- If the stomach is in the field, consider reducing lower border to block stomach at 45 Gy if clinically possible

Dose limitations
- Spinal cord ≤45 Gy at 1.8 Gy/fx
- Lung: limit 70% of both lungs <20 Gy
- Heart: limit 50% of ventricles <25 Gy

COMPLICATIONS
- Acute side effects: esophagitis, weight loss, fatigue, and anorexia
- Esophageal perforation may present with substernal chest pain, increased heart rate, fever, and hemorrhage
- Pneumonitis: subacute, occurs ~26 wks after RT. Presents with cough, dyspnea, hypoxia, & fever. Depending on severity, treat with NSAIDs or steroids
- Late strictures possible, half are due to LR. For benign strictures dilation results in palliation in the majority of patients. For malignant strictures, dilation does not work as well
- Pericarditis, coronary artery disease
- With brachytherapy and/or EBRT, tumor involvement of the trachea can lead to fistula formation during RT (5 to 10%), secondary to tumor necrosis or natural progression of the disease

FOLLOW-UP

- H&P every 4 mo for 1 yr, then every 6 mo for 2 yrs, then annually thereafter. CBC, metabolic panel, CXR, endoscopy, CT chest, and PET should be considered when clinically indicated
- For locally advanced esophageal cancers undergoing combined chemo-RT, metabolic response as determined by FDG-PET imaging before and after treatment is a strong predictor of OS (MS 6–7 mo for non-PET responders vs 16–23 mo for PET responders)

REFERENCES

al-Sarraf M, Martz K, Herskovic A, et al. Progress report of combined chemoradiotherapy versus radiotherapy alone in patients with esophageal cancer: an intergroup study. J Clin Oncol 1997;15: 277–284.

Bates BA, Detterbeck FC, Bernard SA, et al. Concurrent radiation therapy and chemotherapy followed by esophagectomy for localized esophageal carcinoma. J Clin Oncol 1996;14:156–163.

Bosset JF, Gignoux M, Triboulet JP, et al. Chemoradiotherapy followed by surgery compared with surgery alone in squamous-cell cancer of the esophagus. N Engl J Med 1997;337:161–167.

Cooper JS, Guo MD, Herskovic A, et al. Chemoradiotherapy of locally advanced esophageal cancer: long-term follow-up of a prospective randomized trial (RTOG 85-01). Radiation Therapy Oncology Group. JAMA 1999;281:1623–1627.

DiNittis AS. Esophagus. In: Perez CA, Brady LW, Halperin EC, et al., editors. Principles and Practice of Radiation Oncology. 4th ed. Lippincott Williams and Wilkins; 2004. pp. 1282–1304.

Downey RJ, Akhurst T, Ilson D, et al. Whole body 18FDG-PET and the response of esophageal cancer to induction therapy: results of a prospective trial. J Clin Oncol 2003;21:428–432.

Enzinger PC, Mayer RJ. Esophageal cancer. N Engl J Med 2003;349: 2241–2252.

Gaspar LE, Winter K, Kocha WI, et al. A phase I/II study of external beam radiation, brachytherapy, and concurrent chemotherapy for patients with localized carcinoma of the esophagus (Radiation Therapy Oncology Group Study 9207): final report. *Cancer* 2000;88:988–995.

Herskovic A, Martz K, al-Sarraf M, et al. Combined chemotherapy and radiotherapy compared with radiotherapy alone in patients with cancer of the esophagus. N Engl J Med 1992;326:1593–1598.

Kelsen DP, Ginsberg R, Pajak TF, et al. Chemotherapy followed by surgery compared with surgery alone for localized esophageal cancer. N Engl J Med 1998;339:1979–1984.

Minsky BD. Cancer of the esophagus. In: Textbook of Radiation Oncology. 2nd ed. Saunders; 2004. pp. 811–824.

Minsky BD, Pajak TF, Ginsberg RJ, et al. INT 0123 (Radiation Therapy Oncology Group 94-05) phase III trial of combined-modality therapy for esophageal cancer: high-dose versus standard-dose radiation therapy. J Clin Oncol 2002;20:1167–1174.

National Comprehensive Cancer Network. Clinical Practice Guidelines in Oncology: Esophageal Cancer. Available at: http://www.nccn.org/ professionals/physician_gls/PDF/esophageal.pdf. Accessed on May 10, 2005, 2005.

Stahl M, Stuschke M, Lehmann N, et al. Chemoradiation with and without surgery in patients with locally advanced squamous cell carcinoma of the esophagus. J Clin Oncol 2005;23:2310–2317.

Surgical resection with or without preoperative chemotherapy in oesophageal cancer: a randomised controlled trial. Lancet 2002;359: 1727–1733.

Walsh TN, Noonan N, Hollywood D, et al. A comparison of multimodal therapy and surgery for esophageal adenocarcinoma. N Engl J Med 1996;335:462–467.

Wieder HA, Brucher BL, Zimmermann F, et al. Time course of tumor metabolic activity during chemoradiotherapy of esophageal squamous cell carcinoma and response to treatment. J Clin Oncol 2004;22:900–908.

NOTES

Chapter 18
Gastric Cancer

Charlotte Y. Dai

PEARLS

- 22,710 new cases and 11,780 deaths from gastric cancer each year in the U.S.
- Highest death rates are reported in Chile, Costa Rica, Japan, China, and the former Soviet Union
- Median age of diagnosis is 65
- Male:female = 1.5:1
- Etiology and possible risk factors: low fruits & vegetables, high salts & nitrates, salted fish, smoked meats, *H. pylori*, hypochlorohydria, polyps, genetic alterations (p53 mutation, microsatellite instability gene MSI, E-cadherin gene), previous radiation, gastrectomy, pernicious anemia
- Tumor location
  - GE junction, cardia and fundus 35% (diffuse subtype, incidence rising)
  - Body 25%
  - Antrum and distal stomach 40% (intestinal subtype, incidence falling)
- Histology: 90% adenocarcinoma. Others = sarcoma, carcinoid, small-cell, undifferentiated, MALT lymphoma, leiomyosarcoma
- Intestinal subtype: more commonly seen in patients >40 yrs, less aggressive
- Diffuse subtype: affects younger patients, more aggressive
- Borrmann's types:
  - I: polypoid
  - II: ulcerating
  - III: infiltrating and ulcerating
  - IV: infiltrating (linitis plastica)
  - Types I & II have better prognosis than III & IV

Special acknowledgement: We thank Richard M. Krieg, M.D. for his valuable advice in the preparation of this chapter.

219

- Krukenberg tumor = ovarian met
- Sitster Mary Joseph node = peri-umbilical node
- Virchow's node = left SCV
- Irish's node = axillary lymphadenopathy
- Blumer's shelf = metastatic tumor in the pelvic cul-de-sac, frequently palpable on rectal exam

WORKUP

- H&P: dysphagia, indigestion, early satiety, loss of appetite, nausea, abdominal pain, wt loss, obstruction (pyloric lesion), anemia, hematemesis (10–15%), melena. Check for cervical, axillary, SCV, & periumbilical adenopathy
- Labs: CBC, liver and renal function tests, CEA (elevated in 1/3 of cases)
- EGD: allows direct visualization and biopsy
- EUS: assesses the depth of penetration and LN involvement, but study is limited by the degree of obstruction
- CT abdomen: assesses adenopathy and metastasis
- CT or US of the pelvis in women in selected cases
- CXR, CT chest for gastroesophageal junction tumors to rule-out mediastinal LN
- PET scan: may be useful, not routinely done
- Bone scan: recommended if elevated alkaline phosphatase or bone pain
- Laparoscopy: performed prior to open laparotomy to assess extent of disease, peritoneal implants and resectability. Should be performed if pre-op chemo-RT is being considered

STAGING

Primary Tumor (T)	
TX:	Primary tumor cannot be assessed
T0:	No evidence of primary tumor
Tis:	Carcinoma *in situ*: intraepithelial tumor without invasion of the lamina propria
T1:	Tumor invades lamina propria or submucosa
T2:	Tumor invades muscularis propria or subserosa*
:	T2a: Tumor invades muscularis propria
:	T2b: Tumor invades subserosa
T3:	Tumor penetrates serosa (visceral peritoneum) without invasion of adjacent structures**,***
T4:	Tumor invades adjacent structures**,***

Note: A tumor may penetrate the muscularis propria with extension into the gastrocolic or gastrohepatic ligaments, or into the greater or lesser omentum, without perforation of the visceral peritoneum covering these structures. In this case, the tumor is classified T2. If there is perforation of the visceral peritoneum covering the gastric ligaments or the omentum, the tumor should be classified T3.

**Note*: The adjacent structures of the stomach include the spleen, transverse colon, liver, diaphragm, pancreas, abdominal wall, adrenal gland, kidney, small intestine and retroperitoneum

***Note*: Intramural extension to the duodenum or esophagus is classified by the depth of the greatest invasion in any of these sites, including the stomach

Regional Lymph Nodes (N)

NX: Regional lymph node(s) cannot be assessed
N0:   No regional lymph node metastasis*
N1:   Metastasis in 1 to 6 regional lymph nodes
N2:   Metastasis in 7 to 15 regional lymph nodes
N3:   Metastasis in more than 15 regional lymph nodes

Note: A designation of pN0 should be used if all examined lymph nodes are negative, regardless of the total number removed and examined.

Distant Metastasis (M)

MX: Distant metastasis cannot be assessed
M0:   No distant metastasis
M1:   Distant metastasis

Stage Grouping		~3 yr OS by Stage	
0:	TisN0M0	I:	70–100%
IA::	T1N0M0	II:	65–100%
IB::	T1N1M0	III:	60–90%
II::	T1N2M0	IV:	50–70%
	T2a/bN1M0		
	T3N0M0		
IIIA:	T2a/bN2M0		
	T3N1M0		
	T4N0M0		
IIIB:	T3N2M0		
IV:	T4N1-3M0		
	T1-3N3M0		
	Any T, any N, M1		

Used with the permission of the American Joint Committee on Cancer (AJCC), Chicago, Illinois. The original source for this material is the AJCC Cancer Staging Manual, Sixth Edition (2002) published by Springer-Verlag New York, www.springeronline.com.

SURGERY

- General guidelines:
  - For distal (body & antrum): prefer subtotal gastrectomy
  - For proximal (cardia): total or proximal gastrectomy
  - Avoid splenectomy if possible
  - Consider placing feeding jejunostomy-tube
  - ≥5 cm proximal and distal margins whenever possible
  - Remove minimum of 15 LNs
- D1 dissection: includes those lymph nodes adjacent to the stomach
- D2 dissection: also removes those lymph nodes around the celiac axis
- Billroth I = end to end gastrojejunal anastomosis, gastric resection margin used for anastomosis.
- Billroth II = end to side gastrojejunal anastomosis, closure of the duodenal stump and the lesser curvature of the stomach. Gastric resection margin is usually NOT used for anastomosis

TREATMENT RECOMMENDATIONS

Stage	Recommended Treatment
IA IB (T2N0) without extension beyond muscularis propria	Surgery alone
IB (T1N1 or T2N0 with extension beyond muscularis propria)-IV M0 Resectable and operable	Surgery → post-op chemo × 1c → concurrent chemo × 2c + RT (45 Gy) →chemo × 2c [INT 0116]. Chemo = 5-FU + leucovorin
I–IV M0 Unresectable or inoperable	Concurrent chemo-RT (5-FU + 45 Gy) Or, chemo alone (5-FU, cisplatin, oxaliplatin taxane, or irinotecan-based) if patient not RT candidate Or, best supportive care for poor KPS RT alone may provide some palliation, but no survival benefit

Stage	Recommended Treatment
M1	Palliative chemo ± RT (5-FU + 45 Gy). 50–75% pts experience improvement of symptoms such as gastric outlet obstruction, pain, bleeding, or biliary obstruction. Duration of palliation 4–18 mo. Alternatively, palliative surgery

STUDIES

Extent of gastrectomy

■ Gouzi (*Ann Surg* 1989). Distal gastric CA randomized to subtotal vs total gastrectomy. Both arms had similar mobidity (33%), mortality (1.3 vs 3.2%) & 5 yr OS (48%)

Extent of lymphadenectomy

■ Dutch trial (*NEJM* 1999, *JCO* 2004). 711 pts with resectable gastric CA randomized to D1 vs D2 lymph node dissection. D2 dissection led to a significantly higher rate of complications (43% vs 25%, p < 0.001), more post-op deaths (10% vs 4%, p = 0.004), & longer hospital stay (16 d vs 14 d). Similar 11 yr OS (35% vs 30%, p = 0.53) and rate of relapse

■ Japanese trial (*JCO* 2004). 523 pts with resectable gastric CA randomized to standard D2 vs D2 + para-aortic nodal dissection. Overall morbidity was slightly higher in the extended surgery group than the standard surgery group (28.1% vs 20.9%, p = 0.067). There was no difference in the incidence of major complications including anastomotic leak, pancreatic fistula, abdominal abscess, and pneumonia

Pre-op chemo-RT

■ No phase III data

■ Ajani (*JCO* 2004). Phase II study. 34 operable pts with localized gastric CA treated with pre-op chemo × 2c (5-FU/cisplatin/leucovorin) → concurrent chemo (infusional 5-FU) + RT 45 Gy → surgery. 70% R0 resection rate, 30% pCR rate, 24% PR rate, MS 33.7 mo for all pts (63.9 mo for pCR and PR pts)

■ RTOG 9904. Phase II study of pre-op chemo (5-FU/cisplatin/leucovorin) and chemo-RT (5-FU infusion) for potentially resectable adenocarcinoma of the stomach (closed 3/2004)

Post-op chemo-RT

- INT0116/SWOG 9008 (*NEJM* 2001, ASCO abstr., 2004). 556 pts with resected stage IB-IV M0 stomach and gastro-esophageal junction tumors (20%) randomized to observation vs post-op chemo × 1c → concurrent chemo ×2c + RT → chemo × 2c. 54% had D0 dissection & 10% had D2 dissection. Chemo was 5-FU (425 mg/m^2/d, reduced to 400 mg/m^2/d with RT) + leucovorin (20 mg/m^2/d) × 5 days. RT was 45 Gy/25 fx to tumor bed, regional nodes, & 2 cm proximal and distal margin. Median f/u 7.4 yrs. Post-op chemo-RT improved MS (35 vs 26 mo, p = 0.006), DFS (30 vs 19 mo, p < 0.001), & 3 yr OS (50 vs 41%). No difference in DM. 41% grade 3 & 30% grade 4 toxicity in the chemo-RT arm

RADIATION TECHNIQUES
Simulation and field design

- Ensure adequate nutrition prior to radiation. Arrange for a nutrition consult. Recommend at least 1500 Cal/d
- Pt may require feeding tube (preferable if placed at the time of surgery)
- Pt instructed to fast for 3 hrs before simulation & all treatments
- Simulate patient supine with arms up so that lateral fiducials are possible
- Immobilize with wing board or alpha cradle with arms above head
- Use pre-op CT, post-op CT & surgical clips to guide target definition
- Celiac axis is located at approximately T12-L1
- Porta hepatis LN are covered by a field that extends 2 cm to the right of T11-L1
- At UCSF, we use a 3DCRT plan throughout the treatment to help reduce dose to normal tissues such as small bowel, spinal cord, liver, and kidneys
- General target volume: initial tumor bed, remaining stomach (especially for margins <5 cm), adjacent structures (see tables below), anastomotic site, and regional nodes for node positive patients
- Most 3DCRT plans include 3 to 4 fields

- The following are guidelines for target volume definition depending on the site of involvement: (adapted from Tepper, JE, Gunderson, LL. Radiation treatment parameters in the adjuvant postoperative therapy of gastric cancer. Semin Radiat Oncol 2002;12;187–195. Copyright 2002, with permission from Elsevier):

GE junction tumors

Site/Stage	Remaining Stomach	Tumor Bed	Nodes
T2b-3N0	Optional if margin > 5 cm	Medial left hemi-diaphragm, adjacent body of pancreas	None or peri-gastric, peri- esophageal Optional* for T3: mediastinal or celiac
T4N0	Preferable, but optional if margin > 5 cm	As for T3N0 plus sites of adherence with 3–5 cm margin	Nodes related to sites of adherence, +/– peri-gastric, peri-esophageal, mediastinal, celiac
T1-2N+	Preferable	Not indicated for T1 As above for T2b	Peri-esophageal, mediastinal, proximal peri-gastric, celiac
T3-4N+	Preferable	As for T3-4N0	As for T1-2N+ and T4N0

*Optional nodes may be excluded for T2-3N0 if D1 + D2 resection & 10–15 LN have been pathologically examined. Reprinted from *Seminars in Radiation Oncology*,Vol. 12, Tepper JE, Gunderson LL. Radiation treatment paraments in the adjuvant postoperative therapy of gastric cancer, 187–195, 2002, with permission from Elsevier.

Cardia/proximal 1/3 of the stomach tumors

Site/Stage	Remaining Stomach	Tumor Bed	Nodes
T2b-3N0	Optional if margin <5 cm	Medial left hemi-diaphragm, adjacent body of pancreas (+/– tail)	None or perigastric Optional* for T3: peri-esophageal, mediastinal, celiac
T4N0	Preferable, but optional if margin >5 cm	As for T3N0, plus sites of adherence with 3–5 cm margin	Nodes related to sites of adherence, +/– peri-gastric, celiac, peri-esophageal, mediastinal**

Site/Stage	Remaining Stomach	Tumor Bed	Nodes
T1-2N+	Preferable	Not indicated for T1 As above for T2b	Peri-gastric, celiac, splenic, supra-pancreatic, +/− peri- esophageal, pancreacto-duodenal, porta hepatis, mediastinal**
T3-4N+	Preferable	As for T3-4N0	As for T1-2N+ and T4N0

*Optional nodes may be excluded for T2-3N0 if D1 + D2 resection and 10–15 LN have been pathologically examined.

**Pancreatico-duodenal and porta-hepatis LN are at minimal risk if nodal positivity is minimal (i.e., if only 1–2 LN+ & 10–15 LN have been examined, these sites do not need to be irradiated). If there is esophageal extension, peri-esophageal and mediastinal nodes are at risk and should be included.

Reprinted from *Seminars in Radiation Oncology*, Vol. 12, Tepper JE, Gunderson LL, Radiation treatment paramenters in the adjuvant postoperative therapy of gastric cancer, 187–195, 2002, with permission from Elsevier.

Body/middle 1/3 of the stomach tumors

Site/Stage	Remaining Stomach	Tumor Bed	Nodes
T2b-3N0	Yes	Body of pancreas (+/− tail)	None or peri-gastric, optional*: celiac, splenic, supra-pancreatic, pancreato-duodenal, porta-hepatis
T4N0	Yes	Body of pancreas (+/− tail), plus sites of adherence with 3–5 cm margin	Nodes related to sites of adherence, +/− peri-gastric, celiac, supra-pancreatic, splenic, pancreato-duodenal, porta-hepatis
T1-2N+	Yes	Not indicated for T1 As above for T2b	Peri-gastric, celiac, supra-pancreatic, splenic, pancreato-duodenal, porta-hepatis. Optional: splenic hilum

Site/Stage	Remaining Stomach	Tumor Bed	Nodes
T3-4N+	Yes	As for T3-4N0	As for T1-2N+ and T4N0

*Optional nodes may be excluded for T2-3N0 if D1 + D2 resection and 10–15 LN have been pathologically examined. Reprinted from *Seminars in Radiation Oncology*, Vol. 12, Tepper JE, Gunderson LL, Radiation treatment parameters in the adjuvant postoperative therapy of gastric cancer, 187–195, 2002, with permission from Elsevier.

Antrum/pylorus/distal 1/3 of the stomach tumors

Site/Stage	Remaining Stomach	Tumor Bed	Nodes
T2b-3N0	Optional if margin >5 cm	Head of pancreas (+/− body), 1st and 2nd part of the duodenum	None or peri-gastric. Optional*: pancreato-duodenal, porta hepatis, celiac, supra-pancreatic
T4N0	Preferable, but optional if margin >5 cm	Head of pancreas (+/− body), 1st and 2nd part of the duodenum, sites of adherence with 3–5 cm-margin	Nodes related to sites of adherence, +/− peri-gastric, pancreato-duodenal, porta hepatis, celiac, supra-pancreatic
T1–2N+	Preferable	Not indicated for T1 As above for T2b	Peri-gastric, pancreato-duodenal, porta-hepatis, celiac, supra-pancreatic. Optional*: splenic hilum
T3-4N+	Preferable	As for T3-4N0	As for T1-2N+ and T4N0

*Optional nodes may be excluded for T3N0 and T1-2N+ if D1 + D2 dissection with 10–15 LNs have been pathologically examined and 0–2 nodes positive. Reprinted from *Seminars in Radiation Oncology*, Vol. 12, Tepper JE, Gunderson LL, Radiation treatment parameters in the adjuvant postoperative therapy of gastric cancer, 187–195, 2002, with permission from Elsevier.

Dose prescriptions
- 1.8 Gy/fx to 45 Gy

Dose limitations
- Spinal cord ≤45 Gy in 1.8 Gy fractions
- Heart: 50% of ventricles <25 Gy
- Liver: 70% of volume <30 Gy
- Kidneys: 2/3 of each kidney <20 Gy

COMPLICATIONS
- Acute complications include nausea, anorexia, fatigue, and myelosuppression with chemo
- For severe nausea, recommend Ondansetron 8 mg 1 hr before and 3 hrs after RT daily
- 25% of patients have persistent decrease in acid production for >1–5 yrs
- Late complications: dyspepsia, radiation gastritis, and gastric ulcers
- Gastric late effects are rare with 40–52 Gy. Incidence of late effects rises with higher doses

FOLLOW-UP
- H&P every 4 mo for 1st yr, then every 6 mo for 2 yrs, then annually thereafter. CBC, metabolic panel, endoscopies, CT as clinically indicated
- Long term parenteral Vitamin B12 supplementation for all patients who undergo proximal or total gastrectomy

REFERENCES
Ajani JA, Mansfield PF, Janjan N, et al. Multi-institutional trial of pre-operative chemoradiotherapy in patients with potentially resectable gastric carcinoma. *J Clin Oncol* 2004;22:2774–2780.

Hartgrink HH, van de Velde CJ, Putter H, et al. Extended lymph node dissection for gastric cancer: who may benefit? Final results of the randomized Dutch gastric cancer group trial. *J Clin Oncol* 2004;22:2069–2077.

Macdonald JS, Smalley SR, Benedetti J, et al. Chemoradiotherapy after surgery compared with surgery alone for adenocarcinoma of the stomach or gastroesophageal junction. *N Engl J Med* 2001;345:725–730.

Macdonald JS, Smalley SR, Benedetti J, et al. Postoperative combined radiation and chemotherapy improves disease-free survival (DFS) and overall survival (OS) in resected adenocarcinoma of the stomach and gastroesophageal junction: update of the results of Intergroup

Study INT-0116 (SWOG 9008). American Society of Clinical Oncology Gastrointestinal Cancers Symposium, Abstract #6, 2004.

Minsky BD, Wagman RT. Cancer of the stomach. In: Leibel SA, Phillips TL, editors. Textbook of Radiation Oncology. Saunders; 2004. pp. 825–836.

National Comprehensive Cancer Network. Clinical Practice Guidelines in Oncology: Gastric Cancer. Available at: http://www.nccn.org/professionals/physician_gls/PDF/gastric.pdf. Accessed on May 10, 2005.

Sano T, Sasako M, Yamamoto S, et al. Gastric cancer surgery: morbidity and mortality results from a prospective randomized controlled trial comparing D2 and extended para-aortic lymphadenectomy—Japan Clinical Oncology Group study 9501. *J Clin Oncol* 2004;22: 2767–2773.

Soybel DI, Zinner MJ. Stomach and duodenum: operative procedures. In: Zinner MJ, Schwartz SI, Ellis H, editors. Maingot's Abdominal Operations. 10th ed. Appleton and Lange; 1997. pp. 1079–1127.

Tepper JE, Gunderson LL. Radiation treatment parameters in the adjuvant postoperative therapy of gastric cancer. *Semin Radiat Oncol* 2002;12:187–195.

Willett CG, Gunderson LL. Stomach. In: Perez CA, Brady LW, Halperin EC, et al., editors. Principles and Practice of Radiation Oncology. 4th ed. Lippincott Williams and Wilkins; 2004. pp. 1554–1573.

Chapter 19
Pancreatic Cancer

Joy Coleman and Jeanne Marie Quivey

PEARLS

- 5th leading cause of cancer mortality although only the 9th most common cancer
- Found primarily in Western countries. Known risks include tobacco use, diets high in animal fat, ionizing radiation, chemotherapy, & exposure to 2-naphthylamine, benzene, and gasoline. Possible links between alcohol use, coffee use, chronic pancreatitis, and diabetes are less clear
- Four parts: head (including uncinate process), neck, body, and tail. 2/3 cancers present in the head
- Most common presenting symptoms = jaundice (due to common bile duct obstruction), weight loss (due to malabsorption from pancreas exocrine dysfunction), diabetes (related to pancreas endocrine dysfunction), gastric outlet obstruction, & abdominal pain. Jaundice is most common in pts with lesions in the head. Pts with lesions arising in the body or tail typically present with midepigastric or back pain. May infrequently present with Trousseau's sign (migratory thrombophlebitis) or Courvoisier's sign (palpable gallbladder)
- Primary LN drainage includes the pancreaticoduodenal, suprapancreatic, pyloric, & pancreaticosplenic LN with the porta hepatic, infrapyloric, subpyloric, celiac, superior mesenteric, and para-aortic areas being involved in advanced disease
- Most common type is of ductal origin. Cystadenocarcinomas, intraductal carcinomas, and solid and cystic papillary neoplasms (aka *Hamoundi tumors*) have a more indolent course. Acinar cell cancers & giant cell tumors are aggressive & have poor survival. 5% are tumors of the endocrine pancreas – these tumors are rare, slow growing, & have a long natural history

- 70 to 100% contain k-*ras* oncogene. P53 mutation present in approx 50%.
- Peritoneal & liver mets are most common. Lung is most common location outside the abdomen

WORKUP

- Main purpose of the workup is to determine resectability, establish a histologic diagnosis, re-establish biliary-tract outflow, & circumvent gastric outlet obstruction. Various diagnostic approaches exist
- H&P, upper GI, CT scan, US, and ERCP, laparoscopy, or CT-guided biopsy
- Labs: CBC, CEA, CA19-9, glucose, amylase, lipase, bilirubin, alkaline phosphatase, LDH, LFTs
- Endoscopy of the upper GI tract is extremely valuable with endobiliary stent placement. Endoscopic ultrasound can also be performed

STAGING

Primary tumor

TX: Primary tumor cannot be assessed

T0:   No evidence of primary tumor

T*is*:   Carcinoma *in situ* ** this also includes the "PanInIII" classification

T1:   Tumor limited to pancreas, 2 cm or less in greatest dimension

T2:   Tumor limited to pancreas, more than 2 cm in greatest dimension

T3:   Tumor extends beyond pancreas but without involvement of the celiac axis or the superior mesenteric artery

T4:   Tumor involves celiac axis or the superior mesenteric artery (unresectable primary tumor)

Regional lymph nodes

NX: Regional lymph nodes cannot be assessed

N0:   No regional lymph node metastasis

N1:   Regional LN metastases

Metastases

MX: Distant metastasis cannot be assessed

M0:   No distant metastasis

M1:   Distant metastases

STAGE GROUPING			~ SURVIVAL
0:	Tis	N0	M0	
0:	Tis	N0	M0	11 mo without post-op chemo-RT
IA:	T1	N0	M0	21 mo with post-op chemo-RT
IB:	T2	N0	M0	
IIA:	T3	N0	M0	
IIB:	T1-3	N1	M0	
III:	T4	N any	M0	4–6 mo with bypass alone, 10 mo chemo-RT with concurrent chemo-RT
IV:	T any	N any	M1	<6 mo

Used with the permission of the American Joint Committee on Cancer (AJCC), Chicago, Illinois. The original source for this material is the AJCC Cancer Staging Manual, Sixth Edition (2002) published by Springer-Verlag New York, www.springeronline.com.

- For practical purposes, tumors are generally classified as resectable (Stage I, II), unresectable (Stage III), and metastatic (Stage IV)
- Definition of resectabiity varies by institution, but generally includes no encasement of the celiac artery or superior mesenteric artery and patency of portal vein and superior mesenteric vein. Splenic vein involvement does not necessarily mean a tumor is unresectable

TREATMENT RECOMMENDATIONS

Stage	Recommended Treatment
Resectable (5–30% of patients)	Pancreaticoduodenectomy. Mortality <5% when performed by experienced surgeons. Pylorus preserving pancreaticoduodenectomy improves GI function & does not appear to compromise efficacy. Body/tail cancers (when resectable) should have a distal pancreatectomy with en bloc splenectomy

Recommendations about adjuvant treatment are controversial. Most recommend post-op RT with concurrent chemo (5-FU based) ± additional |

Stage	Recommended Treatment
	chemo when possible (gemcitabine based) although some recommend post op chemo alone (5-FU or gemcitabine) and some recommend no post op treatment (see studies below). Consider a clinical trial. Due to post-op complications ~25% of pts do not receive intended post-op therapy. The most common historically used chemo agent is 5-FU (250 mg/m²/d), but other agents & scheduled are being investigated including gemcitabine, capecitabine, tarceva, taxol, and cisplatin either alone or in combination.Gemcitabine, alone or in combination with another agent, may be considered as an alternative to chemoRT, but gemcitabine should be given via slow infusion but not during RT except on protocol due to increased toxicity Open areas of investigation include: 1) IORT, radiosurgery, & brachytherapy for dose escalation 2) Pre-op chemo-RT to decrease treatment toxicity, increase potential for negative margins, decrease risk of intra-op tumor seeding, and ensure operative complications do not require the omission of therapy 3) Role of 5-FU or Gemcitabine chemotherapy preceeding and following course of chemo-RT 4) Prophylactic hepatic irradiation in favorable

Stage	Recommended Treatment
	patients due to the high incidence of liver failure. This has been tested and determined feasible by an RTOG study in pts with unresectable lesions which showed a 13% liver failure rate (lower than historic controls). Other RTOG trials pending 5) Radiosensitizers, radioprotectants, & Yttrium-90 have also been studied
Unresectable	Clinical trial preferred. Other options include treatment with RT & concurrent 5-FU or capecitabine ± adjuvant chemotherapy as above or gemcitabine/gemcitabine combination therapy without RT Palliation with stents or surgical bypass Pre-op chemo-RT infrequently used in an attempt to make an unresectable tumor resectable. Is the subject of a multi-institution cooperative ECOG and RTOG trial
Metastatic	Palliation with stents, surgical bypass, chemo, RT, supportive care, or some combination of the above. Most randomized studies favor the use of gemcitabine over the use of 5-FU based chemo in the treatment of metastatic disease. Celiac nerve block is an effective palliative tool for local pain
Endocrine	Treatment surgical. Chemo for unresectable or metastatic disease. Effects of RT unknown although anecdotal responses exist

STUDIES
Resectable

- <u>GITSG 91–73</u> (*Arch Surg*, 1985). 43 pts with resectable pancreatic cancer were randomized to surgery followed by EBRT (40 Gy split course) with concurrent 5-FU vs surgery alone. Multimodality treatment arm showed increased OS (43% vs 18% at 2 yrs & 14% vs 5% at 5 yrs)
  - Updated (*Cancer*, 1987). Additional 30 nonrandomized patients entered into adjuvant therapy group. 2 year OS 46%
  - Although touted by many as "the Gold Standard", few radiation oncologists currently use this split course regimen
- <u>EORTC 40891</u> (*Ann Surg*, 1999). 218 pts with resectable pancreatic or periampullary cancer status post resection randomized to chemo-RT (40 Gy split course) vs observation. Adjuvant treatment resulted in no significant dif in 2 year PFS or 2 year OS
  - Many consider this study flawed, as only 119 pts had pancreatic cancer, no maintenance therapy was given, & the study included pts with positive margins without stratification. A point of additional concern is the lack of radiation therapy quality assurance in this trial
- <u>ESPAC-1</u> (*Lancet*, 2001). 2 × 2 factorial design. 541 patients with pancreatic or periampullary carcinoma s/p Whipple – not all patients randomized. Arms were chemo-RT (40 Gy split course with 5-FU) ± adjuvant chemo, adjuvant chemo alone (5-FU / leucovorin), & observation alone. Results contradictory when looking at randomized vs nonrandomized pts. For all pts, pts who received chemo had significantly improved median survival (19.7 vs 14 mo). For randomized pts only, chemo had no effect on median survival (17.4 vs 15.9 mo). For all pts and randomized pts only, chemoRT did not significantly affect median survival (~15 mo for chemoRT vs ~17 mo for no chemoRT)
  - Final results (*NEJM* 2004). 2 × 2 factorial design. 289 of the randomized patients from the study above. 47 mo median F/U. Authors concluded that chemo was of benefit while chemo-RT was detrimental. 5 yr survival 20% in two chemo arms & 10% in two RT arms. Only 128 pts with RT details available, of whom only 90 pts got the prescribed dose of 40 Gy. Progressive disease in 19% of pts precluded RT. No RT quality assurance.

- <u>RTOG 9704</u>. Pts with resectable pancreatic cancer s/p Whipple randomized to gemcitabine → concurrent chemo-RT with 5-FU → adjuvant gemcitabine vs 5-FU PVI → chemo-RT with 5-FU → 5-FU. Accrual met, results pending

Unresectable

- <u>GITSG</u> (*Cancer*,1981). 194 pts with unresectable pancreatic cancer were randomized to split course EBRT (40 Gy) with concomitant bolus 5-FU vs split course EBRT (60 Gy) with concomitant bolus 5-FU vs EBRT (60 Gy) alone. Both concomitant chemo arms prolonged median survival vs EBRT alone (42.2 wks, 40.3 wks, 22.9 wks respectively)
- <u>RTOG 9812</u>. Pts with unresectable pancreatic cancer. Phase II study of EBRT 50.4 Gy & weekly paclitaxel. All pts were restaged 6 weeks after completion of chemo/RT. If marked shrinkage, resection was attempted. Median survival 11.2 mo with 1 yr OS 43% and 2 yr OS 13%. 40% grade III & 5% grade IV toxicity with 1 death due to tx
- <u>Tempero</u> (*JCO*, 2003). 92 pts with locally advanced &/or metastatic adenocarcioma of the pancreas randomized to 2,200 mg/m^2 gemcitabine over 30 min or 1, 500 mg/m^2 over 150 min on days 1, 8, and 15 of a 4 week cycle. Slow infusion resulted in increased median survival (5 vs 8 months, p = 0.031) and decreased toxicity

RADIATION TECHNIQUES
Simulation & field design

- Treat tumor (or tumor bed if s/p resection) and nodal groups at risk using pre-op and post-op imaging studies as well as the findings at surgery. 3D planning is necessary to optimize dose distributions while minimizing dose to liver, kidneys, small bowel, and spinal cord
- Sim supine, arms up, with oral contrast. Use gastrografin (proprietary name) oral contrast not barium if CT is planned within 2 days. Give renal contrast or use CT to identify kidneys
- Pancreas lies at L1–L2. Celiac axis is at T12. SMA is at L1
- Lesions at the pancreatic head: treat pancreaticoduodenal, suprapancreatic, and celiac nodes, porta hepatis, the entire duodenal loop, & the tumor with 2–3 cm margin on gross disease

- For lesions in the body/tail: treat pancreatico-duodenal, portal hepatic, lateral suprapancreatic nodes, the nodes of the splenic hilum, & the gross tumor with 2–3 cm margin. Porta hepatis & duodenal bed do not need to be covered
- In general, pts are treated with a 3 or 4 field design – AP (50–80% of dose), two laterals or slightly off axis superior/inferior obliques (20% of dose), plus or minus a posterior field. High energy photon fields (e.g., 18 MV) are useful particularly for the lateral/oblique fields
- In general, for tumors of the pancreatic head treated with AP/PA fields: superior border = T10/T11; inferior border = L3/4; left border = 2 cm to the left of the edge of the vertebral body or 2 cm from the tumor; right border = pre-op location of the duodenum. On the laterals, anterior margin = 1.5–2 cm beyond the gross disease (being sure to include the duodenum); posterior margin = blocks the cord but covers 1.5–2 cm of the vertebral body
- Fluoroscopy is useful at the time of simulation or verification to evaluate organ movement during respiration, which can have an impact on the position of the target volume and the kidneys
- Cone down to gross tumor +2 cm margin at 45 Gy

Dose prescriptions

- Treat to 50.4 Gy with 1.8 Gy/fx with a cone down at 45 Gy
- Experiments are being done with hyperfractionation, brachytherapy, IORT, radiosurgery, & other methods of dose escalation

Dose limitations

- Doses up to 50 Gy are tolerated by small volumes of stomach and intestine. Most common late effects are mucosal ulceration and bleeding. Perforation is rare
- Limit the equivalent of at least one kidney to <20 Gy
- Limit the whole liver to <20 Gy & 70% of liver to <30 Gy to prevent radiation hepatitis. Small volumes of liver can be treated to high doses

COMPLICATIONS

- Critical normal tissues include liver, small bowel, stomach, cord, and kidney.
- Because the pancreas is a gland with both exocrine and endocrine secretions, both can decrease acutely or

chronically following treatment. Adequate monitoring for diabetes is integral to treatment as is supplementation with pancreatic enzymes if exocrine insufficiency is suspected (pancrealipase with each meal)

■ Acute – Nausea & vomiting (use antiemetics, proton pump inhibitor, or H2 blocker). Diarrhea less common. If jaundice develops during RT or following treatment, ascending cholangitis must be considered as a potential etiology

■ Late – Possible side effects include ulceration, stricture formation, obstruction, and (less commonly) perforation of GI tract. Side effects to cord, kidney, liver should not occur if normal tissue tolerances are followed

FOLLOW-UP

■ H&P, labs, & abdominal CT every 2 mo to evaluate for disease recurrence/progression

REFERENCES

Abrams R (2001). Primary Malignancies of the Pancreas, Periampullary Region and Hepatobiliary Tract – Considerations for the Radiation Oncologist (#310). Presented at the American Society of Therapeutic Radiology and Oncology Annual Meeting, San Francisco, CA.

American Society of Therapeutic Radiology and Oncology. Active Protocols. http://www.rtog.org/members/protocols/97-04/97-04.pdf and http://www.rtog.org/members/protocols/98-12/98-12.pdf. Accessed February, 2005.

Crane CH, Evans DB, Wolff RA, Abbruzzese JL, Pisters PWT, Janjan NA. The Pancreas. In: Cox JD, Ang KK, editors. Radiation oncology: rationale, technique, results. 8th ed. St. Louis: Mosby; 2003. pp. 465–480.

Further evidence of effective adjuvant combined radiation and chemotherapy following curative resection of pancreatic cancer. Gastrointestinal Tumor Study Group. Cancer. 1987 Jun 15;59(12): 2006–2010.

Kalser M, Ellenberg S. Pancreatic cancer. Adjuvant combined radiation and chemotherapy following curative resection. Arch Surg. 1985 Aug;120(8):899–903. Erratum in: Arch Surg 1986 Sep;121(9):1045.

Klinkenbijl JH, Jeekel J, Sahmoud T, et al. Adjuvant radiotherapy and 5-fluorouracil after curative resection of cancer of the pancreas and periampullary region: phase III trial of the EORTC gastrointestinal tract cancer cooperative group. Ann Surg. 1999 Dec;230(6):776–782; discussion 782–784.

Lillis-Hearne P. Cancer of the Pancreas. In: Leibel SA, Phillips TL, editors. Textbook of radiation oncology. 2nd ed. Philadelphia: Saunders; 2004. pp. 837–856.

Moertel CG, Frytak S, Hahn RG, et al. Therapy of locally unresectable pancreatic carcinoma: a randomized comparison of high dose (6000 rads) radiation alone, moderate dose radiation (4000 rads + 5-fluorouracil), and high dose radiation + 5-fluorouracil: The Gastrointestinal Tumor Study Group. Cancer. 1981 Oct 15;48(8): 1705–1710.

NCCN Physician Guidelines. Available at http://www.nccn.org/professionals/physician_gls/PDF/pancreatic.pdf and http://nccn.org/about/news/newsinfo.asp?NewsID=70. Accessed May 7, 2006.

Neoptolemos JP, Dunn JA, Stocken DD, et al. Adjuvant chemoradiotherapy and chemotherapy in resectable pancreatic cancer: a randomised controlled trial. Lancet. 2001 Nov 10;358(9293):1576–1585.

Neoptolemos JP, Stocken DD, Friess H, et al. MW; European Study Group for Pancreatic CancerA randomized trial of chemoradiotherapy and chemotherapy after resection of pancreatic cancer. N Engl J Med. 2004 Mar 18;350(12):1200–1210. Erratum in: N Engl J Med. 2004 Aug 12;351(7):726.

Tempero M, Plunkett W, Ruiz Van Haperen V, et al. Randomized phase II comparison of dose-intense gemcitabine: thirty-minute infusion and fixed dose rate infusion in patients with pancreatic adenocarcinoma. J Clin Oncol. 2003 Sep 15;21(18):3402–3408. Epub 2003 Jul 28.

NOTES

Chapter 20
Hepatobiliary Cancer

Laura Millender and Mack Roach, III

GENERAL PEARLS

- Approximately 22,000 cases and 17,000 deaths per year in USA
- Frequency: hepatocellular carcinoma (most common) > gallbladder cancer > extrahepatic cholangiocarcinoma > intrahepatic cholangiocarcinoma (least common)

LIVER (HEPATOCELLULAR)

PEARLS

- 100–250× more common in pts with chronic Hepatitis B
- 3–4× more common in men
- Cirrhosis, Hepatitis C, and aflatoxin B exposure are also risk factors
- Prevention: Hepatitis B vaccine
- Screening tools frequently used in high risk pts: serum alpha-fetoprotein, liver ultrasound

WORKUP

- Labs: CBC, LFTs, chemistries, coagulation panel, serum AFP (10–15% false negative), hepatitis B/C panels
- Abdominal CT scan (special contrast protocol)
- FNA can be performed but is not always needed

STAGING: LIVER (INCLUDING INTRAHEPATIC BILE DUCTS)

Primary Tumor (T)	
TX	Primary tumor cannot be assessed
T0	No evidence of primary tumor
T1	Solitary tumor without vascular invasion
T2	Solitary tumor with vascular invasion or multiple tumors none more than 5 cm
T3	Multiple tumors more than 5 cm or tumor involving a major branch of the portal or hepatic vein(s)

T4   Tumor(s) with direct invasion of adjacent organs other than the gallbladder or with perforation of visceral peritoneum

Regional Lymph Nodes (N)
NX   Regional lymph nodes cannot be assessed
N0   No regional lymph node metastasis
N1   Regional lymph node metastasis

Distant Metastasis (M)
MX   Distant metastasis cannot be assessed
M0   No distant metastasis
M1   Distant metastasis

Stage Grouping		~5 yr OS by Stage	
I	T1N0M0	I	50–60%
II	T2N0M0	II	30–40%
IIIA	T3N0M0	III	10–20%
IIIB	T4N0M0	IV	<10%
IIIC	Any T, N1, M0		
IV	Any T, Any N, M1		

Used with the permission of the American Joint Committee on Cancer (AJCC), Chicago, Illinois. The original source for this material is the AJCC Cancer Staging Manual, Sixth Edition (2002) published by Springer-Verlag New York, www.springeronline.com.

TREATMENT RECOMMENDATIONS

Presentation	Recommended Treatment
Resectable	1. Partial hepatectomy 2. Liver transplant
Unresectable, medically inoperable	1. Ablation (radiofrequency, cryotherapy, alcohol) 2. Chemoembolization 3. Conformal RT 4. RT with concurrent chemotherapy 5. Chemotherapy alone 6. Supportive care

Surgery
- Partial hepatectomy is treatment of choice if tumor can be resected with negative margins and pt has enough functional reserve to tolerate procedure
  - 5 year overall survival ~35–40%

- Total hepatectomy with liver transplant is an option for pts with advanced cirrhosis and tumors smaller than 5 cm without vascular invasion
  - 5 year overall survival as high as ~70% in selected patients
- Local failure is common
- Role of adjuvant and neoadjuvant therapy unclear

Ablative procedures/other interventions

- Radiofrequency ablation best for deep tumors with diameter of 3 cm or less
- Cyroablation can treat tumors up to 6 cm in size but requires laparotomy
- Alcohol injection is commonly used because inexpensive, but limited to small tumors and may require several injections to be effective
- Chemoembolization and intrahepatic artery chemotherapy have response rates of 40–50% but may not improve survival
- Systemic chemotherapy not useful, response rates <20%, no survival benefit
- Anti-viral therapy for pts with chronic hepatitis

Radiation therapy

- **EBRT definitive**
  - Option for unresectable tumors
  - Use local field for each lesion
  - High doses may improve survival, use conformal techniques
  - Consider addition of concurrent FUDR hepatic arterial chemotherapy
- **EBRT palliative**
  - Whole liver
  - Consider for pts with multiple small lesions and liver related symptoms who are not candidates for other therapies
- **^{131}I Lipiodol**
  - Intraarterial injection
  - May decrease recurrences and improve overall survival
- **Yttrium microspheres**

STUDIES

- Borgelt (*IJROBP* 1981). Whole liver RT can relieve symptoms of abdominal pain, nausea, vomiting, fever, night sweats, ascites, anorexia, abdominal distention, weakness, fatigue

- <u>Russell</u> (*IJROBP* 1993). RTOG whole liver fractionation paper. Pts treated with 1.5 bid with dose escalation 27 Gy → 30 Gy → 33 Gy. No liver injury at 27 & 30 Gy. 5/51 pts had toxicity at 33 Gy. Authors suggest that 21 Gy may be insufficient radiation dose
- <u>Dawson</u> (*JCO* 2000). University of Michigan method for treating with high-dose 3DCRT. 68% response rate. Survival improved with tumor doses of 70 Gy or higher
- <u>Dawson</u> (*IJROBP* 2002). Liver tolerance histograms. No radiation induced liver disease (RILD) with mean liver dose <31 Gy. Whole organ TD_{50} for mets 45.8 Gy, for primary hepatobiliary 39.8 Gy
- <u>Lau</u> (*Lancet* 1999). Pts randomized to intraarterial lipiodol vs no adjuvant therapy. Pts receiving lipiodol had fewer recurrences (59% vs 29%) & improved DFS (57 mo vs 14 mo)

RADIATION TECHNIQUES
Simulation and field design
- Supine with arms above head (out of field)
- Use wingboard to immobilize arms and alpha cradle to stabilize torso
- Whole liver (palliation only)
  - AP/PA, chose borders based on CT scan
  - 3DCRT reasonable because permits generation of kidney and lung DVHs
- Partial liver (definitive option)
  - 3D treatment planning
  - Give contrast with planning CT scan to visualize tumor
  - CTV = gross tumor + 1 cm in all directions
  - PTV = CTV + 0.5 cm for set-up error + 0.3–3 cm for organ motion error secondary to breathing (determined using fluoroscopy)
  - Stereotactic radiosurgery investigational

Dose prescriptions
- Whole liver: 21 Gy/7 fx
- Partial liver: determined individually
  - Prescribe dose that gives 10% risk of RILD based on NTCP model

- Limit isocenter dose to 90 Gy even if risk of RILD is less than 10%
- 1.5 Gy bid with at least 6 hrs between fractions

Dose limitations
- Whole liver
  - TD 5/5: 30 Gy/15 fx
  - TD 50/5: 42 Gy/21 fx
- 2/3 of liver TD 5/5: 50.4 Gy/28 fx
- 1/3 of liver TD 5/5: 68.4 Gy/38 fx

COMPLICATIONS
- Refer to Dawson paper (above) to estimate risk of RILD
- RILD occurs 2–8 weeks after treatment
- Signs/symptoms include fatigue, RUQ pain, ascites, hepatomegally
- Alkaline phosphatase and transaminase levels are frequently markedly elevated while bilirubin levels remain near normal

FOLLOW-UP
- Office visit, CT scan, and labs (LFTs, AFP) every 3 months for 2 years, then every 6 months

GALLBLADDER

PEARLS
- Chronic gallbladder inflammation (usually from gallstones) increases risk of development of gallbladder cancer
- Generally considered to have poor prognosis, frequently advanced stage at presentation
- Usually undiagnosed before cholecystectomy

WORKUP
- Labs: CBC, LFTs, chemistries, coagulation panel, serum CEA, CA 19-9
- Right upper quadrant US and/or abdominal CT scan and/or MRI
- ERCP or percutaneous needle biopsy for diagnosis

STAGING

Primary Tumor (T)

TX	Primary tumor cannot be assessed
T0	No evidence of primary tumor
Tis	Carcinoma *in situ*
T1	Tumor invades lamina propria or muscle layer
T1a	Tumor invades lamina propria
T1b	Tumor invades muscle layer
T2	Tumor invades perimuscular connective tissue; no extension beyond serosa or into liver
T3	Tumor perforates the serosa (visceral peritoneum) and/or directly invades the liver and/or one other adjacent organ or structure, such as the stomach, duodenum, colon, or pancreas, omentum or extrahepatic bile ducts
T4	Tumor invades main portal vein or hepatic artery or invades multiple extrahepatic organs or structures

Regional Lymph Nodes (N)

NX	Regional lymph nodes cannot be assessed
N0	No regional lymph node metastasis
N1	Regional lymph node metastasis

Distant Metastasis (M)

MX	Distant metastasis cannot be assessed
M0	No distant metastasis
M1	Distant metastasis

Stage Grouping

0	TisN0M0
IA	T1N0M0
IB	T2N0M0
IIA	T3N0M0
IIB	T1N1M0, T2N1M0, T3N1M0
III	T4, Any N, M0
IV	Any T, Any N, M1

TREATMENT RECOMMENDATIONS

Presentation	Recommended Treatment
Incidental finding on cholecystectomy pathology, T1a	Cholecystectomy is adequate surgery. No adjuvant therapy
Incidental finding on cholecystectomy pathology, T1b or more advanced	1. Additional resection with Lymphadenectomy 2. Adjuvant treatment with RT and concurrent 5-FU based chemo
Mass on imaging or jaundice, resectable	1. Surgery with lymphadenectomy 2. Adjuvant treatment with RT and concurrent 5-FU based chemo
Mass on imaging or unresectable	1. Biliary decompression if needed 2. RT with concurrent 5-FU based chemo 3. Gemcitabine or 5-FU based chemo alone 4. Supportive care

SURGERY

- Cholecystectomy possible in ~30% of patients
- Radical cholecystectomy with partial hepatectomy for node negative pts with invasion of perimuscular connective tissue
- Palliation

ADJUVANT THERAPY

- Role of EBRT and chemo-RT unclear, but generally recommended for residual disease after surgery

STUDIES

- Cubertafond (*Hepatogastroenerol* 1999). Review of surgical data for 724 pts. 5 yr survival: Tis 93%, T1 18%, T2 10%. No 3 yr survivors with T3/4 cancer
- North (*Am Surg* 1998). Review of surgical data for 162 pts. Median survival: complete resection 67 mo, microscopic residual disease 9 mo, gross residual disease 4 mo. Some pts received chemo and/or RT

RADIATION TECHNIQUES
Simulation and field design
- Supine with arms above head (out of field)
- Use wingboard to immobilize arms and alpha cradle to stabilize torso
- CT scan for treatment planning
- Cover tumor bed and any areas of involved nodes

Dose prescription
- 45 Gy/25 fx

Dose limitations
- Small bowel <45–50.4 Gy/25–28 fx
- Spinal cord <45 Gy/25 fx
- Liver (see previous sections, use NTCP model)
- Kidney ≤20 Gy

COMPLICATIONS
- RILD
- Small bowel obstruction
- Fistula formation

FOLLOW-UP
- See liver section above

BILE DUCT

PEARLS
- Divided into intrahepatic (IHCC) & extrahepatic (EHCC) cholangiocarcinoma
- Klatskin (hilar) tumor is located at birufication of common hepatic duct and is classified as extrahepatic
- History of primary sclerosisng cholangitis gives 10% life-time risk of developing cholangiocarcinoma
- Cholecystectomy decreases risk of cholangiocarcinoma
- ~55% of pts are lymph node positive at diagnosis

WORKUP
- Labs: CBC, LFTs, chemistries, coagulation panel, CA19-9, CEA, hepatitis B/C
- Right upper quadrant US and/or abdominal CT scan and/or MRI
- ERCP with biopsy

STAGING: EXTRAHEPATIC BILE DUCTS

Primary Tumor (T)

TX   Primary tumor cannot be assessed

T0   No evidence of primary tumor

Tis   Carcinoma *in situ*

T1   Tumor confined to bile duct histologically

T2   Tumor invades beyond wall of bile duct

T3   Tumor invades the liver, gallbladder, pancreas snd/or unilateral branches of the portal vein (right or left) or hepatic artery (right or left)

T4   Tumor invades any of the following: main portal vein or its branches bilaterally, common hepatic artery, or other adjacent structures, such as the colon, stomach, duodenum, or abdominal wall

Regional Lymph Nodes (N)

NX   Regional lymph nodes cannot be assessed

N0   No regional lymph node metastasis

N1   Regional lymph node metastasis

Distant Metastasis (M)

MX   Distant metastasis cannot be assessed

M0   No distant metastasis

M1   Distant metastasis

Stage Grouping

0   TisN0M0

IA   T1N0M0

IB   T2N0M0

IIA   T3N0M0

IIB   T1N1M0, T2N1M0, T3N1M0

III   T4, Any N, M0

IV   Any T, Any N, M1

Used with the permission of the American Joint Committee on Cancer (AJCC), Chicago, Illinois. The original source for this material is the AJCC Cancer Staging Manual, Sixth Edition (2002) published by Springer-Verlag New York, www.springeronline.com.

STAGING: INTRAHEPATIC BILE DUCTS, please see Liver and intraheaptic bile duct staging

TREATMENT RECOMMENDATIONS
Intrahepatic cholangiocarcinoma

Presentation	Recommended Treatment
Resectable. No residual disease	Observation
Resectable. Residual disease	1. Repeat resection 2. Ablative procedure 3. RT with concurrent 5-FU based chemo 4. Gemcitabine based chemo alone
Unresectable	1. Ablative procedure 2. RT with concurrent 5-FU based chemo 3. 5-FU or gemcitabine based chemo alone 4. Supportive care

Extrahepatic cholangiocarcinoma

Presentation	Recommended Treatment
Resectable. No residual disease	1. Observation 2. RT with concurrent 5-FU based chemo
Resectable. Residual disease	RT with concurrent 5-FU based chemo
Unresectable.	1. RT with concurrent 5-FU based chemo (consider brachytherapy boost) 2. 5-FU or gemcitabine based chemo alone 3. Supportive care

SURGERY

- Complete surgical resection is the most effective treatment
- Surgical procedure depends on tumor location and extent of disease
    - Partial hepatectomy or lobectomy for intrahepatic tumors
    - Roux-en-y hepaticojejunostomy for hilar tumors
    - Pancreaticoduodenectomy for distal lesions
    - Liver transplant
- Palliative Options – biliary enteric bypass, percutaneous transhepatic biliary drainage, stents

ADJUVANT THERAPY

- Not studied prospective
- Adjuvant RT and chemotherapy may improve overall survival

STUDIES

- Todoroki (*IJROBP* 2000). 63 patients. Treatment: surgical resection. RT given to 28/47 with microscopic disease & 13/14 with gross residual disease. 5 yr OS with RT 32 mo vs surgery alone 13.5 mo. RT group OS: IORT + EBRT 39%, IORT alone 17%, EBRT alone 0%. LRC with RT 79% vs with surgery alone 31.2%. IORT dose recommendations – 20 Gy, 8 MeV electrons, 6 cm cone
- Schoenthaler (*Ann Surg* 1994). UCSF experience. 129 pts, retrospective, extrahepatic ducts only. Treatment: 62 pts surgery alone, 45 pts surgery + conventional RT (46 Gy median), 22 pts surgery + charged particles (60 GyE median). MS: 6.5 mo with surgery, 11 mo with surgery + EBRT, 14 mo with surgery + particles; 7 mo with gross residual disease, 19 mo with microscopic residual disease, & 39 mo with negative margins
- Alden (*IJROBP* 1994). Unresectable disease. Higher RT doses improve survival. MS: 44 Gy = 4.5 mo, 45–54 Gy = 18 mo, >54 Gy = 24 mo. Recommended dose is 45 Gy EBRT with a 25 Gy intraluminal brachytherapy boost
- Crane (*IJROBP* 2002). 52 pts, locally advanced, unresectable treated with RT + chemo (73% of pts, PVI 5-FU). Median time to local progression: 9 mo after 30 Gy, 11 mo after 36–50.4 Gy, 15 mo after 54–85 Gy (p = ns). MS 10 mo. Grade 3 toxicity similar in all groups

RADIATION TECHNIQUES

Simulation and field design

- Supine with arms above head (out of field)
- Use wingboard to immobilize arms and alpha cradle to stabilize torso
- CT scan for treatment planning
- Cover tumor bed, porta hepatis, celiac axis + 1.5 cm margins
- Consider extending field 3–5 cm into liver to cover additional intrahepatic bile duct length for margin
- Add additional margins as needed to account for organ motion secondary to breathing, determined using fluoroscopy

Dose prescription

- 45 Gy/25 fx to large field described above
- Additional boost dose should be given. Options include: EBRT with cone down to tumor bed to 60 Gy total; ^{192}Ir intraluminal brachytherapy (20–25 Gy); IORT at time of surgery

Dose Limitations

- See liver and gallbladder sections

COMPLICATIONS

- RILD rare, as much of the liver can be excluded from the field
- Cholangitis after brachytherapy
- Small bowel damage (ulcer, bleeding, obstruction)

FOLLOW-UP

- See liver section above

REFERENCES

Alden ME, Mohiuddin M. The impact of radiation dose in combined external beam and intraluminal Ir-192 brachytherapy for bile duct cancer. Int J Radiat Oncol Biol Phys 1994;28:945–951.

Bartlet DL, Carr BI, Marsh JW. Cancer of the Liver. In: DeVita VT, Hellman S, Rosenberg SA, editors. Cancer, Principles and Practice of Oncology. 7th ed. Philadelphia: Lippincott Willaims & Wilkins, 2005. 986–1009.

Borgelt BB, Gelber R, Brady LW, et al. The palliation of hepatic metastases: results of the Radiation Therapy Oncology Group Pilot Study. Int J Radiat Oncol Biol Phys 1981;7:587–591.

Cheng SH, Huang AT. Liver and hepatobiliary tract. In: Perez CA, Brady LW, Halperin EC, et al., editors. Principles and Practice of Radiation Oncology. 4th ed. Philadelphia: Lippincott Williams & Wilkins; 2004. pp. 1589–1606.

Crane CH, MacDonald KO, Vauthey JN, et al. Limitations of conventional doses of chemoradiaion for unresectable biliary cancer. Int J Radiat Oncol Biol Phys 2002;53:969–974.

Cubertafond P, Mathonnet M, Gainant A, et al. Radical surgery for gallbladder cancer. Results of the French Surgical Association Survey. Hepatogastroenerology 1999;46:1567–1571.

Dawson LA, McGinn CJ, Normolle D, et al. Escalated focal liver radiation and concurrent hepatic artery flourodeoxyuridine for unresectable intrahepatic malignancies. J Clin Oncol 2000;18:2210–2218.

Dawson LA, Normolle D, Balter JM, et al. Analysis of radiation-induced liver disease using the Lyman NTCP model. Int J Radiat Oncol Biol Phys 2002;53:810–821.

Fritz P, Brambs HJ, Schraube P, et al. Combined external beam radiotherapy and intraluminal high dose rate brachytherapy on bile duct carcinomas. Int J Radiat Oncol Biol Phys 1994;29:855–861.

Greene FL, American Joint Committee on Cancer, American Cancer Society. AJCC Cancer Staging Manual. 6th ed. New York: Springer-Verlag; 2002.

Lau WY, Leung TW, Ho SK, et al. Adjuvant intra-arterial iodine-131-labelled for resectable hepatocellular carcinoma: a prospective randomised trial. Lancet 1999;353:797–801.

Morganti AG, Trodella L, Valentini V, et al. Combined modality treatment in unresectable extrahepatic biliary carcinoma. Int J Radiat Oncol Biol Phys 2000;46:913–919.

National Comprehensive Cancer Network. Clinical Practice Guidelines in Oncology: Hepatobiliary Cancers. Available at: http://www.nccn.org/professionals/physician_gls/PDF/hepatobiliary.pdf. Accessed on March 19, 2005.

North JH, Pack MS, Hong C, et al. Prognostic factors for adenocarcinoma of the gallbladder: an analysis of 162 cases. Am Surg 1998;64:437–440.

Robertson JM, Lawrence TS. Hepatobiliary Tumors. In: Gunderson LL, Tepper JE, editors. Clinical Radiation Oncology. 1st ed. Philadelphia: Churchill Livingstone; 2000. pp. 707–719.

Russell AH, Clyde C, Wasserman TH, et al. Accelerated hyperfractionated hepatic irradiation in the management of patients with liver metastases: results of the RTOG Dose Escalating Protocol. Int J Radiat Oncol Biol Phys 1993;27:117–123.

Schoenthaler R, Phillips TL, Efrid JT, et al. Carcinoma of the extrahepatic bile ducts, the University of California at San Francisco experience. Ann Surg 1994;219:267–274.

Stevens, KR. The liver and biliary system. In: Cox JD, Ang KK, editors. Radiation Oncology: Rationale, Technique, Results. 8th ed. St. Louis: Mosby; 2003. pp. 481–496.

Todoroki T, Ohara K, Kawamoto T, et al. Benefits of adjuvant radiotherapy after radical resection of locally advanced main hepatic duct carcinoma. Int J Radiat Oncol Biol Phys 2000;46:581–587.

Urego M, Flickinger JC, Carr BI. Radiotherapy and multimodality management of cholangiocarcinoma. Int J Radiat Oncol Biol Phys 1999;44:121–126.

Wagman R, Schoenthaler R. Cancer of the liver, bile duct, and gallbladder. In: Leibel SA, Phillips TL, editors. Textbook of Radiation Oncology. 2nd ed. Philadelphia: Saunders; 2004. pp. 857–884.

NOTES

Chapter 21
Colorectal Cancer

Kavita K. Mishra

PEARLS

- Third most frequently diagnosed cancer in U.S. men and women
- Rectum begins at the rectosigmoid junction at level of S3 vertebra. It is divided into three ~5 cm segments by transverse folds: upper, mid, lower rectum. Cancer of rectum is defined as those straddling or inferior to the peritoneal reflection
- Rectal nodal drainage: superior half rectum drains to pararectal, sacral, sigmoidal, inferior mesenteric; inferior half rectum drains to internal iliacs; lower rectum & tumors extending to anal canal may drain to superficial inguinal nodes
- Rectal metastases travel along portal drainage to liver via superior rectal vein, as well as systemic drainage to lung via middle and inferior rectal veins
- Colon nodal drainage: left colon to inferior mesenteric; right colon to superior mesenteric. Periaortic nodes at risk if cancer invades retroperitoneum. External iliac nodes at risk if cancer invades adjacent pelvic organs
- Hematochezia most common presentation in rectal and lower sigmoid CA; abdominal pain common with colon CA

SCREENING

- Average risk persons (age ≥50 yrs, asymptomatic, no FH): colonoscopy q 10 yr (preferred) or FOBT q 1 yr + flexible sigmoidoscopy q 5 yr or double-contrast barium enema q 5 yr

Special acknowledgement: We thank Richard M. Krieg, M.D. for his valuable advice in the preparation of this chapter.

- Inflammatory bowel disease: colonoscopy q 1–2 yrs, initiate 8 yrs after symptom onset if pancolitis or 15 yrs after symptom onset if L-sided colitis
- Family Hx (non-FAP/HNPCC): colonoscopy q 1–5 yrs, initiate at age 40 yrs or 10 yrs prior to earliest cancer diagnosis in family
- Familial adenosis polyposis (lifetime cancer risk ~100% by age 50): APC gene testing, early screening, colectomy or proctocolectomy after onset of polyposis
- Hereditary nonpolyposis colorectal cancer: colonoscopy q 1–2 yrs, initiate at age 20–25 or 10 yrs younger than earliest cancer diagnosis in family

WORKUP

- H&P including DRE and complete pelvic exam in women
- Labs including CBC, LFTs, CEA
- Endoscopic biopsy, pathology review
- Colonoscopy, CT chest/abdomen/pelvis
- Endorectal US to assess tumor extension and nodal status

STAGING

<u>Primary tumor</u>
TX: Primary tumor cannot be assessed
T0:   No evidence of primary tumor
Tis: Carcinoma in situ: intraepithelial or invasion of lamina propria
T1:   Tumor invades submucosa
T2:   Tumor invades muscularis propria
T3:   Tumor invades through the muscularis propria into the subserosa, or into non-peritonealized pericolic or perirectal tissues
T4:   Tumor directly invades other organs or structures, and/or perforates visceral peritoneum
<u>Regional lymph nodes</u>
NX: Regional lymph nodes cannot be assessed
N0:   No regional lymph node metastasis
N1:   Metastasis in 1 to 3 regional lymph nodes
N2:   Metastasis in 4 or more regional lymph nodes
<u>Metastases</u>
MX: Distant metastasis cannot be assessed
M0:   No distant metastasis
M1:   Distant metastasis

Stage Grouping		Dukes	Modified Aster-Coller	~5 yr OS	
0:	TisN0M0	–	–		
I:	T1N0M0	A	A	I:	80–95%
	T2N0M0	A	B1		
IIA:	T3N0M0	B	B2	II:	50–90%
IIB:	T4N0M0	B	B3		
IIIA:	T1-2N1M0	C	C1	III:	30–60%
IIIB:	T3-4N1M0	C	C2/C3		
IIIC:	Any T, N2, M0	C	C1/C2/C3		
IV:	Any T, Any N, M1		D	IV:	<5%

Used with the permission of the American Joint Committee on Cancer (AJCC), Chicago, Illinois. The original source for this material is the AJCC Cancer Staging Manual, Sixth Edition (2002) published by Springer-Verlag New York, www.springeronline.com.

TREATMENT RECOMMENDATIONS

Stage	Rectal Cancer
I	APR (low lesions); LAR (mid-upper lesions). Consider local excision for favorable tumors (<3 cm size, <30% circumference, within 8 cm of anal verge, well-moderately differentiated; margin >3 mm, no LVSI/PNI). After local excision, favorable T1 lesions may be observed, while T2 lesions should receive adjuvant 5-FU/RT
II & III (locally resectable)	Pre-op 5-FU/RT → transabdominal resection → adjuvant 5-FU based therapy* × 3 cycles (preferred) If pt treated with surgery initially, then pt should receive adjuvant 5-FU × 2 cycles → concurrent chemo-RT → 5-FU × 2 cycles
III (T4/locally unresectable)	5-FU/RT → resection if possible. Consider IORT for microscopic disease (after 50 Gy EBRT, give IORT 12.5–15 Gy to 90% IDL) or brachytherapy for macroscopic disease → adjuvant 5-FU based therapy*

Stage	Rectal Cancer
IV	Individualized options, including combination 5-FU based chemo alone, or chemo ± resection ± RT
Recurrent	Individualized options. If no prior RT, then consider chemo-RT, followed by surgery ± IORT or brachytherapy. If prior RT, then chemo → surgery ± IORT or brachytherapy as appropriate.

*Consider post-op 5-FU ± leucovorin vs FOLFOX (infusional 5-FU/leucovorin/oxaliplatin) vs FOLFIRI (infusional 5-FU/leucovorin/irinotecan).

Stage	Colon Cancer**
I	Colectomy + LND
IIA	Colectomy + LND. For adverse pathologic features, consider adjuvant chemo
IIB	Colectomy + LND. Consider adjuvant chemo
III	Colectomy + LND → adjuvant chemo
IV	Consider resection and neoadjuvant/adjuvant chemo

**No clear OS/LC benefit with RT in colon CA. May consider post-op RT in setting of node-negative disease if close/+ margins & tumor bed can be clearly identified.

STUDIES
Rectal

- Dutch Colorectal Cancer Group (*NEJM* 2001, ASCO abstr. 2002). 1861 pts with resectable rectal CA randomized to pre-op RT (25 Gy/5 fx) and surgery vs surgery alone. Pre-op RT improved 2 yr LR (2% vs 8%); 5 yr LR (6% vs 12%)

- German Rectal Cancer Study Group (*NEJM* 2004). 823 pts with T3/4 or N+ rectal CA randomized to pre-op vs post-op chemo-RT. Both arms had 50.4 Gy with concurrent 5-FU; post-op arm had additional 5.4 Gy boost. Pre-op chemo-RT improved 5 yr LR rate (6% vs 13%); increased rate of sphincter saving procedures

(39% vs 19%); and decreased grade 3–4 toxicity (27% vs 40%)

- GITSG 7175 (*Radiother Oncol* 1988). 227 pts with stage B2-C rectal CA randomized postoperatively to no adjuvant therapy vs chemo alone vs RT alone vs concurrent chemo-RT. Chemo-RT arm improved 5 yr DFS and OS over control

- O'Connell (*NEJM* 1994). 660 pts with stage II or III rectal CA randomized to postoperative bolus 5-FU vs PVI 5-FU during post-op pelvic RT. Chemo given ± semustine. PVI 5-FU improved 4 yr OS (70% vs 60%) and relapse-free rate (63% vs 53%). No benefit with semustine

- RTOG 89-02 (*IJROBP* 2000). 65 pts in phase II trial of sphincter-sparing local excision for low-lying rectal tumors ≤4 cm, ≤40% circumference, mobile, N0 status. 51 higher-risk pts also received post-op chemo-RT. RT dose 45–50 Gy with boost to total 50–65 Gy. 5 yr OS 78%, 11 pts failed. LRF correlated with T stage (T1 4%, T2 16%, T3 23%) and % rectal circumference involved. DM correlated with T stage

- Swedish Rectal Cancer Trial (*NEJM* 1997). 1168 pts with resectable rectal CA randomized to pre-op RT (25 Gy/5 fx) and surgery vs surgery alone. Pre-op RT improved 5 yr LR (11% vs 27%) and 5 yr OS (58% vs 48%)

- Tepper (*JCO* 2002). 1695 pts with T3/4 or N+ rectal CA randomized to postoperative bolus 5-FU vs 5-FU and leucovorin vs 5-FU and levamisole vs 5-FU, leucovorin and levamisole. All received concurrent pelvic RT 50.4–54 Gy. No difference in 7 yr OS (~56%), DFS (~50%) between 4 chemo arms

Colon

- Andre (*NEJM* 2004). 2246 pts with stage II or III colon CA randomized to postoperative 5-FU/leucovorin vs 5-FU/leucovorin/oxaliplatin. Oxaliplatin improved 3 yr DFS (78% vs 73%)

- Twelves (*NEJM* 2005). 1987 pts with resected stage III colon CA randomized to oral capecitabine vs bolus 5-FU/LV. Capecitabine had at least equivalent DFS, with improved RFS with fewer adverse events

- INT0130 Trial (*JCO* 2004). 222 pts with resected T3N1-N2 or T4 colon CA randomized to chemo vs chemo-RT. RT given as 45 Gy/25 fx ± 5.4 boost to tumor bed. No difference in survival or local recurrence

- Moertel (*NEJM* 1990) 1296 pts with resected colon cancer that either was locally invasive (Stage B2-3) or had regional nodal involvement (Stage C), were randomized to observation vs treatment for one year with levamisole and fluorouracil. Overall death rate was reduced by 33% in chemo treatment arm

RADIATION TECHNIQUES: RECTAL CANCER
Simulation and field design
- Prone position; radiopaque markers include anal, vaginal, rectal, perineal skin; wire perineal scar if present; small bowel contrast, ensure bladder full
- Rectal field designed to cover tumor with margin, presacral, & internal iliac nodes (if T4, external iliac nodes also)
- Whole pelvis (PA field) borders: superior = L5-S1; inferior = 3 cm below initial tumor volume or inferior obturator foramen, whichever most inferior; lateral = 1.5 cm outside pelvic inlet
- Whole pelvis (lateral fields) borders: posterior = behind bony sacrum; anterior = posterior pubic symphysis if T3 vs anterior pubic symphysis if T4. Corner blocks as needed
- Avoid flashing posterior skin, unless s/p APR then include perineal scar in all fields
- Tumor bed boost borders: tumor + 2–3 cm margin superior/inferior/anterior; posterior border includes sacral hollow. Corner blocks used to protect small bowel
- IORT: consider for close/+ microscopic margins, especially for T4 or recurrent CA
- Brachytherapy: consider for macroscopic residual after pre-op chemoRT and resection
- Chemo: concurrent PVI 5-FU based therapy with RT given as 5-FU 225 mg/m^2 over 24 h 7 d/wk during RT. Use of oral 5-FU is becoming common

Dose prescriptions
- Whole pelvis: 3 field with PA + opposed laterals; use lateral wedges as appropriate. 45 Gy (1.8 Gy × 25 fx) then boost. Use high-energy photon beams for lateral fields. Choose appropriate energy photon beam for PA field based on depth of sacral hollow

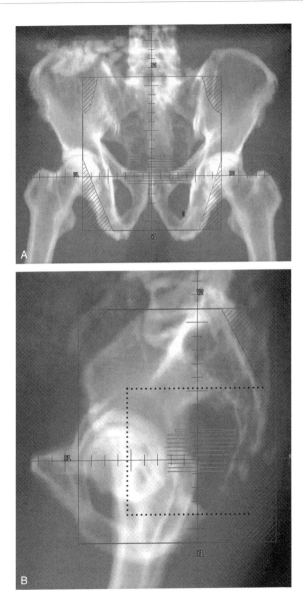

FIGURE 21.1. (A) and (B) lateral DRRs of fields used to treat a T3NO rectal primary. The lateral boost field is indicated by the black dotted line. Note: radiopaque markers not shown.

- Boost: opposed laterals only; 5.4 Gy (1.8 Gy × 3 fx), to total dose 50.4 Gy. Consider second boost to 54 Gy if all small bowel is out of field
- If no planned surgical intervention, definitive RT dose is 45 Gy to whole pelvis, then tumor boost including primary and sacral hollow to 50.4 Gy as above. Then second boost to primary tumor, off small bowel, with additional 10 Gy

Dose limitations (at standard fractionation)
- Small bowel 45–50 Gy
- Femoral head and neck 42 Gy
- Bladder 65 Gy
- Rectum 60 Gy

RADIATION TECHNIQUES: COLON CANCER
- No clear evidence of survival benefit with RT. However, RT may be useful in the setting of node-negative disease with close/+ microscopic margins at the primary site, where a target can be clearly demarcated. If RT is included in treatment regimen, field should include margin around tumor bed based on pre-op imaging and/or surgical clips
- Dose 45–50 Gy in 25–28 fx

COMPLICATIONS
- Potential side effects include diarrhea, dysuria, fatigue, skin irritation, and hematologic toxicity. Long-term GI complications include change in bowel habits, rectal urgency, diarrhea, small bowel obstruction
- Check weekly CBC and skin reaction on treatment

FOLLOW-UP
- H + P, CEA every 3 mo × 2 yrs, then every 6 mo × 5 yrs
- Consider CT scan if high risk of recurrence approximately every 4–6 mo. Recurrence commonly occurs within 2 yrs after initial therapy. However, late failures even beyond 5 yrs have been noted after local excision
- Colonoscopy in 1 yr, then every 2–3 yrs if negative

REFERENCES
Andre T, Boni C, Mounedii-Boudiaf L, et al. Oxaliplatin, fluorouracil, and leucovorin as adjuvant treatment for colon cancer. N Engl J Med 2004;350:2343–2351.

Gunderson LL, Sargent DJ, Tepper JE, et al. Impact of T and N stage and treatment on survival and relapse in adjuvant rectal cancer: A pooled analysis. J Clin Oncol 2004;22:1785–1796.

Janjan NA, Delclos ME, Ballo MT, et al. The colon and rectum. In: Cox JD, Ang KK, editors. Radiation Oncology: Rationale, Technique, Results. 8th ed. St. Louis: Mosby; 2003. pp. 497–536.

Kapiteijn E, Marijnen CAM, Nagtegaal ID, et al. Preoperative radiotherapy combined with total mesorectal excision for resectable rectal cancer. N Engl J Med 2001;345:638–646.

Martenson Jr JA, Willet CG, Sargent DJ, et al. Phase III study of adjuvant chemotherapy and radiation therapy compared with chemotherapy alone in the surgical adjuvant treatment of colon cancer: results of Intergroup protocol 0130. J Clin Oncol 2004;22:3277–3283.

Minsky BD. Cancer of the colon. In: Leibel SA, Phillips TL, editors. Textbook of Radiation Oncology. 2nd ed. Philadelphia: Saunders; 2004. pp. 885–895.

Minsky BD. Cancer of the rectum. In: Leibel SA, Phillips TL, editors. Textbook of Radiation Oncology. 2nd ed. Philadelphia: Saunders; 2004. pp. 897–912.

Moertel CG, Fleming TR, Macdonald JS, et al. Levamisole and fluorouracil for adjuvant therapy of resected colon carcinoma. N Engl J Med 1990;322:352–358.

Myerson RJ. Colon and rectum. In: Perez CA, Brady LW, Halperin EC, et al., editors. Principles and Practice of Radiation Oncology. 4th ed. Philadelphia: Lippincott Williams & Wilkins; 2004. pp. 1607–1629.

National Comprehensive Cancer Network. Clinical Practice Guidelines in Oncology: Colon Cancer. Available at: http://www.nccn.org/professionals/physician_gls/PDF/colon.pdf. Accessed on January 18, 2005.

National Comprehensive Cancer Network. Clinical Practice Guidelines in Oncology: Rectal Cancer. Available at: http://www.nccn.org/professionals/physician_gls/PDF/rectal.pdf. Accessed on January 24, 2005.

O'Connell MJ, Martenson JA, Wieand HS, et al. Improving adjuvant therapy for rectal cancer by combining protracted-infusion fluorouracil with radiation therapy after curative surgery. N Engl J Med 1994;331:502–507.

Pahlman L, Glimelius B, et al. Improved survival with preoperative radiotherapy in resectable rectal cancer: Swedish Rectal Cancer Trial. N Engl J Med 1997;336:980–987.

Russell AH, Harris J, Rosenberg PJ, et al. Anal sphincter conservation for patients with adenocarcinoma of the distal rectum: long term results of Radiation Therapy Oncology Group Protocol 89-02. Int J Radiat Oncol Biol Phys 2000;46:313–322.

Sauer R, Becker H, Hohenberger W, et al. Preoperative versus postoperative chemoradiotherapy for rectal cancer. N Engl J Med 2004;351:1731–1740.

Tepper JE, O'Connell M, Niedzwiecki D, et al. Adjuvant therapy in rectal cancer: analysis of stage, sex, and local control – final report of Intergroup 0114. J Clin Oncol 2002;20:1744–1750.

Tepper JE, O'Connell MJ, Petroni GR, et al. Adjuvant postoperative fluorouracil-modulated chemotherapy combined with pelvic radiation therapy for rectal cancer: initial results of Intergroup 0114. J Clin Oncol 1997;15:2030–2039.

Thomas PR, Lindblad AS. Adjuvant postoperative radiotherapy and chemotherapy in rectal carcinoma: a review of the Gastrointestinal Tumor Study Group experience. Radiother Oncol 1988;13:245–252.

Twelves C, Wong A, Nowacki MP, et al. Capecitabine as adjuvant treatment for stage III colon cancer. N Engl J Med 2005;352: 2696–2704.

Chapter 22
Anal Cancer

Amy Gillis

PEARLS

- 3900 new cases in 2002
- Majority are SCC (75–80%), others are adenocarcinoma or melanoma
- HPV: strongly associated with SCC, may be requisite for disease formation. High grade intraepithelial lesions are precursors. In particular HPV-16, 18 as in cervical cancer
- AIDS is associated with anal cancer, likely through an association with immunodeficiency in the setting of HPV co-infection. Increased risk if CD4 <200
- Additional risk factors: >10 sexual partners, history of anal warts, history of anal intercourse <age 30 or with multiple partners, history of STDs
- Anatomy: anal canal is 3–4 cm long. Extends from anal verge to the dentate line. Anal margin is 5 cm ring on skin around the anus. Use CT to measure depth of femoral vessels for inguinal node location: large variations exist (Koh, *IJROBP* 1993)
- Anal margin tumors: may behave like skin cancers, and can be treated as skin cancer as long as there is no involvement of the anal sphincter, tumor <2 cm, moderately or well differentiated
- Adenocarcinoma: higher local and distant recurrence rates with chemo-RT compared to SCC. Use 5-FU chemo-RT pre-op followed by APR. (Papagikos, *IJROBP* 2003)
- Lymph node drainage: superiorly (above dentate line) along hemorrhoidal vessels to perirectal and internal iliac

Special acknowledgement: We thank Richard M. Krieg, M.D. for his valuable advice in the preparation of this chapter.

nodes; inferior canal (below dentate line) & anal verge to inguinal nodes
- <u>Presentation</u>: bleeding, anal discomfort, pruritis, rectal urgency

WORKUP
- H&P. Note anal sphincter tone
- Labs: CBC, HIV test if any risk factors
- Proctoscopy with biopsy
- May biopsy inguinal nodes if clinically suspicious. Only FNA, avoid open biopsy
- CXR. CT abdomen and pelvis or MRI
- Transanal ultrasound (considered optional, but may be helpful to visualize perirectal nodes)

STAGING

<u>Primary Tumor (T)</u>

TX:	Primary tumor cannot be assessed
T0:	No evidence of primary tumor
Tis:	Carcinoma *in situ*
T1:	Tumor 2 cm or less in greatest dimension
T2:	Tumor more than 2 cm but not more than 5 cm in greatest dimension
T3:	Tumor more than 5 cm in greatest dimension
T4:	Tumor of any size invades adjacent organ(s), e.g., vagina, urethra, bladder*

Note: Direct invasion of the rectal wall, perirectal skin, subcutaneous tissue, or the sphincter muscle(s) is not classified as T4.

<u>Regional Lymph Nodes (N)</u>

NX:	Regional lymph nodes cannot be assessed
N0:	No regional lymph node metastasis
N1:	Metastasis in perirectal lymph node(s)
N2:	Metastasis in unilateral internal iliac and/or inguinal lymph node(s)
N3:	Metastasis in perirectal and inguinal lymph nodes, and/or bilateral internal iliac and/or inguinal lymph nodes

<u>Distant Metastasis (M)</u>

MX:	Distant metastasis cannot be assessed
M0:	No distant metastasis
M1:	Distant metastasis

Stage Grouping	~5 yr survival	~Local Failure rates by T stage (Peiffert, *Int J Radiat Oncol Biol Phys* 1997)
0: TisN0M0		
I: T1N0M0	I: 90–95%	T1: 11%
II: T2-3N0M0	II: 70–80%	T2: 24%
IIIA: T1-3N1M0, T4N0M0	IIIA: 40–50%	T3: 45%
		T4: 45%
IIIB: T4N1M0, Any T N2-3M0	IIIB: 40–50%	
IV: Any T any N M1	IV: 10%	

Used with the permission of the American Joint Committee on Cancer (AJCC), Chicago, Illinois. The original source for this material is the AJCC Cancer Staging Manual, Sixth Edition (2002) published by Springer-Verlag New York, www.springeronline.com.

TREATMENT RECOMMENDATIONS

Situation	Recommended Treatment
T1, small, well differentiated	Local excision ■ Consider only if small, <2 cm, well-differentiated and superficially invasive, negative margins on excision ■ Not to be used if sphincter involved or if >40% of circumference (would cause loss of continence, so use chemo-RT) ■ Consider only in very compliant pts as close follow up is needed. Better if anal dysplasia clinic available for close follow-up ■ With proper selection, control >90% ■ [Boman, *Cancer* 1984. Greenall, *Br J Surg* 1985]
I-III	Concurrent chemo-RT ■ CR ~50–90% depending on stage ■ Colostomy for salvage
IV	Individualized treatment depending on case
Salvage, or if prior pelvic RT	APR – salvage rate after chemo-RT failure is ~50%

TRIALS

Chemo-RT vs RT

- UKCCCR (*Lancet* 1996). 585 pts. RT: 45 Gy + boost (15 Gy EBRT or 25 Gy brachy) +/– 5-FU + mitomycin. 6 wk break in RT. Chemo-RT improved 3 yr LC (59% vs 36%) but no significant change in 3 yr OS (65% vs 58%). Poorer results with RT alone may be due to mandatory 6 wk break
- EORTC (Bartelink, *JCO* 1997). 110 pts. T3-4N0-3 or T1-2N1-3. RT (45 Gy + 15–20 Gy boost) + concurrent chemo (bolus 5-FU + mitomycin) vs RT alone. 6 wk break in RT, prior to boost. Chemo-RT improved CR rate (80% vs 54%), 5 yr LC (68% vs 50%), colostomy free survival (72% vs 40%), & PFS (61% vs 43%). No difference in OS (57% vs 52%). Poorer results with RT alone may again be due to mandatory 6 wk break
- RTOG 87-04 (Flam, *JCO* 1996). 291 pts. 45 Gy + 5-FU +/– mitomycin. If no CR at 6 weeks, gave 9 Gy boost + 5-FU/cisplatin. 5-FU given bolus × 4 d starting d1, d29 (1000 mg/m^2/d). Mitomycin given as 10 mg/m^2 bolus d1, d29. Mitomycin improved CR rate (92% vs 85%) & decreased 4 yr colostomy rate (9% vs 22%). No difference in 4 yr OS (75% vs 70%)
- RTOG 92-08 (John, *Cancer J Sci Am* 1996). Dose escalation, phase II. 5-FU + mitomycin + 59.6 Gy. 2 week break included. Closed early. Colostomy rate at 2 years: 30%. Higher colostomy rate may be due to 2 week break.

Role of cisplatin

- Cisplatin has been tested in phase II trials with 5-FU & RT (Martenson, *IJROBP* 1996). However, no published randomized data available directly comparing cisplatin vs mitomycin combined with 5-FU & RT

HIV

- Hoffman (*IJROBP* 1999). 17 HIV + pts. 9 had CD4 ≥200: no hospitalization or colostomy. 8 had CD4 <200: 4 hospitalized, 4 colostomies

Neo-adjuvant chemo

- Consider for advanced disease, T3-T4, often with 5-FU/cisplatin (CALGB 9281)
- Consider for pts with abscess or fistula
- Currently under study (RTOG 98-11)

Brachytherapy

- Higher complication rates. Not frequently used in North America due to risk of necrosis. 6% complication requiring surgery (Ng, *IJROBP* 1988). Rates of necrosis in the range of 7–15% (Sandhu, *IJROBP* 1998, Gerard *Radiother Oncol* 1998)

Posttreatment biopsy

- Cummings (*IJROBP* 1991). No benefit to routine re-biopsy at 6 weeks post chemo-RT. Continued regression of tumor for up to 12 mo, mean time to regression 3 mo
- Follow pts clinically. Biopsy for clinically suspicious lesions

Salvage APR

- Ellenhorn (*Ann Surg Oncol* 1994). Retrospective review of 38 pts treated with RT + 5-FU + mitomycin. Overall, 5 yr OS was 44% when salvage APR used for chemo-RT failure

RADIATION TECHNIQUES
General points

- No randomized data of chemo-RT vs surgery alone, but chemo-RT produces better survival with sphincter preservation as compared to historical controls
- Chemotherapy is concurrent 5-FU/cisplatin or 5-FU/mitomycin
- Plan to treat inguinal nodes
- Minimize breaks (try to keep under 2 weeks)
- HIV + patients with CD4 <200
  a. Smaller field: superior border of initial pelvic field is usually the bottom of SI joints
  b. Increased morbidity (Hoffman, *IJROBP* 1999)
  c. Final tumor dose may need to be decreased to 50 Gy
- IMRT is currently being investigated for use in anal cancer

UCSF Field design A

Used for smaller lesions, ≤3 cm, below dentate line, & clinical/radiologic N0 (and therefore low risk for iliac nodes)

SIMULATION

- Simulate patient prone with arms up
- Anal marker in place

- Wire posterior skin surface of buttocks
- Wire inguinal node regions
- If possible, treat with full bladder to minimize small bowel toxicity
- Inguinal nodes are treated in the exit beam of the PA field and boosted with an anterior electron field (with patient in supine position). This technique decreases the dose to anterior structures (genitals and bladder)
- Pelvis, PA field: 6 MV. Superior border = bottom of SI joints. Inferior border = 3 cm below tumor or anal verge (choose that which is more inferior). Lateral border = include inguinal nodes in exit beam (to edge of greater trochanter)
- Pelvis, lateral fields: 18 MV. Superior & inferior borders = same as above. Posterior border = minimum 3 cm around tumor and to include sacrum/coccyx. Use posterior skin surface wire as guide to avoid flashing the buttock skin if clinically possible. Anterior border = Minimum 3 cm margin on anterior border of tumor
- Electron boost to inguinal nodes: Reposition pt in the supine position & use anterior fields. Electron energy depends on node depth. 5% IDL of anterior electron fields should not overlap the anterior border of the lateral field. If there is an overlap, use Field Design B (below).
- Final photon boost to primary: Pt treated prone. Small bowel contrast used to ensure that if there is small bowel in the field, tolerance is not exceeded. Single PA field over the primary anal lesion only. Energy depends on the depth of the primary tumor. Margins are 3 cm around primary tumor

Dose prescriptions
- Use 1.8 Gy/fx. Pelvis (PA + laterals) to 36 Gy.
- Electron boost to bring inguinal nodes to total 36 Gy. Must take into account exit dose from PA field into inguinal nodes
- At 36 Gy, use final photon PA boost to bring total tumor dose to 55–60 Gy. If only microscopic disease in primary area, treat to 50 Gy

UCSF Field design B
Used for larger lesions >3 cm, lesions at or above the dentate line, or clinical/radiographic N+ (iliac and inguinal nodes at risk)

Simulation

- Patient supine, alpha cradle
- Anal marker in place
- Wire inguinal node regions, & wire nodes if palpable
- If possible, treat with full bladder to minimize small bowel toxicity
- Tip of penis aimed cranially at all times to avoid bolus effect over scrotum
- <u>Whole pelvis, AP field</u>: 18 MV. Superior border = L5/S1. Inferior border = 3 cm below tumor or anal verge (choose that which is more inferior). Lateral border = include inguinal nodes (to edge of greater trochanter). 1 cm bolus over inguinal regions
- <u>Whole pelvis, PA field</u>: 6 MV. Borders as above
- <u>Lateral boost field</u>: re-simulate in the prone position. Small bowel contrast to ensure that if there is small bowel in field, small bowel tolerance is not exceeded. Anal marker, rectal marker. Wire inguinal regions, to ensure that anterior border does not overlap with the

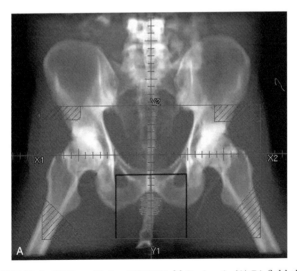

FIGURE 22.1. DRRs utilizing UCSF Field Design A. (A) PA field shown in blue, to 36 Gy. Final PA photon boost to primary shown by black line, to total tumor dose of 55–60 Gy (B) Electron boost fields performed in supine position, shown in red (C) Lateral fields. Arrow shows inguinal wires. It is critical to ensure there is no overlap between electron exit beam and anterior border of lateral photon field.

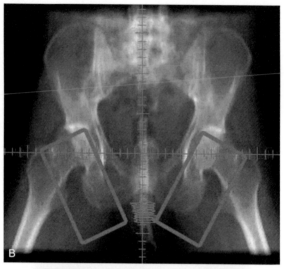

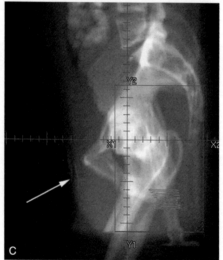

FIGURE 22.1. (b) (c) (*Continued*)

anterior electron field if inguinal nodes need boost. 18 MV opposed laterals. Margins are 2–3 cm around primary tumor

■ <u>Electron boost to inguinal nodes</u>: boost inguinal nodes with electrons if clinically positive. This is done while the patient is receiving lateral boost, but flip to the supine position. 5% IDL of anterior electron field should not overlap with anterior border of lateral field

Dose Prescriptions

■ Use 1.8 Gy/fx. Treat whole pelvis (AP/PA) with superior border at L5/S1 to 30.6 Gy, then drop superior border to bottom of SI joints, & take to 36 Gy

■ Then, use lateral boost to give dose to primary tumor 55–60 Gy. If only microscopic disease in primary area, treat to 50 Gy

■ Tumor dose is measured at midplane on lateral fields, but is measured at the posterior exit for AP/PA fields (because the anus is not at midplane)

■ If clinical/radiographic N+, use electrons to boost inguinal nodes beyond 36 Gy, to 50–60 Gy

RTOG Technique

■ Initial large field (all pts) treated AP/PA 1.8/30.6 Gy. Borders: Superior = L5/S1. Inferior = 2.5 cm margin on anus & tumor. Lateral (AP field) = includes lateral inguinal nodes. Lateral (PA field) = 2 cm lateral to greater sciatic notch. Supplementary RT delivered to inguinal nodes with anterior electron fields matched with exit of PA field

■ Reduced field #1 (all pts) drops AP/PA superior border to inferior border of sacroiliac joints and is treated 1.8/14.4 Gy (total 45 Gy). If N0, field reduced off inguinal nodes after 36 Gy

■ Reduced field #2 (for T3–T4, N+, & T2 lesions with residual disease after 45 Gy). Boost original tumor plus 2–2.5 cm margin 2/10–14 Gy (total 55–59 Gy) using either a multi-field technique or a direct photon or electron perineal field. Involved pelvic LN should be included if small bowel can be avoided. Involved inguinal LN also boosted with 2–2.5 cm margin 2/10–14 Gy (total 55–59 Gy) with electrons

■ For further details see http://www.rtog.org/members/protocols/98-11/9811.pdf

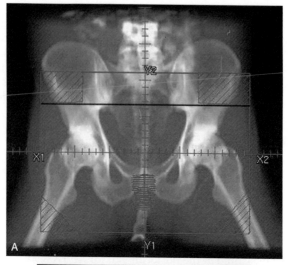

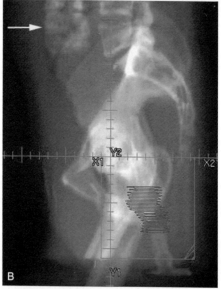

FIGURE 22.2. DRRs utiliazing UCSF Field Design B. (A) AP/PA fields with conedown at 30.6 Gy (black line) to 36 Gy. (B) Lateral boost field. Arrow depicts small bowel contrast.

Dose limitations
- Small bowel: 45–50 Gy

COMPLICATIONS
- Acute complications: skin reaction/desquamation, leukopenia, thrombocytopenia, proctitis, diarrhea, cystitis
- Subacute and late complications include chronic diarrhea, rectal urgency, sterility, impotence, vaginal dryness, vaginal fibrosis, and possibly decreased testosterone

FOLLOW-UP
- H&P and anoscopy every 6 wks until CR, then every 3 mo for 1st yr , every 4 mo for 2nd yr , every 6 mo for 3rd yr , then annually
- On exam if mass increases in size, or new clinical symptoms develop (pain, bleeding, incontinence) → biopsy. If + → salvage APR
- If tumor decreasing in size, continue to follow. Median time to regression ~3 mo, but may take 12 mo
- Most recurrences occur within 2 yrs. Most are at primary site

REFERENCES

Radiation Therapy Oncology Group. RTOG 98-11. A phase III randomized study of 5-fluorouracil, mitomycin-C, and radiotherapy versus 5-fluorouracil, cisplatin and radiotherapy in carcinoma of the anal canal. Available at http://www.rtog.org/members/protocols/98-11/9811.pdf. Accessed on May 3, 2006.

Bartelink H, Roelofsen F, et al. Concomitant radiotherapy and chemotherapy is superior to radiotherapy alone in the treatment of locally advanced anal cancer: results of a phase III randomized trial of the European Organization for Research and Treatment of Cancer Radiotherapy and Gastrointestinal Cooperative Groups. *J Clin Oncol* 1997;15:2040–2049.

Boman BM, Moertel CG, et al. Carcinoma of the anal canal. A clinical and pathological study of 188 cases. *Cancer* 1984;54:114–125.

Chao KC, Perez CA, Brady LW, editors. Radiation Oncology Management Decisions. 2nd ed. Philadelphia: Lippincott Williams & Wilkins; 2002. pp. 407–417.

Cummings BJ, Keane TJ, O'Sullivan B, et al. Epidermoid anal cancer: treatment by radiation alone or by radiation and 5-fluorouracil with and without mitomycin-c. *Int J Radiat Oncol Biol Phys* 1991; 21(5):1115–1125.

Ellenhorn JDI, Enker WE, Quan SH. Salvage Abdominoperineal resection following combined chemotherapy and radiotherapy for epidermoid carcinoma of the anus. *Ann Surg Oncol* 1994;1:105–110.

Flam M, Madhu J, et al. Role of mitomycin in combination with fluoro-uracil and radiotherapy, and of salvage chemoradiation in the definitive nonsurgical treatment of epidermoid carcinoma of the anal canal: results of a phase III randomized intergroup study. *J Clin Oncol* 1996;14:2527–2539.

Gerard JP, Ayzac L, et al. Treatment of anal canal carcinoma with high dose radiation therapy and concomitant fluorouracil-cisplatinum. Long-term results in 95 patients. *Radiother Oncol* 1998;46(3): 249–256.

Greenall MJ, Quan HQ, Decosse JJ. Epidermoid cancer of the anus. *Br J Surg* 1985;72:S97.

Hoffman R, Welton ML, et al. The significance of pretreatment CD4 count on the outcome and treatment tolerance of HIV-positive patients with anal cancer. 1999;44:127–131.

Janjan NA, Ballo MT, et al. The anal region. In: Cox JD, Ang KK, editors. Radiation Oncology: Rationale, Technique, Results. 8th ed. St. Louis: Mosby; 2003. pp. 537–556.

John M, Pajak T, et al. Dose escalation in chemoradiation for anal cancer: preliminary results of RTOG 92-08. *Cancer J Sci Am* 1996;2(4):205.

Koh WJ, Chiu M, Stelzer KJ, et al. Femoral vessel depth and the implications for groin node radiation. *Int J Radiat Oncol Biol Phys* 1993;27:969–974.

Martenson JA, Lipsitz SR, et al. Initial results of a phase II trial of high dose radiation therapy, 5-fluorouracil, and cisplatin for patients with anal cancer (E4292): an Eastern Cooperative Oncology Group study. *Int J Radiat Oncol Biol Phys* 1996;35(4):745–749.

Minsky BD. Cancer of the Anal Canal. In: Leibel SA, Phillips TL, editors. Textbook of Radiation Oncology. 2nd ed. Philadelphia: Saunders; 2004. pp. 913–922.

Ng Ying Kin NY, Pigneux J, et al. Our experience of conservative treatment of anal canal carcinoma combining external irradiation and interstitial implants. *Int J Radiat Oncol Biol Phys* 1988;14:253–259.

Papagikos M, Crane CH, et al. Chemoradiation for adenocarcinoma of the anus. *Int J Radiat Oncol Biol Phys* 2003;55:669–678.

Papillon J, Montbarbon JF. Epidermoid carcinoma of the anal canal. A Series of 276 cases. *Dis Colon Rectum* 1987;30:324–333.

Peiffert D, Bey P, Pernot M, et al. Conservative treatment by irradiation of epidermoid carcinomas of the anal margin. *Int J Radiat Oncol Biol Phys* 1997;39:57–66.

Sandhu APS, Symonds RP, et al. Interstitial Iridium-192 implantation combined with external radiotherapy in anal cancer: ten years experience. *Int J Radiat Oncol Biol Phys* 1998;40:575–581.

UKCCCR Anal Cancer Trial Working Party. Epidermoid anal cancer: results from the UKCCCR randomized trial of radiotherapy alone versus radiotherapy, 5-fluorouracil, and mitomycin. *Lancet* 1996; 348:1049–1054.

NOTES

Chapter 23
Renal Cell Carcinoma

James Rembert and Alexander R. Gottschalk

PEARLS

- 3% all new cancers diagnosed in U.S. (31,900 new cases 2003)
- Steady increase in incidence not explained by incidental diagnoses (~7% of cases) made from increased diagnostic imaging
- M:F 1.5:1
- Most common in 4th to 6th decades, peak incidence 6th decade
- 95% diagnoses made with imaging – characteristic solid, hypervascular mass
- Metastatic disease in 30% at diagnosis, and eventually in 50% (lung, liver, bone, distant LN, adrenal, brain, opposite kidney, soft tissue)
- Stage at diagnosis is the most important prognostic factor
- Predominant histologic type: adenocarcinoma arising from tubular epithelium
- Variants: clear cell (85%), granular, sarcomatoid (1–6%; poor prognosis)
- Risk factors: urban environmental toxins (cadmium/asbestos/petrols), tobacco, obesity, high dietary fat intake, acquired cystic renal disease from renal failure (premalignant condition with 4–9% incidence RCC; US surveillance q 2 yrs)
- von Hippel-Lindau disease: autosomal dominant, loss 3p, >70% chance developing RCC (almost all clear cell histology), also associated with multiple other benign & malignant tumors (retinal angiomas, CNS hemangioblastomas, pheochromocytoma, pancreatic cancer)
- Two large cancer database studies suggest association with lymphoma

- RCC has low response rates to traditional chemotherapy (~6–7%); response rates to immunotherapy (IL-2, interferon alpha) slightly higher (~10–15%)

WORKUP

- H&P
  - Common signs and symptoms: hematuria (60%), flank pain (45%), flank mass (40%), classic triad of prior three only present in 10%, normocytic/normochromic anemia, fever, weight loss
  - Less common signs and symptoms: hepatic dysfunction without mets, polycythemia, hypercalcemia (occurs in 25% of patients with RCC mets)
- Labs: CBC, LFT, BUN/Cr, LDH, urinalysis
- Imaging: CT abdomen. MRI abdomen if CT suggests IVC involvement
- Metastatic evaluation: CXR. Bone scan or MRI brain only if clinically indicated

STAGING (AJCC 6TH EDITION, 2002)

Primary tumor

TX:	Primary tumor cannot be assessed
T0:	No evidence of primary tumor
T1:	Tumor 7 cm or less in greatest dimension, limited to the kidney
	T1a: Tumor 4 cm of less in greatest dimension, limited to the kidney
	T1b: Tumor more than 4 cm but not more than 7 cm in greatest dimension, limited to the kidney
T2:	Tumor more than 7 cm, limited to the kidney
T3:	Tumor extends into major veins or invades adrenal gland or perirenal and/or renal sinus fat but not beyond Gerota's fascia
	T3a: Tumor directly invades adrenal gland or perirenal and/or renal sinus fat but not beyond Gerota's fascia
	T3b: Tumor grossly extends into the renal vein or its segmental (muscle-containing) branches, or vena cava below the diaphragm
	T3c: Tumor grossly extends into vena cava above diaphragm or invades the wall of the vena cava
T4:	Tumor invades beyond Gerota's fascia

Regional lymph nodes*

NX:	Regional lymph nodes cannot be assessed
N0:	No regional lymph node metastasis
N1:	Metastases in a single regional lymph node

N2: Metastasis in more than one regional lymph node

*Laterality does not affect the N classification

Regional lymph nodes: renal hilar, paracaval, aortic (para-aortic, peri-aortic, lateral aortic), Retroperitoneal NOS

Note: If a lymph node dissection is performed, then pathologic evaluation would ordinarily include at least eight nodes.

Distant metastasis
MX: Distant metastasis cannot be assessed
M0: No distant metastasis
M1: Distant metastasis

Stage Grouping		~5 yr OS by Stage	
0:	TisN0M0	I:	~85–90%
I:	T1N0M0	II:	~65–85%
II:	T2N0M0	III:	~40–60%%
III:	T3N0M0, T1-3N1M0	IV:	~30% if only 1 metastatic site <10% if> 1 metastatic site
IV:	T4N0-1M0, AnyTN2M0 Any M1		

Staging portion of the above table used with the permission of the American Joint Committee on Cancer (AJCC), Chicago, Illinois. The original source for this material is the AJCC Cancer Staging Manual, Sixth Edition (2002) published by Springer-Verlag New York, www.springeronline.com.

TREATMENT RECOMMENDATIONS

Stage	Recommended Treatment
I-III	Nephrectomy ■ Open radical nephrectomy, but laparoscopic gaining popularity. Nephron sparing surgery via partial nephrectomy, if possible (open or laparoscopic) ■ Possible to spare adrenal gland in ~75% cases No role for adjuvant chemo/immunotherapy No widely accepted role for adjuvant radiotherapy. Retrospective data suggests possible utility in select cases: ■ Positive surgical margins

Stage	Recommended Treatment
	■ Locally advanced disease with perinephric fat invasion & adrenal invasion (IVC/ renal vein extension alone does not increase local recurrence significantly) ■ LN+ ■ Unresectable (pre-op RT)

IV	1) *Cytoreductive nephrectomy,* Improved survival with nephrectomy followed by interferon alpha vs interferon alpha alone
	(Flanigan et al. *NEJM* 345:1655–1659, 2001)
	2) *Systemic therapy*
	■ Clinical trial (if available)
	■ Immunotherapy (IL-2, interferon alpha, or combination)
	  ■ High-dose IL-2 only FDA approved treatment for stage IV RCC
	■ As second line, after immunotherapy consider chemo or biologic agent
	  ■ Gemcitabine +/– 5-FU or capecitabine
	  ■ Bevacizumab
	3) *Focal palliation of metastases*
	■ RT alone
	■ Metastasectomy
	■ Combination of both

TRIALS

■ Two prospective randomized trials (Finney, *Br J Urol* 1973; Kjaer, *IJROBP* 1987) showed no benefit to adjuvant radiotherapy, yet these trials did not select a patient population that was likely to benefit from adjuvant RT. LR in radical nephrectomy series is ~5%. These excellent results are driven mainly by completely resected stage I/ II tumors. However, with incomplete resection or +LN, LR rises dramatically to ~20–30%, suggesting a role for adjuvant RT in these patients. The following two studies, retrospectively, analyze patients at high risk for local recurrence and support a role for adjuvant RT in select patients

- <u>Kao</u> (*Radiology* 1994). Retrospective, 12 consecutive patients with locally advanced RCC (perinephric invasion or +margins) who received adjuvant RT 41-63 Gy (1.8–2 Gy fx) – 100% 5 yr LC, with 5 yr actuarial DFS 75% compared with 30% in 12 consecutive patients of similar stage treated with surgery alone
- <u>Stein</u> (*Radiother Oncol* 1992). Retrospective, 147 pts, post-op RT median 46 Gy, given to 56 patients, in the T3N0 patients LR 10% (4/37) vs 37% (11/30) favoring adjuvant RT. Also, 3/19 recurrences at the scar

RADIATION TECHNIQUES: SIMULATION AND FIELD DESIGN
Primary site

- Supine, arms-up to allow visualization of lateral isocenter marks, immobilize with wing-board or alpha cradle, wire scar, planning CT scan
- <u>Volume:</u> nephrectomy bed, (involved kidney if pre-op), lymph-node drainage sites, surgical clips; scar failures reported [Stein], so if not possible to include scar in treatment volume treat it with electrons to full dose

Metastatic site (non-CNS)

- Proper immobilization depending on site, planning CT if 3DRT needed to spare normal tissue
- <u>Volume:</u> focal treatment of metastasis with 2–3 cm margin
- Chapter 40 for management of CNS metastases

Dose prescriptions

- Pre-op: 40–50 Gy (1.8–2 Gy/fx)
- Post-op: 45–50 Gy with 10–15 Gy boost to micro/gross disease; total 50–60 Gy
- Metastases: 45–50 Gy in 3–4.5 wks

Dose limitations

- Contralateral kidney: limit to ≤20 Gy in 2–3 wks
- Liver: limit to <30% receiving >36–40 Gy
- Spinal cord: <45 Gy
- Small bowel: <40 Gy

FOLLOW-UP (NCCN 2005 RECOMMENDATIONS)

- Stage I-II: Every 6 mo × 2 yrs then every 1 yr × 5 yrs – H&P, CXR, Labs w/LDH; CT abdomen/pelvis at 4–6 mo then as indicated
- Stage III: Every 4 mo × 2 yrs then every 6 mo × 3 yrs, then every 1 yr – H&P, CXR, Labs with LDH; CT abdomen/pelvis at 4–6 mo then every 1 yr

REFERENCES

Buskirk SJ, Smalley SR, Zincke H. Kidney and ureteral carcinoma. In: Gunderson L, Tepper J, editors. Clinical Radiation Oncology. 1st ed. Philadelphia: Churchill Livingstone; 2000. pp. 863–878.

Finney R. The value of radiotherapy in the treatment of hypernephroma – a clinical trial. Br J Urol 1973;45(3):258–269.

Flanigan RC, Salmon SE, Blumenstein BA, et al. Nephrectomy followed by interferon alfa-2b compared with interferon alfa-2b alone for metastatic renal-cell cancer. N Engl J Med 2001;345(23):1655–1659.

Greene FL. American Joint Committee on Cancer, American Cancer Society. AJCC Cancer Staging Manual. 6th ed. New York: Springer-Verlag; 2002.

Kao GD, Malkowicz SB, Whittington R, et al. Locall advanced renal cell carcinoma: low complication rate and efficacy of postnephrectomy planned with CT. Radiology 1994;193(3):725–730.

Kjaer M, Frederiksen PL, Engelholm SA. Postoperative radiotherapy in stage II and III renal adenocarcinoma. A randomized trial by the Copenhagen Renal Cancer Study Group. Int J Radiat Oncol Biol Phys 1987;13(4):665–672.

Michalski JM. Kidney, Renal pelvis, and ureter In: Perez CA, Brady LW, Halperin EC, et al., editors. Principles and Practice of Radiation Oncology. 4th ed. Philadelphia: Lippincott Williams and Wilkins; 2004. pp. 757–775.

National Comprehensive Cancer Network. Clinical Practice Guidelines in Oncology: Kidney Cancer. Available at: http://www.nccn.org/professionals/physician_gls/PDF/kidney.pdf. Accessed on January 1, 2005.

Redman BG, Kawachi M, Hurwitz M. Urothelial and kidney cancers. In: Pazdur R, Coia L, Hoskins W, Wagman L, editors. Cancer Management: A Multidisciplinary Approach. 8th ed. New York: CMP Healthcare Media; 2004. pp. 403–418.

Schefter T, Rabinovitch R. Cancer of the Kidney In: Leibel SA, Phillips TL, editors. Textbook of Radiation Oncology. 2nd ed. Philadelphia: Saunders; 2004. pp. 923–938.

Stein M, Kuten A, Halpern J, et al. The value of postoperative irradiation in renal cell cancer. Radiother Oncol 1992;24(1):41–44.

Chapter 24
Bladder Cancer

Brian Lee and Joycelyn L. Speight

PEARLS

- Risk factors: smoking, napthylamines, benzidines, amino biphenyl, cytoxan exposure. Chronic irritation with bladder stones/foley catheters
- Lymphatics: bladder lymphatics drain via 3 pathways (anterior, posterior, trigone). Anterior/posterior ducts → Internal iliacs + common iliacs; trigone duct → external iliacs
- Tumors tend to be multifocal in nature
- TCC constitutes 93% of cases in U.S. TCC with squamous or glandular features behaves like pure TCC
- SCC constitutes 5% of cases (in Egypt this is the majority due to Schistosoma)
- Adenocarcinoma = 1–2% (most often in urachus)
- Three layers of bladder wall = epithelium/subepithelial connective tissue, muscularis, perivesical fat
- Most common sites = trigone (inferiorly below uretero-vesical junctions), lateral & posterior wall, and bladder neck
- Hematuria (gross or microscopic) = initial presentation for 75% of cases
- Vesical irritation = initial presentation for 25% of cases
- Majority have urinary frequency, urgency, dysuria, microscopic hematuria eventually. Advanced cases – pelvic pain, ureteral obstruction, hydronephrosis, rectal obstruction
- 75% bladder CA cases are Ta, Tis, or T1
- Probability of LN involvement (~20% all cases): pT1 5%, pT2-T3a 30%, pT3b 64%, pT4 50% (Skinner et al.)
- DM = 8% of cases at diagnosis: lung, bone, liver

WORKUP

- Urine cytology: identifies 50–80% of poorly differentiated CA but only 20% of well-differentiated CA
- Cystoscopy & EUA

- TURBT with random biopsies of normal appearing mucosa to exclude CIS. If in trigone, biopsy prostatic urethra
- Labs: CBC, alkaline phosphatase
- CT A/P. Historically, IVP used
- If invasive, then CXR, & bone scan if alkaline phosphatase elevated
- MRI valuable pre-op for depth of invasion, staging

STAGING

Primary tumor		Regional lymph nodes	
TX	Primary tumor cannot be assessed	N1:	Metastasis in single lymph node, 2 cm or less in greatest dimension
T0	No evidence of primary tumor		
Ta:	Non-invasive papillary carcinoma	N2:	Metastasis in single lymph node, more than 2 cm but not more than 5 cm in greatest dimension; or multiple lymph nodes, none more than 5 cm in greatest dimension
Tis:	Carcinoma in situ: "flat tumor"		
T1:	Tumor invades subepithelial connective Tissue		
T2:	Tumor invades muscle		
pT2a:	Tumor invades superficial muscle (inner half)	N3:	Metastasis in a lymph node, more than 5 cm in greatest dimension
pT2b:	Tumor invades deep muscle (outer half)	Metastases	
T3a:	Perivesical tumor, microscopic	MX:	Distant metastasis cannot be assessed
T3b:	Perivesical tumor, macroscopic	MO:	No distant metastasis
T4a:	Invades prostate, uterus, vagina	M1:	Distant metastases
T4b:	Invades pelvic wall, abdominal wall		

Stage Grouping		Survival (5 yr OS)	
0a:	TaN0M0	Ta:	95%
0is:	TisN0M0	T1 (G3):	50–80%
I:	T1N0M0	T2:	Cystectomy = 60–80%, bladder preservervation = 60%
II:	T2aN0M0		
	T2bN0M0		
III:	T3aN0M0	T3b-T4:	Cystectomy = 20–40%, bladder preservervation = 40%
	T3bN0M0		
	T4aN0M0		
IV:	T4bN0M0	pN+:	Cystectomy = 15–30%
	Any T N1 M0		
	Any T N2 M0	M1:	Untreated MS <6 mo, 13 mo with chemo
	Any T N3 M0		
	Any T Any N M1		

Used with the permission of the American Joint Committee on Cancer (AJCC), Chicago, Illinois. The original source for this material is the AJCC Cancer Staging Manual, Sixth Edition (2002) published by Springer-Verlag New York, www.springeronline.com.

TREATMENT RECOMMENDATIONS

Stage	Recommended Treatment
Non-muscle invasive (Ta, Tis, T1)	■ TURBT alone → 30% recurrence ■ Indications for adjuvant treatment: persistent tumor on urine cytology, multifocal, grade II/III, Tis, T1, or subtotal resection ■ TURBT + BCG × 6 wks (other adjuvant options = mitomycin, doxorubicin) ■ Disease persistence 6 mo s/p BCG → use another agent with BCG × 3 wks q 6 mo × 2 yrs ■ Disease persistence >1 yr or multiple recurrences → radical cystectomy (can consider RT but tolerance may be poor secondary to preexisting chronic irritation after multiple resections /intravesical therapy)

Stage	Recommended Treatment
Muscle invasive	■ Treatment options: radical cystectomy, partial cystectomy, or bladder preservation w/chemo-RT ■ Small tumors in the dome without CIS may be treated with partial cystectomy ■ Unifocal T2-T3a, <5 cm, no hydronephrosis or hydroureter, good initial bladder function and visibly complete TURBT → bladder preserving treatment. In general, 5 yr OS = 50–60%; 40–50% of surviving patients have intact functioning bladder. 60% of pts w/CR to chemo-RT remain free of any recurrence including superficial ■ Multifocal T2-T3a, T3b-T4, hydroureter/hydronephrosis, subtotal resection → Radical cystectomy +/− RT ■ T3b-T4 → Consider pre-op chemo; cystectomy + LN dissection + adjuvant chemo
Local recurrence	■ LR s/p cystectomy → cisplatin + RT to 40–45 Gy to true pelvis, 50–54 Gy to sidewall if clinical recurrence, 60–64 Gy to local recurrence ■ 10–20% of pts with CR to chemo-RT develop invasive LR → treat with cystectomy

Treatment	Description
Bladder preservation	■ Maximal TURBT → induction EBRT to 40 Gy with concomitant chemo – 4 wks later cystoscopy with multiple biopsies +/– cytology. ~70–80% of pts have CR. If residual tumor, radical cystectomy. If CR, consolidation EBRT boost to primary (24 Gy) with concomitant chemo → 4 wks later cystoscopy with biopsy. If CR after all RT → adjuvant chemo. If superficial disease persistence → BCG or radical cystectomy. If invasive disease persistence → radical cystectomy
Radical cystectomy	■ En bloc removal of bladder, perivesical tissue, urethra, (prostate, seminal vesicles / uterus, fallopian tubes, ovaries, anterior vaginal wall) ■ Local recurrence after cystectomy = 5–10% for pT2-T3a, but 30–50% w/ T3b-T4 ■ If (+) margins, post-op chemo, or post-op RT + concurrent cisplatin. Problem w/ post-op RT = 20–40% GI complications ■ Pre-op RT unlikely to benefit T2-T3a because low risk of LR & LN, but recommended for T3b-T4 by MD Anderson based on review of 338 pts treated with 2/50 Gy pre-op. 65% down-staging, 40% pCR, 90% LC, 5 yr OS 45%, DM 45%, no change in surgical morbidity ■ Neoadjuvant chemo before cystectomy provides 5% OS advantage @ 5 yrs based on meta-analysis

STUDIES

- No randomized trials of cystectomy vs bladder preservation

Bladder preservation

- NCIC (*JCO* 1996). 99 pts T2-4. (RT alone or pre-op RT) +/– concurrent cisplatin × 3. Concurrent chemo decreased LRF but no change OS
- RTOG 8512 (*IJROBP* 1993). 42 pts T2-T4N0-2. Phase II = WP 2/40 Gy + cisplatin ×2. Restage 2 wks after with cystoscopy, biopsy, EUA, CT. If CR, 2/24 Gy with 3rd cycle cisplatin. No CR = cystectomy. F/U = cystoscopy q 3 mo. Results: 67% CR. 5 yr OS = 52%. All LC = 42%. Invasive only LC = 50%. 5 yr LF = 25%
- RTOG 8802 (*JCO* 1996). 91 pts. Phase II neoadjuvant MCV (methotrexate, cisplatin, vinblastine) then RT + cisplatin same as RTOG 8512. Results: 75% CR, 5 yr OS 62%
- RTOG 8903 (*JCO*, 1998). 123 pts T2-4aNx s/p maximal TURBT. Phase III. Randomized to [neoadjuvant MCV ×2c → concurrent cisplatin ×2c + WP 1.8/39.6 Gy] vs [same but no MCV]. Both, restage 4 wks later with cystoscopy, biopsy, EUA, cytology. If CR, 1.8/25.2 Gy boost (total dose = 64.8 Gy) + cisplatin ×1c. Stopped early due to MCV toxicity (14% died). Results: No significant change in CR, OS or DMFS
- RTOG 9506 (*Oncologist*, 2000). 34 pts T2-T4aNx without hydronephrosis. Phase II = TURBT → WP 3 Gy (bid)/24 Gy + concurrent 5-FU + cisplatin. Re-stage 4 wks later. If CR, 2.5 Gy (bid)/20 Gy + concurrent 5-FU + cisplatin. No CR = cystectomy. Results: 67% CR. 3 yr OS 83%, with intact bladder = 66%. 20% grade 3/4 toxicity. In follow-up, 45% superficial recurrence
- RTOG 9706 (*IJROBP* 2003). 52 pts T2-T4aN0. TURBT → within 6 wks, WP 1.8 Gy qAM + bladder 1.6 Gy qPM × 13 d (= WP 21.6 Gy, bladder 40.8 Gy) + concurrent cisplatin. Re-stage at 4 wks with biopsy & cytology. If CR, bid RT × 8 d (total WP 45.6, bladder 64.8) + concurrent cisplatin. If no CR, cystectomy. All got MCV × 3. Results: similar to 8903 but more toxic. 75% CR. 3 yr OS 61%, with intact bladder 48%. Only 45% of pts completed MCV ×3. 3 yr LRF = 27%, DM = 29%
- MGH (*Urology*, 2002). RTOG 8903 style technique. 190 pts. 6.7 yr follow-up. Results: Only 35% needed cystectomy (including salvage for recurrence). 5 yr OS 54% (T2 = 62%, T3-4a = 47%). 5 yr DSS 63% (T2 = 74%, T3-4a = 53%). 5 yr

DSS with intact bladder 46% (T2 57%, T3-4a 35%). Hydronephrosis not significant

- <u>Meta-analysis of neoadjuvant chemo trials</u> (*Lancet* 2003). Neoadjuvant multiagent cisplatin based chemo gives 5% OS @ 5 yrs. No data to support single agent cisplatin

RADIATION TECHNIQUES
Simulation and field design
- Need CT and bladder map from cystoscopy
- Simulate supine with immobilization and bladder emptied by pt
- Double-contrast cystogram = introduce via Foley typically 25–30 cc radiopaque contrast + 10–15 cc air. May need more contrast to equal PVR volume
- Rectal tube for non-3D simulation. 50 cc rectal barium (for lateral sim films) administered <u>after</u> AP field film
- Planning CT scan
- Whole pelvis AP/PA borders = bottom sacroiliac joint, 2 cm below inferior extent of tumor (or 1.5 cm below obturator foramen), 2 cm lateral to bony pelvis. Block femoral heads (45 Gy)
- Whole pelvis lateral borders = 2 cm anterior to air bubble of bladder (often in front of symphysis), 2.5 cm posterior to bladder or tumor mass, same inferior and superior borders. Block rectum, small bowel
- Treat with empty bladder
- PTV = at least 2 cm around bladder
- Boost volumes = entire bladder or partial bladder. CTV = GTV + 0.5 cm. PTV = CTV + 1.5 cm

Dose prescriptions
- Bladder preservation: 40 Gy with concurrent cisplatin + 24 Gy boost (if CR)
- LR s/p cystectomy → cisplatin + RT to 40–45 Gy to true pelvis, 50–54 Gy to sidewall if clinical recurrence, 60–64 Gy to local recurrence.

Dose limitations
- Whole bladder 50 Gy = 5–10% late grade 3–4 effects
- Whole bladder 60 Gy = 10–40% late grade 3–4 effects
- <1/3 bladder: 60 Gy = 5–10% late effects; 70 Gy = 20%
- 60–70 Gy causes urethral stricture in 5–10% of pts
- Chemo-RT trials = 0–13% late sequelae

COMPLICATIONS

- Urinary tract infection; treat with antibiotic
- Acute bladder spasm. Use terazosin or tamsulosin
- Acute dysuria. Treat with ibuprofen or pyridium
- 75% of late bladder symptoms present within 3 yrs = frequency, dysuria, intermittent hematuria. 70% will resolve within 2–3 yrs
- 5–15% late bowel complications

FOLLOW-UP

- Follow-up with urine cytology & cystoscopy every 3 mo × 1 yr, every 6 mo × 2 yr, then annually. CT abdomen & pelvis every 1–2 yr

REFERENCES

Coppin CM, Gospodarowicz MK, James K, et al. Improved local control of invasive bladder cancer by concurrent cisplatin and preoperative or definitive radiation. The National Cancer Institute of Canada Clinical Trials Group. J Clin Oncol 1996;14:2901–2907.

Hagan MP, Winter KA, Kaufman DS, et al. RTOG 97-06: initial report of a phase I-II trial of selective bladder conservation using TURBT, twice-daily accelerated irradiation sensitized with cisplatin, and adjuvant MCV combination chemotherapy. Int J Radiat Oncol Biol Phys 2003;57:665–672.

Kaufman DS, Winter KA, Shipley WU, et al. The initial results in muscle-invading bladder cancer of RTOG 95-06: phase I/II trial of transurethral surgery plus radiation therapy with concurrent cisplatin and 5-fluorouracil followed by selective bladder preservation or cystectomy depending on the initial response. Oncologist 2000; 5:471–476.

Milosevic MF GM. The urinary bladder. In: Cox JD, Ang KK, editors. Radiation Oncology: Rationale, Technique, Results. 8th ed. St. Louis: Mosby; 2003. pp. 575–602.

Petrovich Z SJ, Jozsef G, Formenti SC. Bladder. In: Perez CA, Brady LW, Halperin ED, Schmidt-Ullrich RK, editors. Principles and Practice of Radiation Oncology. 4th ed. Philadelphia: Lippincott Williams & Wilkins; 2004. pp. 1664–1691.

Shipley WU, Winter KA, Kaufman DS, et al. Phase III trial of neoadjuvant chemotherapy in patients with invasive bladder cancer treated with selective bladder preservation by combined radiation therapy and chemotherapy: initial results of Radiation Therapy Oncology Group 89-03. J Clin Oncol 1998;16:3576–3583.

Shipley WU, Kaufman DS, Zehr E, et al. Selective bladder preservation by combined modality protocol treatment: long-term outcomes of 190 patients with invasive bladder cancer. Urology 2002;60:62–67; discussion 67–68.

Tester W, Porter A, Asbell S, et al. Combined modality program with possible organ preservation for invasive bladder carcinoma: results of RTOG protocol 85-12. Int J Radiat Oncol Biol Phys 1993; 25:783–790.

Tester W, Caplan R, Heaney J, et al. Neoadjuvant combined modality program with selective organ preservation for invasive bladder cancer: results of Radiation Therapy Oncology Group phase II trial 8802. J Clin Oncol 1996;14:119–126.

Zelefsky MJ RJ, Small EJ. Cancer of the bladder. In Leibel SA, Phillips TL, editors. Textbook of Radiation Oncology. 2nd ed. Philadelphia: Saunders; 2004. pp. 939–957.

Chapter 25
Prostate Cancer

Eric K. Hansen and Mack Roach III

PEARLS

■ Prostate cancer is the #1 non-cutaneous cancer in men (~234,000 estimated cases in the U.S. in 2006), & is estimated to be the #3 cause of cancer mortality (~27,350 deaths in 2006) after lung cancer (~90,330 deaths) & colorectal cancer (~27,870 deaths)

■ Median age at diagnosis previously was 72, but with increased screening more younger men are being diagnosed

■ Due to its long natural history, many men may not benefit from treatment if their life expectancy is short (<5–10 yrs) & if they have early-stage, low-grade disease

■ Screening recommendations from the ACS include annual PSA & DRE beginning at age 50 if life expectancy is >10 yrs. Men with a +FH & African Americans may begin screening at 40–45 yrs

■ Risk of finding prostate cancer on biopsy is related to PSA level: ~5-25% for PSA <4, ~15–25% for PSA 4–10, & up to ~50–67% for PSA >10. For PSA <4, a rule-of-thumb is risk of Gleason score (GS) 7–10 prostate cancer is 2× the PSA level

■ Prostate gland consists of the peripheral zone (70% of glandular prostate & site of nearly all cancers), the central zone (25% of the glandular prostate), the transition zone (surrounding the urethra & the site of BPH), & the anterior fibromuscular stroma

■ ~50–80% of tumors involve the prostate apex & ~85% of pts have multifocal disease in the prostate

■ At the apex, the capsule is not well-defined & true ECE is difficult to recognize

■ ECE is most common at the posterior lateral portion of the prostate (associated with regions penetrated by nerves)

■ >95% of prostate cancers are adenocarcinomas

- GS represents the sum of the major and minor glandular patterns (ranging from slight disorganization (1) to anaplastic (5))
- LN drainage is primarily to the internal iliac obturator, external iliac, & presacral nodes, but disease also may spread to perirectal, common iliac, & paraaortic nodes
- Most frequently used prognostic factors are GS, clinical stage, & pretreatment PSA (including PSA velocity, doubling-time, &/or slope)
- The % of + cores is related to risk of recurrence (>50% + cores behaves more aggressively)
- Many risk-stratification schemes exist & they predict for different outcomes (e.g., pathologic stage, bPFS, DFS, OS, etc.). Risk-classification schemes & nomograms are used to help guide treatment decisions. Each have their own advantages & disadvantages. See Table below
- PSA velocity >2 ng/ml in the yr before radical prostatectomy (RP) or EBRT may be associated with increased risk of death from prostate cancer (D'Amico, *NEJM* 2004; D'Amico, *JAMA* 2005)

WORKUP

- H&P (including American Urology Association (AUA) symptom scores, baseline erectile function, bony pain, & DRE)
- Labs include PSA, testosterone, CBC, & LFTs
- TRUS-guided biopsy is used for pathologic diagnosis (>8 separate cores is recommended, & the highest GS is used).
- Bone scan & pelvic CT or MRI are usually ordered for T3-T4 or GS ≥8 or PSA >20
- MR spectroscopy shows decreased citrate & increased choline with prostate cancer, but its role in routine management has not been studied
- Prostascint (an In-111 labeled monoclonal Ab) has limited sensitivity (60–70%), but may be useful for staging high-risk disease, nodes, and/or sites of recurrence

STAGING

Primary tumor (Clinical)	Regional lymph nodes
TX: Primary tumor cannot be assessed	NX: Regional lymph nodes were not assessed
T0: No evidenct of primary tumor	N0: No regional lymph node metastasis
T1: Clinically inapparent tumor neither palpable nor visible on imaging	N1: Regional lymph node metastasis
T1a: Tumor incidental histologic finding in 5% or less of tissue resected	Metastases MX: Distant metastasis cannot be assessed (not evaluated by any modality)
T1b: Tumor incidental histologic finding in more than 5% of tissue resected	M0: No distant metastasis M1: Distant metastasis M1a: Non-regional lymph node(s)
T1c: Tumor identified by needle biopsy (e.g., because of elevated PSA)	M1b: Bone(s) M1c: Other site(s) with or without bone disease
T2: Tumor confined within the prostate	Grade
T2a: Tumor involves $^1/_2$ of one lobe or less	GX: Grade cannot be assessed G1: Well-differentiated (slight anaplasia, Gleason 2–4)
T2b: Tumor involves more than $^1/_2$ of one lobe but not both lobes	G2: Moderately-differentiated (moderate anaplasia, Gleason 5–6)
T2c: Tumor involves both lobes	G3-4: Poorly-differentiated/ undifferentiated (marked Gleasou 7–10)
T3: Tumor extends through prostate capsule	
T3a: Extracapsular extension (unilateral or bilateral)	Stage Grouping I: T1aN0M0 G1
T3b: Tumor invades seminal vesicle(s)	II: T1aN0M0 G2-4, T1-2N0M0 any G
T4: Tumor is fixed or invades adjacent structures other than seminal vesicles: bladder neck, external sphincter, rectum, levator muscles, and/or pelvic wall	III: T3N0M0 any G IV: T4N0M0; any TN1M0; any T any N M1

RISK CLASSIFICATION SCHEMES

D'Amico & MD Anderson Groups	5/10yr bPFS after EBRT
Predict bPFS & CSS	
<u>Low</u>: T1-2a & GS ≤6 & PSA ≤10	
<u>Intermediate</u>: T2b (MD Anderson T2b-T2c) &/or GS 7 &/or PSA 10–20. Low-intermediate risk: ≤50% + biopsies; high-intermediate risk: >50% + biopsies	~85–90%/80– 85% ~70%/65%
<u>High</u>: ≥T2c (MD Anderson T3-4) or GS 8–10 or PSA >20	~40%/35%

Memorial Sloan-Kettering/Seattle Risk Groups – predict bPFS
<u>Low</u>: T1-T2b & GS ≤6 & PSA ≤10
<u>Intermediate</u>: ≥T2c or GS 7–10 or PSA >10 (one intermediate risk factor)
<u>High</u>: 2–3 intermediate risk factors

Mt. Sinai Risk Groups – predict bPFS
<u>Low</u>: T1-T2a & GS ≤6 & PSA ≤10
<u>Intermediate</u>: ≥T2b or GS 7 or PSA 10–20
<u>High</u>: 2–3 intermediate risk factors or ≥T2c or GS 8–10 or PSA >20

RTOG Meta-Analysis Risk Groups – predict DSS & OS	10yr DSS
I: T1–2 & GS ≤6 (low)	86%
II: T1–2 & GS 7, or T3 or N1 with GS ≤6 (intermediate)	75%
III: T1–2 & GS 8–10, or T3 or N1 with GS 7 (high)	62%
IV: T3 or N1 with GS 8–10 (very high)	34%

Partin Nomograms predict pathologic stage (organ confined, ECE, seminal vesicle invasion, or LN involvement) based on T stage, GS, & pre-treatment PSA

Roach Formulas predict pathologic stage based on original Partin data

$$ECE = 3/2 \times PSA + 10 \times (GS-3)$$
$$\text{Seminal vesicle involvement} = PSA + 10 \times (GS-6)$$
$$\text{LN involvement} = 2/3 \times PSA + 10 \times (GS-6)$$

Kattan Nomograms are computerized & predict primarily PSA recurrence, but some also predict PFS (based on biochemical & clinical failure) as well as prostate cancer specific mortality after radical prostatectomy, 3DCRT, or brachytherapy. (Online access: http://www.mskcc.org/mskcc/html/10088.cfm)

TREATMENT RECOMMENDATIONS

Stage	Recommended Treatment
Low risk	For life expectancy <10 yrs, expectant management or definitive RT (3DCRT, IMRT, or brachytherapy) For life expectancy ≥10 yrs, RT alone (3DCRT, IMRT, or brachytherapy), radical prostatectomy (RP) ± pelvic LN dissection, or expectant management. If RP + margins → adjuvant RT (preferred) or expectant management
Intermediate risk	For life expectancy <10 yrs, expectant management or definitive RT ± short-term hormone therapy (HT) For life expectancy ≥10 yrs, RT + short-term HT (4–6 mo) (preferred), high-dose RT alone, or RP ± pelvic LN dissection. RT may be 3DCRT or IMRT ± brachytherapy boost. Consider whole pelvic RT If RP + margins → adjuvant RT ± short-term HT (preferred) or expectant management. If RP + LN → androgen ablation ± RT or expectant management
High risk	RT (3DCRT or IMRT ± brachytherapy boost) + long term HT (≥2 yrs). Consider whole pelvic RT
Node +	RT (3DCRT or IMRT ± paraaortic RT) + long-term HT (≥2 yrs), or androgen ablation alone
Metastatic	Androgen ablation ± palliative RT ± bisphosphonates. For hormone-refractory disease, docetaxel + prednisone or estramustine prolongs survival vs mitoxantrone + prednisone

Stage	Recommended Treatment
Residual disease or recurrence after RP	If persistent local disease or high risk of local residual disease → RT ± HT. If no evidence of persistent local disease or high-risk of metastases → HT or observation ± RT
Residual disease or recurrence after RT	If biopsy + & no evidence (or low risk) of metastases, surgery or salvage brachytherapy. If metastatic or not a candidate for local therapy, androgen ablation or observation

STUDIES
Watchful waiting (WW)
- Swedish trial (*NEJM* 2002, 2005). Randomized 695 pts with T1b-T2 to WW vs RP. RP significantly improved 10 yr DSS (85→90%, p = 0.01), reduced DM (25→15%, p = 0.004) & local progression (44→19%, p < 0.001), & increased OS (68→73%, p = 0.04). On subgroup analysis, 10 yr death from prostate cancer was highest among men <65 yrs with WW (19%) compared to men >65 yrs or men treated with RP (9–12%)
- Klotz (*J Urol* 2004). Phase II study of 299 pts with low-risk or intermediate-risk disease (if >70 yrs) treated with active surveillance with delayed intervention for PSA DT ≤2 yrs or grade progression on re-biopsy. 8 yr DSS & OS were 99% & 85%, respectively

EBRT & dose
- Kuban (*IJROBP* 2003). Multi-institutional analysis of 4839 pts with T1b-2N0 treated with EBRT alone. The greatest risk failure was 1.5–3.5 yrs after treatment. Doses >72 Gy reduced PSA failure in the intermediate- & high-risk groups, but not the low-risk group. By 10 yrs, 1/3 of low-risk pts developed PSA failure. 40–60% of intermediate- to high-risk pts failed at 8 yrs despite >72 Gy. The 5 yr bPFS was similar to pooled results after RRP when doses >72 Gy were used
- Thames (*IJROBP* 2003). Multi-institutional analysis of 4839 pts with T1b-2N0 treated with EBRT alone compared

the ability of 102 definitions of biochemical failure to predict clinical failure. The ASTRO definition had a sensitivity 0.61 & specificity 0.8. The best definitions were PSA $\geq$ absolute nadir +2 ng/ml, PSA $\geq$ current nadir +2–3 ng/ml, & 2 rises backdated each $\geq$0.5 ng/ml (sensitivity 0.66–0.74, specificity 0.82–0.87). The worst definitions were PSA >0.2 or >0.5 (sensitivity 0.9–0.91, specificity 0.09–0.26). Backdating methods underestimate bPFS during the 1st 5 yrs after treatment

- Pollack (*JCO* 2000). Randomized 301 pts with T1–3N0 to 70 Gy vs 78 Gy EBRT (isocenter dose). RT was initially a 4-field box to 46 Gy $\rightarrow$ field size reduction for 70 Gy group & conformal boost for 78 Gy group. 78 Gy improved 6 yr freedom from clinical &/or biochemical failure for pts with pre-treatment PSA >10 (43$\rightarrow$62%) but not for pts with PSA <10 (~75%). 78 Gy reduced DM for pts with PSA >10 (12$\rightarrow$2%). There was no difference in OS. Rectal toxicity was higher with 78 Gy (12$\rightarrow$26%), but bleeding was reduced if <25% of the rectum received >70 Gy

- Zietman (*JAMA* 2005). 393 pts with T1b-T2b & PSA <15 treated with 50.4 Gy photons to prostate & seminal vesicles + margin randomized to proton boost to prostate + margin of 19.8 GyE (total 70.2 GyE) or 28.8 GyE (total 79.2 GyE). Median f/u 5.5 yrs, median PSA 6.3, 58% low-risk, 33% intermediate-risk, 8% high-risk. No pt received HT. 5 yr freedom from biochemical failure rates were higher with 79.2 GyE for both low-risk (60% vs 81%) & intermediate-risk pts (63% vs 81%). No difference in OS (96–97%) or grade $\geq$3 acute GU/GI toxicity

- Sathya (*JCO* 2005). Randomized 104 pts with stage T2–3N0 (by pelvic lymphadenectomy) to EBRT 2/66 Gy vs Ir-192 implant 35 Gy (over 2 d) $\rightarrow$ EBRT 2/40 Gy two wks later. EBRT covered the prostate + seminal vesicles + 2 cm margin, but there was no CT planning. Ir-192 implant improved 5 yr bPFS (29$\rightarrow$61%). Of 87 pts with post-RT biopsy, Ir-192 reduced + biopsy rate (51$\rightarrow$24%). 5 yr OS was not different (92–94%)

RT + short-term HT

- RTOG 8610 (Pilepich, *IJROBP* 2001). Randomized 456 pts with palpable (>25 cm^3) T2–4N0 to RT $\pm$ HT (goserelin & flutamide) for 2 mo before & 2 mo during RT. RT was 44–

46 Gy to whole pelvis (WP) → prostate boost to 65–70 Gy. HT improved 8 yr DFS (23→31%) & reduced DM (45→ 34%). OS was not different among all pts, but it was improved for pts with GS 2–6 (52→70%)

- <u>RTOG 9413</u> (Roach, *JCO* 2003). Randomized 1323 pts with PSA <100 with a risk of LN involvement >15% (by the Roach formula) to one of 4 arms comparing WP RT to prostate-only RT (PO), & neoadjuvant & concurrent HT (N&CHT) to adjuvant HT (AHT). WP RT was 50.4 Gy; the final prostate RT dose was 70.2 Gy. HT was goserelin or leuprolide & flutamide. N&CHT was 2 mo before & 2 mo during RT, & AHT was 4 mo after RT (=2 mo bias in favor of AHT because PFS was defined from time of randomization). Median pre-treatment PSA was 23. WP-RT improved 4 yr PFS vs PO-RT overall (40→56%), & WP-RT + N&CHT improved PFS (61%) vs the other 3 arms (45–49%). Results suggest that when using WP-RT, N&CHT improves PFS vs AHT. In contrast, when using PO-RT, there is no sequence dependence for the timing of HT. There were no differences in 4 yr OS

- <u>D'Amico</u> (*JAMA* 2004). Randomized 206 pts with T1b-T2b PSA 10–40 GS 7–10, or pts with lower PSA or GS with ECE or seminal vesicle invasion on MRI to 3DCRT alone or 3DCRT + HT for 2 mo before, during, & after RT (total 6 mo). RT was 45 Gy to prostate + seminal vesicles + 1.5 cm margin → boost to prostate + 1.5 cm margin to 70 Gy iso-center dose. HT was leuprolide or goserelin & flutamide. 24% of pts had GS <6 & PSA 10–20, & ~15% had GS 8–10. Adding HT improved 5 yr OS (78→88%), CSS, & survival free of salvage HT (57→82%)

- <u>Laverdiere</u> (*J Urol* 2004). reported 2 successive randomized studies of 486 pts with T2–3N0. Median PSA was 12. In the 1st study, pts were randomized to EBRT alone, 3 mo NHT → EBRT, or N&CHT → adjuvant HT (total 10 mo). In the 2nd study, pts were treated with N&CHT (total 5 mo) vs N&CHT → adjuvant HT (total 10 mo). HT was an LHRH agonist + an antiandrogen. In study 1, adding HT improved 7 yr bPFS (66–69%) vs EBRT alone (42%), but there was no difference between the HT arms. In study 2, 4 yr bPFS was not different between arms (65%). The authors conclude that short course NHT improves bPFS but adding short-course AHT provides no further advantage

- Roach (*IJROBP* 2000). performed a meta-analysis of pts treated on RTOG 7506, 7706, 8531, & 8610 to determine DFS & OS when stratified by RTOG risk groups (listed in the table above). Long-term HT improved 8 yr OS by ~20% for risk groups 3 & 4 compared to RT alone. Short-term HT improved 8 yr DSS by ~15% for risk group 2 compared to RT alone

- Crook (*IJROBP* 2004). Randomized 378 pts with T1c-4N0 to 3 mo vs 8 mo of goserelin + flutamide before RT. RT was 66–67 Gy to prostate (+WP 45–46 Gy if risk of LN >10–15%). 26% of pts were low risk, 43% intermediate risk, & 31% high risk. There was no difference in biochemical, local, or distant failure in the two arms, although there was a trend for improved 5 yr DFS for high-risk pts with 8 mo HT (39→52%)

- TROG 96.01 (Denham, *Lancet Oncol* 2005). Randomized 818 pts with T2b-T4N0 treated with 2/66 Gy to prostate & seminal vesicle to HT (goserelin & flutamide) for 0 mo, 3 mo (starting 2 mo before RT), or 6 mo (starting 5 mo before RT). Median age 68, median PSA ~15, ~84% high-risk, ~14% intermediate-risk. Compared to no HT, 3 mo & 6 mo HT improved LF, bFFS, DFS, & freedom from salvage treatment. 6 mo HT also reduced DM & improved prostate-cancer specific survival compared to no HT, & it further improved freedom from salvage treatment compared to only 3 mo HT

RT + long-term HT

- RTOG 8531 (*JCO* 1997 & 2005, *IJROBP* 2005). Randomized 945 pts with LN+, cT3, or pT3 to RT ± goserelin indefinitely (starting the last wk of RT). RT was 50 Gy to WP → prostate boost to 65–70 Gy. HT improved 10 yr OS (39→49%), LF (38→23%), DM (39→24%), & DSS (16→22%). On subset analysis, OS benefit seen for GS 7–10 but not GS 2–6

- EORTC (Bolla, *Lancet* 2002). Randomized 415 pts with T1–2N0 WHO grade 3 (GS ≥7) or T3–4N0 any grade to RT ± goserelin for 3 yrs starting from the 1st day of RT. RT was 50 Gy to the whole pelvis (WP) → prostate boost to 70 Gy. HT improved 5 yr OS (62→78%) & DFS (40→74%) for all pts

- RTOG 9202 (*JCO* 2003). Randomized 1554 pts with T2c-T4 PSA <150 to RT +4 mo goserelin & flutamide (2 mo before & 2 mo during RT) ± 2 yrs adjuvant goserelin. RT was

44–50 Gy to WP → prostate boost to 65–70 Gy. Adjuvant HT improved 5 yr DFS (28→46%) & reduced DM (17→11%), local progression (12→5%), & biochemical failure (56→28%), but there was no difference in OS, except for pts with GS 8–10 (71→81%)

LDR brachytherapy

- Grimm (*IJROBP* 2001). Reviewed 125 consecutive pts with T1-T2b treated with I-125 brachytherapy monotherapy from 1988 to 1990. The 10 yr bPFS (modified ASTRO definition with 2 PSA rises) was 87% for Seattle low-risk pts & 85% overall. PSA declined over time (80% of pts had PSA <2 after 18 mo & 80% had PSA <0.2 after 6 yrs). Absolute PSA & bPFS curves merged at 10 yrs
- Sylvester (*IJROBP* 2003). Reviewed 232 pts treated with EBRT to 45 Gy to a limited pelvic field → LDR implant with I-125 (120 Gy) or Pd-103 (90 Gy). Using Seattle risk-groups, 10 yr bPFS for low-risk pts was 85%, for intermediate-risk 77%, & for high-risk 45%. Using D'Amico risk-groups, bPFS was 86%, 90%, & 48%. Using Mt Sinai risk groups, bPFS was 84%, 93%, & 57%

HDR brachytherapy

- Galalae (*IJROBP* 2004). Reviewed 611 pts on 3 studies treated with EBRT (45–50 Gy to prostate, seminal vesicles, & pelvic LN) with a HDR boost of 2–4 fractions during EBRT. Included 177 pts treated with short-course N&CHT. 5 yr bPFS/CSS for low-risk (≤T2a & GS ≤6 & PSA ≤10) = 96/100%, intermediate-risk (one factor: ≥T2b or GS ≥7 or PSA ≥10) = 88/99%, & high-risk (≥2 intermediate risk factors) = 69/95%. Predictors of failure were risk group, stage, PSA, & GS. Short-course N&CHT did not improve outcome. 5 yr OS for all groups was 85–88%
- Grills (*J Urol* 2004). Review of 65 consecutive pts treated with HDR monotherapy (Ir-192, 9.5 Gy bid × 2 d) & 84 pts treated with LDR monotherapy (Pd-103, 120 Gy) at William Beaumont Hospital. The majority had T1c-T2a, GS ≤6, & PSA <10; 36% received neoadjuvant HT. 3 yr biochemical control (ASTRO definition) was 98% for HDR & 97% for LDR. HDR was associated with reduced acute grade 1–3 dysuria, urinary frequency/urgency, & rectal pain, as well as late urinary frequency/urgency & impotence

Comparison of modalities

- Kupelian (*IJROBP* 2004). Compared 2991 consecutive pts treated at Cleveland Clinic & Memorial Sloan Kettering with RP, EBRT <72 Gy, EBRT >72 Gy, permanent seed implant (PPI), & combined PPI + EBRT. Pts treated with RP were younger & had more favorable tumor characteristics. ≤6 mo neoadjuvant HT was used in 21% of pts (mainly the RT groups). bPFS was defined as PSA >0.2 for RP or 3 consecutive rises for all others. The 5 yr bPFS was: RP 81%, EBRT <72 Gy 51%, EBRT >72 Gy 81%, PPI 83%, PPI+EBRT 77%. Only EBRT <72 Gy was worse. Pretreatment PSA, GS, & yr of therapy predicted bPFS, but T stage & HT did not

- D'Amico (*JAMA* 1998). Reviewed 1872 pts treated at University of PA or the Joint Center in Boston with RP, EBRT, or LDR implant ± neoadjuvant HT. Using the ASTRO PSA failure definition & D'Amico risk groups, there was no difference in bPFS for low-risk pts. For intermediate-risk pts, there was no difference between RP, EBRT, implant + neoadjuvant HT. For high-risk pts, implants (±NHT) had lower bPFS than RP or EBRT

- Beyer & Brachman (*Radiother Oncol* 2000). Reviewed >2200 pts with T1–2 disease treated with either EBRT (n = 1527) or PPI (n = 695) at a single institution. There was no difference in 5 yr FFS for T1 or T2 disease with GS <7 and PSA <10. For pts with GS 8–10 or PSA >10–<20, EBRT provided improved FFS

- Pickett (*IJROBP* 2006). Compared MRSI results for 50 pts with low-risk disease treated with EBRT (≥72 Gy) or PPI (144 Gy). Median time to resolution of spectroscopic abnormalities and time to nadir PSA were faster after PPI, & more PPI pts achieved complete metabolic atrophy

Adjuvant & salvage RT after RP

- EORTC 22911 (Bolla, *JCO* 2005). Randomized 1005 pN0M0 pts treated with RRP who had ECE, + margins, or SVI to observation or post-op RT (median 60 Gy). Post-op RT improved 5 yr bPFS (53→74%) & clinical PFS (77→85%), & reduced LRF (15→5%). Grade 3 toxicity was 2.6–4.2% in both groups. No difference in OS (92–93%), but more prostate cancer deaths in wait-and-see group. In wait-and-see group, ~50% of relapsing pts eventually received RT

- <u>SWOG 8794</u> (Swanson, ASTRO 2005 abstr #1). 473 pts with pathologic ECE, + margins, &/or seminal vesicle involvement randomized to 60–64 Gy EBRT vs observation. Median f/u 9.7 yrs. RT significantly improved 10 yr bDFS (23→47%) & there was a trend for improved DM-free survival (61→83%) & OS (63→74%). In observation group, 32% ultimately received RT. Subsequent HT was instituted in 39% of RT group at 12 yrs vs 50% of observation group at 10 yrs. Although acute toxicity was worse with RT, by 2 yrs there was no difference in GI or GU toxicity or QOL
- <u>Valicenti</u> (*Semin Radiat Oncol* 2003). Reviewed the literature on post-op EBRT & recommended adjuvant RT after RP for pts with high-risk of local recurrence, including ECE, + margin, & high volume GS 8–10. EBRT dose >64 Gy was recommended
- <u>Quinn</u> (*JCO* 2001). Reviewed 732 pts treated with RP to determine clinicopathologic features as predictors of DFS. Adjuvant RT for pts with multiple + margins reduced relapse
- <u>Stephenson</u> (*JAMA* 2004). Reviewed 501 pts at 5 centers treated with salvage EBRT for rising PSA after RP to determine prognostic variables associated with response. Predictors of progression after salvage RT were GS 8–10, pre-RT PSA >2, negative margins, PSA doubling time <10 mo, and seminal vesicle invasion. After salvage RT, the 4 yr PFS was 45% overall & 77% for pts without adverse features. Even pts with GS 8–10 or short PSA-DT could achieve CR if RT was given early
- <u>Beyer</u> (*Semin Radiat Oncol 2003*). Reviewed the literature on salvage brachytherapy after EBRT & noted that 5 yr freedom from 2nd relapse after salvage brachytherapy is ~50% overall, but with careful selection may be as high as 83%. Pts most likely to benefit include those with histologically confirmed local recurrence, no evidence of distant disease, adequate urinary function, >5–10 yr life expectancy, >2 yr disease-free interval after EBRT, PSAdt >6–9 mo, GS ≤6, & PSA <10 at time of recurrence

Node + disease

- <u>Messing</u> (*NEJM* 1999). 98 pts who had a RP who were found to have + nodes were randomized to immediate goserelin or bilateral orchiectomy vs observation. At 7 yr, 77% of pts were alive & NED with treatment vs only 18% with observation

- Zagars (*Urology* 2001). 255 node + pts were treated with early androgen ablation (AA) alone or with 70 Gy EBRT to the prostate. Adding EBRT improved 10 yr OS (46→67%) & freedom from relapse or rising PSA (25→ 80%)

- RTOG 8531 (*IJROBP* 1997). Showed that the addition of early HT to RT improved OS, DSS, & bPFS for N+ pts

Metastatic disease

- MRC (*Br J Urol* 1997). 934 pts with T2–4 or asymptomatic M1 disease were randomized to immediate androgen ablation (AA) (LHRH analogue or orchiectomy) vs deferred AA. Early treatment decreased local & metastatic disease progression & increased OS & CSS (mostly among M0 pts)

- SWOG 99-16 (*NEJM* 2004). Randomized 770 pts with androgen-independent prostate cancer (AIPC) to docetaxel/estramustine (D/E) vs mitoxantrone/prednisone (M/P). D/E increased MS (15→18 mo), & median time to progression (3→6 mo)

- Tannock (*NEJM* 2004). Randomized 1000 pts with AIPC to docetaxel/prednisone (D/P) vs M/P. D/P q 3 wk increased MS (16.5→19 mo) & increased pain response (22→35%)

RADIATION TECHNIQUES
EBRT

- At UCSF, pts are treated supine with alpha cradle immobilization

- Alternatively, pts may be treated prone with thermoplastic shell immobilization. A randomized trial by Bayley (*Radiother Oncol* 2004), however, noted that there was significantly less prostate motion in the supine position & that prone position resulted in increased dose to critical structures

- Pts are instructed to have a full bladder & empty rectum (following an enema) for simulation

- At UCSF, a daily electronic portal imaging device (EPID) is used to monitor prostate position. Gold marker seeds are placed in the base & apex of the prostate 7–10 d prior to simulation. If EPIDs are unavailable, transabdominal US-based daily imaging may be used

- If gold seeds are not placed, retrograde urethrography is used in conjunction with CT for identifying the inferior border of the prostate. The prostate apex is assumed to be 1–1.5 cm superior to the point at which the dye narrows. Retrograde urethrography is particularly useful in the post-op setting

- Planning is CT-based. The prostate appears larger inferiorly & posteriorly on non-contrast CT images compared to TRUS or MRI

- Indications for whole-pelvic RT at UCSF include + nodes, + seminal vesicle involvement, a calculated risk of lymph node involvement >15% (using the Roach formula), pts with T3 GS 6 disease, & pts with high intermediate risk (>50% + biopsies) or high-risk disease

- Indications for seminal vesicle irradiation include + biopsy, + TRUS, + MRI, or calculated risk >15% (using the Roach formula)

- For traditional whole pelvic RT, initial field borders are: superior = L5/S1; inferior = 0.5–1 cm below the area where the dye narrows on the urethrogram (or 1–1.5 cm below in the post-op setting); lateral = 1.5 cm lateral to the bony margin of the true pelvis. On the AP/PA fields, corners are blocked to decrease dose to the femoral heads, bowel, & bone marrow. On the lateral fields, the anterior border is anterior to the pubic synthesis. The posterior border splits the sacrum to S2/3 and a beam's eye view is generated with CT contours of the rectum present in order to draw the rectal bloc excluding the posterior rectum. "Mini-pelvic" fields are not recommended

- For the conedown on the prostate + seminal vesicles or the prostate alone, non-uniform field edge margins of 0.5–1.5 cm are used in order to account for set-up error, movement error, & beam penumbra

- With daily EPID imaging, the margins are reduced to 0.5–1 cm

- Weekly port films are obtained throughout treatment

- Alternatively, IMRT may be used for both whole pelvic and boost portions of treatment. With whole-pelvic IMRT, careful review of lymph node mapping is recommended (Shih, *IJROBP* 2005; Taylor, *IJROBP* 2005; Chao, *IJROBP* 2002)

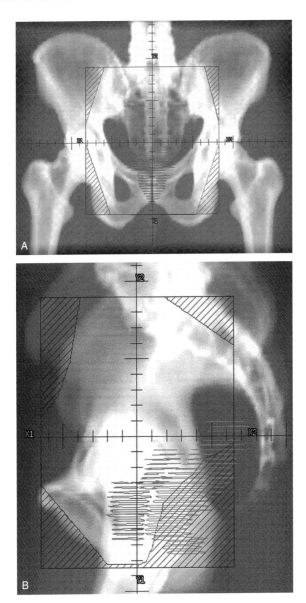

FIGURE 25.1. DRRs of whole pelvic fields used to treat a T3b Gleason 8 adenocarcinoma of the prostate with a pre-treatment PSA of 19. (A) AP field and (B) lateral field.

EBRT dose

- Prophylactic dose to the whole pelvis is 1.8 Gy/fx to 45 Gy prescribed to the 92–95% isodose line. Prophylactic dose to the seminal vesicles is 54 Gy. Documented seminal vesicle disease receives full-dose. Involved nodes receive 54–56 Gy (or higher with IMRT)
- Conedown boosts using 3DCRT or IMRT are prescribed at 1.8 Gy/fx to 72 Gy to the 92–95% isodose line (range 90–100%). The minimum central axis dose for low-risk pts is 78 Gy
- The volume of the rectum receiving ≥70 Gy is limited to ≤20%

LDR brachytherapy

- Contraindications include metastases, gross seminal vesicle involvement, & large T3 disease that cannot be easily implanted due to geometrical impediments. Pts unlikely to cope well with a temporary exacerbation of obstructive symptoms may be better served with EBRT or RP (e.g., significant pre-treatment urinary obstructive symptoms (AUA score >15)). Other relative contraindications are prostate size (>50 ml) – related to pubic arch interference, prostatitis, & median lobe hypertrophy
- Implants are typically pre-planned from TRUS images of the prostate taken in the lithotomy position at 5 mm intervals from the base through the apex ≤7 days before the implant. Recently intra-operative planning based on intra-operative TRUS image capture has been used
- The goal of treatment planning is to cover the prostate + a 3–5 mm margin to cover potential ECE
- Pre-op bowel preparation is necessary. Spinal, epidural, or general anesthesia is generally used, but local anesthesia is used at some centers
- In the OR, a catheter or aerated gel is used to visualize the urethra. TRUS frequencies of 5–7 MHz are used. The TRUS is supported on an adjustable 0.5 cm stepping unit mounted to the table. If using a pre-plan, match the intra-op images to the pre-op images using the seminal vesicles and the base of the gland. Needles are inserted through the template holes until they are viewed in the desired plane. Rotating the needle allows two distinct

lines to be seen, corresponding to the bevel. Seeds are deposited from pre-loaded needles or the Mick applicator. Seeds may be single or suture-mounted. An extended lithotomy position may help reduce pubic arch interference

LDR dose

- Brachytherapy monotherapy doses: I-125 144 Gy; Pd-103 125 Gy
- After 40–50 Gy EBRT: I-125 110 Gy; Pd-103 90 Gy
- I-125: source activity 0.2–0.9 mCi, half-life 60 d, photon energy 28 keV
- Pd-103: source activity 1.1–2.5 mCi, half-life 17 d, photon energy 21 keV
- Review isodose overlays to determine significance of under- & over-dosed regions
- V100 is the percent of the post-implant prostate volume covered by 100% of the prescription dose (desire ≥90%)
- D90 is the dose that covers 90% of the post-implant prostate volume (desire >90% of the prescribed dose)
- Limit ≥40% of the urethra to ≤150% of the prescription dose

HDR brachytherapy

- Generally, HDR implants are performed less frequently than LDR implants
- HDR after-loading catheters are inserted under TRUS guidance & secured into position. A CT scan captures the catheter position into the treatment planning system. Each catheter is sequentially loaded with Ir-192 by computer driven stepping motors. The treatment planning software determines the optimal loading & duration of the source in a given position in order to accomplish a desired dose distribution
- Temporary implants are usually administered using multiple fractionated treatments delivered over 1–3 out-patient or in-patient visits

HDR dose

- After EBRT, HDR is given as 9.5 Gy × 2 fractions in 1 implant
- As monotherapy, HDR dose is 9.5 Gy bid × 2 d with 1 implant

COMPLICATIONS

Acute EBRT Complications	Incidence	Time of Onset	Management
Dysuria, urgency, frequency, nocturia	Most	2 wk	NSAID, alpha-blockers, pyridium Catheter
Urinary retention	Rare	>1 wk	
Diarrhea	25–75%	2 wk	Diet, anti-diarrheals, sitz baths, rectal steroids
Rectal irritation, pain, bleeding	<10–20%	2–6 wk	
Fatigue	Most	>3 wk	Reassurance

- Perioperative brachytherapy complications include pain, dysuria, urinary retention, hematuria, & urinary frequency. Obstructive symptoms occur in ~10% of pts & tend to resolve 6–12 mo after the implant. Retention usually resolves in 1–3 d. Rectal injury is technique related & occurs in about 1–5% of pts
- Decreased volume of ejaculate is seen with both EBRT & brachytherapy
- In a meta-analysis by Robinson (*IJROBP* 2002), post-treatment impotence rates were: brachytherapy alone 24%, brachytherapy + EBRT 40%, EBRT alone 45%, nerve-sparing RP 66%, non-nerve sparing RP 75%, & cryosurgery 87%
- Complications of hormone therapy include hot flashes, impotence, liver dysfunction (due to antiandrogen), anemia, & osteoporosis

FOLLOW-UP

- H&P with DRE & PSA every 6 mo for 5 yrs then annually. In the first 1–3 yrs after definitive RT, PSA may be ordered more frequently (e.g., every 3–6 mo)
- The definition of PSA failure following surgery is controversial & values ≥0.2, ≥0.3, & ≥0.4 ng/ml have been used
- The 1996 ASTRO definition of PSA failure following EBRT is 3 consecutive PSA rises, with the time of failure backdated to the midpoint between the PSA nadir & the first rising PSA or any rise great enough to provoke initiation of salvage therapy; a minimum follow-up of 2 yrs was recommended for presentation or publication of data

- The new Phoenix/ASTRO/RTOG definition of PSA failure after EBRT, with or without short-term HT, is defined as a rise by ≥ 2 ng/ml above the nadir PSA (defined as the lowest PSA achieved), with the date of failure "at call" & not backdated. Pts who undergo salvage therapy (e.g., with HT, RP, brachytherapy, or cryosurgery) are declared failures at the time of + biopsy or salvage therapy administration (whichever comes first). Alternatively, for pts treated with EBRT alone, a modified stricter version of the ASTRO definition may continue to be used. For presentations & publications, the stated date of control should be listed as 2 yrs short of the median follow-up
- The PSA nadir after RP is ~3 wks, after EBRT ~2–3 yrs (but can be up to 4–5 yrs), & after brachytherapy ~3–4 yrs
- PSA "bounce" consists of transient PSA rises usually <2 ng/ml) after RT with a subsequent fall in the value. After brachytherapy, ~90% of blips occur within 3 yrs, & 15–30% of all pts have a bounce after brachytherapy. The median time to bounce after EBRT is ~9 mo & ~12% of pts have a bounce. Risk factors for PSA bounce after brachytherapy include age <65, higher implant dose, sexual activity & larger prostate volume. PSA bounce after brachytherapy or EBRT does not predict PSA failure

REFERENCES

Bayley AJ, Catton CN, Haycocks T, et al. A randomized trial of supine vs. prone positioning in patients undergoing escalated dose conformal radiotherapy for prostate cancer. Radiother Oncol 2004;70: 37–44.

Beyer DC. Brachytherapy for recurrent prostate cancer after radiation therapy. Semin Radiat Oncol 2003;13:158–165.

Beyer DC, Brachman DG. Failure free survival following brachytherapy alone for prostate cancer: comparison with external beam radiotherapy. Radiother Oncol 2000;57:263–267.

Bill-Axelson A, Holmberg L, Ruutu M, et al. Radical prostatectomy versus watchful waiting in early prostate cancer. N Engl J Med 2005;352:1977–1984.

Bolla M, Collette L, Blank L, et al. Long-term results with immediate androgen suppression and external irradiation in patients with locally advanced prostate cancer (an EORTC study): a phase III randomised trial. Lancet 2002;360:103–106.

Bolla M, Van Poppel H, Collette L, et al. Postoperative radiotherapy after radical prostatectomy: a randomised controlled trial (EORTC 22911). Lancet 2005;366:572–578.

Cagiannos I, Karakiewicz P, Eastham JA, et al. A preoperative nomogram identifying decreased risk of positive pelvic lymph nodes in patients with prostate cancer. J Urol 2003;170:1798–1803.

Chao KS, Lin M. Lymphangiogram-assisted lymph node target delineation for patients with gynecologic malignancies. Int J Radiat Oncol Biol Phys 2002;54:1147–1152.

Crook J, Ludgate C, Malone S, et al. Report of a multicenter Canadian phase III randomized trial of 3 months vs. 8 months neoadjuvant androgen deprivation before standard-dose radiotherapy for clinically localized prostate cancer. Int J Radiat Oncol Biol Phys 2004;60:15–23.

D'Amico AV, Chen MH, Roehl KA, et al. Preoperative PSA velocity and the risk of death from prostate cancer after radical prostatectomy. N Engl J Med 2004;351:125–135.

D'Amico AV, Keshaviah A, Manola J, et al. Clinical utility of the percentage of positive prostate biopsies in predicting prostate cancer-specific and overall survival after radiotherapy for patients with localized prostate cancer. Int J Radiat Oncol Biol Phys 2002;53:581–587.

D'Amico AV, Manola J, Loffredo M, et al. 6-month androgen suppression plus radiation therapy vs radiation therapy alone for patients with clinically localized prostate cancer: a randomized controlled trial. JAMA 2004;292:821–827.

D'Amico AV, Renshaw AA, Cote K, et al. Impact of the percentage of positive prostate cores on prostate cancer-specific mortality for patients with low or favorable intermediate-risk disease. J Clin Oncol 2004;22:3726–3732.

D'Amico AV, Renshaw AA, Sussman B, et al. Pretreatment PSA velocity and risk of death from prostate cancer following external beam radiation therapy. JAMA 2005;294:440–447.

D'Amico AV, Whittington R, Malkowicz SB, et al. Biochemical outcome after radical prostatectomy, external beam radiation therapy, or interstitial radiation therapy for clinically localized prostate cancer. JAMA 1998;280:969–974.

D'Amico AV, Whittington R, Malkowicz SB, et al. Clinical utility of the percentage of positive prostate biopsies in defining biochemical outcome after radical prostatectomy for patients with clinically localized prostate cancer. J Clin Oncol 2000;18:1164–1172.

Denham JW, Steigler A, Lamb DS, et al. Short-term androgen deprivation and radiotherapy for locally advanced prostate cancer: results from the Trans-Tasman Radiation Oncology Group 96.01 randomised controlled trial. Lancet Oncol 2005;6:841–850.

Galalae RM, Martinez A, Mate T, et al. Long-term outcome by risk factors using conformal high-dose-rate brachytherapy (HDR-BT) boost with or without neoadjuvant androgen suppression for localized prostate cancer. Int J Radiat Oncol Biol Phys 2004;58:1048–1055.

Gleason DF, Mellinger GT. Prediction of prognosis for prostatic adenocarcinoma by combined histological grading and clinical staging. J Urol 1974;111:58–64.

Gottschalk AR, Roach M, 3rd. The use of hormonal therapy with radiotherapy for prostate cancer: analysis of prospective randomised trials. Br J Cancer 2004;90:950–954.

Greene FL, American Joint Committee on Cancer, American Cancer Society. AJCC Cancer Staging Manual. 6th ed. New York: Springer-Verlag; 2002.

Grills IS, Martinez AA, Hollander M, et al. High dose rate brachytherapy as prostate cancer monotherapy reduces toxicity compared to low dose rate palladium seeds. J Urol 2004;171:1098–1104.

Grimm PD, Blasko JC, Sylvester JE, et al. 10-year biochemical (prostate-specific antigen) control of prostate cancer with (125)I brachytherapy. Int J Radiat Oncol Biol Phys 2001;51:31–40.

Grossfeld GD, Latini DM, Lubeck DP, et al. Predicting disease recurrence in intermediate and high-risk patients undergoing radical prostatectomy using percent positive biopsies: results from CaPSURE. Urology 2002;59:560–565.

Hanks GE, Lu J, Machtay M, et al. RTOG protocol 92-02: a phase III trial of the use of long term androgen supression following neoadjuvant hormonal cytoreduction and radiotherapy in locally advanced carcinoma of the prostate. Int J Radiat Oncol Biol Phys 2000;48(3 Suppl 1):112.

Hanks GE, Pajak TF, Porter A, et al. Phase III trial of long-term adjuvant androgen deprivation after neoadjuvant hormonal cytoreduction and radiotherapy in locally-advanced carcinoma of the prostate: The Radiation Therapy Oncology Group Protocol 92-02. J Clin Oncol 2003 21:3972–3978.

Holmberg L, Bill-Axelson A, Helgesen F, et al. A randomized trial comparing radical prostatectomy with watchful waiting in early prostate cancer. N Engl J Med 2002;347:781–789.

Immediate versus deferred treatment for advanced prostatic cancer: initial results of the Medical Research Council Trial. The Medical Research Council Prostate Cancer Working Party Investigators Group. Br J Urol 1997;79:235–246.

Jemal A, Siegel R, Ward E, et al. Cancer Statistics, 2006. CA Cancer J Clin 2006;56:106–130.

Kattan MW, Karpeh MS, Mazumdar M, et al. Postoperative nomogram for disease-specific survival after an R0 resection for gastric carcinoma. J Clin Oncol 2003;21:3647–3650.

Kattan MW, Zelefsky MJ, Kupelian PA, et al. Pretreatment nomogram that predicts 5-year probability of metastasis following three-dimensional conformal radiation therapy for localized prostate cancer. J Clin Oncol 2003;21:4568–4571.

Klein EA, Thompson IM, Lippman SM, et al. SELECT: the next prostate cancer prevention trial. Selenum and Vitamin E Cancer Prevention Trial. J Urol 2001;166:1311–1315.

Klotz L. Active surveillance with selective delayed intervention: using natural history to guide treatment in good risk prostate cancer. J Urol 2004;172:S48–50; discussion S50–41.

Kuban DA, Thames HD, Levy LB, et al. Long-term multi-institutional analysis of stage T1-T2 prostate cancer treated with radiotherapy in the PSA era. Int J Radiat Oncol Biol Phys 2003;57:915–928.

Kupelian PA, Potters L, Khuntia D, et al. Radical prostatectomy, external beam radiotherapy <72 Gy, external beam radiotherapy > or =72 Gy, permanent seed implantation, or combined seeds/external beam radiotherapy for stage T1-T2 prostate cancer. Int J Radiat Oncol Biol Phys 2004;58:25–33.

Langen KM, Pouliot J, Anezinos C, et al. Evaluation of ultrasound-based prostate localization for image-guided radiotherapy. Int J Radiat Oncol Biol Phys 2003;57:635–644.

Laverdiere J, Nabid A, De Bedoya LD, et al. The efficacy and sequencing of a short course of androgen suppression on freedom from biochemical failure when administered with radiation therapy for T2-T3 prostate cancer. J Urol 2004;171:1137–1140.

Lawton CA, Winter K, Byhardt R, et al. Androgen suppression plus radiation versus radiation alone for patients with D1 (pN+) adenocarcinoma of the prostate (results based on a national prospective randomized trial, RTOG 85-31). Radiation Therapy Oncology Group. Int J Radiat Oncol Biol Phys 1997;38:931–939.

Lawton CA, Winter K, Grignon D, et al. Androgen suppression plus radiation versus radiation alone for patients with stage d1/pathologic node-positive adenocarcinoma of the prostate: updated results based on national prospective randomized trial radiation therapy oncology group 85-31. J Clin Oncol 2005;23:800–807.

Lawton CA, Winter K, Murray K, et al. Updated results of the phase III Radiation Therapy Oncology Group (RTOG) trial 85-31 evaluating the potential benefit of androgen suppression following standard radiation therapy for unfavorable prognosis carcinoma of the prostate. Int J Radiat Oncol Biol Phys 2001;49:937–946.

Martinez AA, Pataki I, Edmundson G, et al. Phase II prospective study of the use of conformal high-dose-rate brachytherapy as monotherapy for the treatment of favorable stage prostate cancer: a feasibility report. Int J Radiat Oncol Biol Phys 2001;49:61–69.

Messing EM, Manola J, Sarosdy M, et al. Immediate hormonal therapy compared with observation after radical prostatectomy and pelvic lymphadenectomy in men with node-positive prostate cancer. N Engl J Med 1999;341:1781–1788.

National Cancer Institute. Prostate Cancer (PDQ): Treatment. Available at: http://cancer.gov/cancertopics/pdq/treatment/prostate/healthprofessional/. Accessed on January 19, 2005.

National Comprehensive Cancer Network. Clinical Practice Guidelines in Oncology: Prostate Cancer. Available at: http://www.nccn.org/professionals/physician_gls/PDF/prostate.pdf. Accessed on January 19, 2005.

Partin AW, Mangold LA, Lamm DM, et al. Contemporary update of prostate cancer staging nomograms (Partin Tables) for the new millennium. Urology 2001;58:843–848.

Petrylak DP, Tangen CM, Hussain MH, et al. Docetaxel and estramustine compared with mitoxantrone and prednisone for advanced refractory prostate cancer. N Engl J Med 2004;351:1513–1520.

Pickett B, Kurhanewicz J, Coakley F, et al. Use of MRI and spectroscopy in evaluation of external beam radiotherapy for prostate cancer. Int J Radiat Oncol Biol Phys 2004;60:1047–1055.

Pickett B, Kurhanewicz J, Coakley F, et al. Efficacy of external beam radiotherapy compared to permanent prostate implant in treating low risk prostate cancer based on endorectal magnetic resonance spectroscopy imaging and PSA. Int J Radiat Oncol Biol Phys 2004;60(1; Suppl 1):S185–S186.

Pickett B, Ten Haken RK, Kurhanewicz J, et al. Time to metabolic atrophy after permanent prostate seed implantation based on magnetic resonance spectroscopic imaging. Int J Radiat Oncol Biol Phys 2004;59:665–673.

Pilepich MV, Caplan R, Byhardt RW, et al. Phase III trial of androgen suppression using goserelin in unfavorable-prognosis carcinoma of the prostate treated with definitive radiotherapy: report of Radiation Therapy Oncology Group Protocol 85-31. J Clin Oncol 1997;15:1013–1021.

Pilepich MV, Winter K, John MJ, et al. Phase III radiation therapy oncology group (RTOG) trial 86-10 of androgen deprivation adjuvant to definitive radiotherapy in locally advanced carcinoma of the prostate. Int J Radiat Oncol Biol Phys 2001;50:1243–1252.

Pisansky TM, Lee WR, Lawton CA, et al. Prostate cancer. In: Gunderson LL, Tepper JE, editors. Clinical Radiation Oncology. 1st ed. Philadelphia: Churchill Livingstone; 2000. pp. 762–818.

Pollack A, Zagars GK, Smith LG, et al. Preliminary results of a randomized radiotherapy dose-escalation study comparing 70 Gy with 78 Gy for prostate cancer. J Clin Oncol 2000;18:3904–3911.

Pollack A. The prostate. In: Cox JD, Ang KK, editors. Radiation Oncology: Rationale, Technique, Results. 8th ed. St. Louis: Mosby; 2003. pp. 629–680.

Quinn DI, Henshall SM, Haynes AM, et al. Prognostic significance of pathologic features in localized prostate cancer treated with radical prostatectomy: implications for staging systems and predictive models. J Clin Oncol 2001;19:3692–3705.

Roach III M, Wallner K. Cancer of the prostate. In: Leibel SA, Phillips TL, editors. Textbook of Radiation Oncology. 2nd ed. Philadelphia: Saunders; 2004. pp. 959–1030.

Roach M, 3rd, DeSilvio M, Lawton C, et al. Phase III trial comparing whole-pelvic versus prostate-only radiotherapy and neoadjuvant versus adjuvant combined androgen suppression: Radiation Therapy Oncology Group 9413. J Clin Oncol 2003;21:1904–1911.

Roach M, 3rd, Lu J, Pilepich MV, et al. Predicting long-term survival, and the need for hormonal therapy: a meta-analysis of RTOG prostate cancer trials. Int J Radiat Oncol Biol Phys 2000;47:617–627.

Roach M, 3rd. Hormonal therapy and radiotherapy for localized prostate cancer: who, where and how long? J Urol 2003;170:S35–40; discussion S40–31.

Roach M, Lu J, Pilepich MV, et al. Four prognostic groups predict long-term survival from prostate cancer following radiotherapy alone on Radiation Therapy Oncology Group clinical trials. Int J Radiat Oncol Biol Phys 2000;47:609–615.

Robinson JW, Moritz S, Fung T. Meta-analysis of rates of erectile function after treatment of localized prostate carcinoma. Int J Radiat Oncol Biol Phys 2002;54:1063–1068.

Sathya JR, Davis IR, Julian JA, et al. Randomized trial comparing iridium implant plus external-beam radiation therapy with external-beam radiation therapy alone in node-negative locally advanced cancer of the prostate. J Clin Oncol 2005;23:1192–1199.

Shih HA, Harisinghani M, Zietman AL, et al. Mapping of nodal disease in locally advanced prostate cancer: Rethinking the clinical target volume for pelvic nodal irradiation based on vascular rather than bony anatomy. Int J Radiat Oncol Biol Phys 2005;63:1262–1269.

Stephenson AJ, Shariat SF, Zelefsky MJ, et al. Salvage radiotherapy for recurrent prostate cancer after radical prostatectomy. JAMA 2004;291:1325–1332.

Stock RG, Stone NN, Cesaretti JA. Prostate-specific antigen bounce after prostate seed implantation for localized prostate cancer: descriptions and implications. Int J Radiat Oncol Biol Phys 2003;56:448–453.

Storey MR, Pollack A, Zagars G, et al. Complications from radiotherapy dose escalation in prostate cancer: preliminary results of a randomized trial. Int J Radiat Oncol Biol Phys 2000;48:635–642.

Sylvester JE, Blasko JC, Grimm PD, et al. Ten-year biochemical relapse-free survival after external beam radiation and brachytherapy for localized prostate cancer: the Seattle experience. Int J Radiat Oncol Biol Phys 2003;57:944–952.

Tannock IF, de Wit R, Berry WR, et al. Docetaxel plus prednisone or mitoxantrone plus prednisone for advanced prostate cancer. N Engl J Med 2004;351:1502–1512.

Taylor A, Rockall AG, Reznek RH, & Powell ME. Mapping pelvic lymph nodes: guidelines for delineation in intensity-modulated radiotherapy. Int J Radiat Oncol Biol Phys 2005;63:1604–1612.

Thames H, Kuban D, Levy L, et al. Comparison of alternative biochemical failure definitions based on clinical outcome in 4839 prostate cancer patients treated by external beam radiotherapy between 1986 and 1995. Int J Radiat Oncol Biol Phys 2003;57:929–943.

Thompson IM, Goodman PJ, Tangen CM, et al. The influence of finasteride on the development of prostate cancer. N Engl J Med 2003; 349:215–224.

Thompson IM, Pauler DK, Goodman PJ, et al. Prevalence of prostate cancer among men with a prostate-specific antigen level < or =4.0 ng per milliliter. N Engl J Med 2004;350:2239–2246.

Valicenti RK, Gomella LG, Perez CA. Radiation therapy after radical prostatectomy: a review of the issues and options. Semin Radiat Oncol 2003;13:130–140.

Zagars GK, Pollack A, von Eschenbach AC. Addition of radiation therapy to androgen ablation improves outcome for subclinically node-positive prostate cancer. Urology 2001;58:233–239.

Zietman AL, DeSilvio M, Slater JD, et al. Comparison of conventional-dose vs high-dose conformal radiation therapy in clinically localized adenocarcinoma of the prostate. JAMA 2005;294:1233–1239.

Zelefsky MJ, Valicenti RK, Goodman K, et al. Prostate cancer. In: Perez CA, Brady LW, Halperin EC, et al., editors. Principles and Practice of Radiation Oncology. 4th ed. Philadelphia: Lippincott Williams & Wilkins; 2004. pp. 1692–1762.

NOTES

Chapter 26
Cancer of the Penis

Alice Wang-Chesebro and Alexander R. Gottschalk

PEARLS

- Penile cancer is rare in Western countries, (<1% of cancers in men), but accounts for 10–20% of male malignancies in Africa, Asia, & South America
- LN drainage: skin of penis – bilateral superficial inguinal nodes; glans penis – bilateral inguinal or iliac nodes; penis corporal tissue – bilateral deep inguinal and iliac; 20% chance of LN+ at surgery if clinically node negative
- Risk factors: uncircumcised status, phimosis, poor local hygiene, HPV-16
- Pathology: 95% squamous cell; others very rare-melanoma, lymphoma, basal cell, Kaposi's sarcoma

WORKUP

- H&P with careful palpation and exam; if deep, consider cystourethroscopy with biopsy; bimanual exam under anesthesia
- Labs: CBC, chemistries, BUN, Cr, LFTs including alkaline phosphatase
- Imaging: Ultrasound (penis) or MRI for extent of local extension; pelvic/abdominal CT for nodes; CXR for all, bone scan if advanced/suspicious
- Needle biopsy for suspicious nodes

STAGING (AJCC)

Primary tumor

TX:	Primary tumor cannot be assessed
T0:	No evidence of primary tumor
Tis:	Carcinoma in situ
Ta:	Non-invasive verrucous carcinoma
T1:	Tumor invades subepithelial connective tissue
T2:	Tumor invades corpus spongiosum or cavernosum
T3:	Tumor invades urethra or prostate
T4:	Tumor invades other adjacent structures

Regional lymph nodes
NX: No regional lymph node metastasis cannot be assessed
N0:   No regional lymph node metastasis
N1:   Metastasis in single, superficial, inguinal node
N2:   Metastasis in multiple or bilateral superficial inguinal lymph
      nodes
N3:   Metastasis in deep inguinal or pelvic lymph node(s), unilateral
      or bilateral

Distant metastasis
MX: Distant metastasis cannot be assessed
M0:   No distant metastasis
M1:   Distant metastasis

Stage Grouping		~3 yr OS by Stage	
0:	TisN0M0, TaN0M0		
I:	T1N0M0	I:	70–100%
II:	T2N0M0, T1-2N1M0	II:	65–100%
III:	T3N0-1M0	III:	60–90%
	T1-3N2M0		
IV:	T4 Any N M0	IV	50–70%
	Any T N3 M0		
	Any T Any N M1		

Used with the permission of the American Joint Committee on Cancer (AJCC), Chicago, Illinois. The original source for this material is the AJCC Cancer Staging Manual, Sixth Edition (2002) published by Springer-Verlag New York, www.springeronline.com.

TREATMENT RECOMMENDATIONS

Stage	Recommended Treatment
CIS	Circumcision, local excision, or Moh's surgery
Early limited lesions (For RT alone lesions should be T1-2, <4 cm size)	Options: penectomy noted to have high psychosocial morbidity; therefore, organ preservation is gaining popularity ■ Penis preservation: circumcise first, then EBRT or brachytherapy alone, or chemo-RT ■ EBRT: 40 Gy to whole penile shaft, then 20 Gy boost to primary lesion +2 cm margin

Stage	Recommended Treatment
	■ Brachytherapy alone: Contraindicated if >1 cm invasion into corpus cavernosa or >4 cm size. Two methods: radioactive mold 60 Gy to tumor, 50 Gy to urethra; or interstitial with Ir-192 to 65 Gy (treatment of choice in Europe ■ Chemo-RT: gaining popularity based on data from anal and cervical cancers ■ Consider prophylactic inguinal node RT ■ Surgery: from circumcision to local excision to radical penectomy. Recommend >1.5–2 cm margin. For clinically node negative, consider prophylactic inguinal node dissection (controversial) with tumors extending onto shaft of penis or poorly differentiated. If no node dissection, requires very close monitoring. Post-op RT for LN+ based on vulvar cancer data
More advanced lesions	Options ■ EBRT: 60 Gy in 2 Gy fractions. Chemo-RT preferred to RT alone based on data from other cancers; include pelvic & bilateral inguinal nodes; consider LND for bulky nodes ■ Surgery: save for salvage; partial to radical penectomy; consider prophylactic inguinal node dissection with tumors extending onto shaft of penis/poorly differentiated; if node positive, need inguinal and pelvic LND; post-op RT for LN+ based on vulvar cancer data

Stage	Recommended Treatment
	■ <u>Investigational</u>: neoadjuvant chemo to render unresectable disease resectable; chemo (various regimens) for +LN or metastatic disease

STUDIES

- There are no randomized trials for primary penile cancers
- Selected results for early penile cancer treated with EBRT
  - Grabstald et al. (*Urology* 1980) report of 10 pts with stage I–II treated with EBRT; at 6–10 yrs follow-up, LC 90% & DFS 90%, OS 90%
  - McLean (IJROBP 1993). 26 pts with stage I–II treated with "radical" EBRT, range 35–50 Gy, most 50 Gy in 20 fx with cobalt-60; median f/u 9.7 yrs; 5 yr OS 62% (for N0-79%, for N + 12%), 5yr CSS 69%, 5 yr DFS 50%
- Selected results for early penile cancer treated with brachytherapy
  - Crook et al. (IJROBP 2005). 49 pts with T1 (51%), T2 (33%), and T3 (8%) penile SCC treated with Ir-192 to 55–65 Gy; median f/u 33 mo.; 5y OS 78%, 5y CSS 90%, 5y FFS 64%, 5y LF 15%, 5y penile preservation rate 86.5%, 5y soft tissue necrosis rate 16%, urethral stenosis rate 12%
  - Mazeron et al. (*IJROBP* 1984). 50 pts with T1-T3 treated with Ir-192 to median dose 65 (60–70 Gy); LC-78%, penis conservation 74%
- Selected series with all stages of penile cancer
  - Krieg et al. (*Urology* 1981). 17 pts with stage I–IV treated with surgery ± LND and 12 pts with stage I–III treated with EBRT alone (dose 50–65 Gy, no prophylactic node RT); LC 88% with surgery; 75% with RT alone and 92% with surgical salvage; 88% (8/9) of pts not treated prophylactically to groin did not develop pelvic/inguinal node recurrence; 2 pts developed stricture, 1 developed penile necrosis (66 Gy)
  - Sarin et al. (*IJROBP* 1997). 101 pts with stages I–IV, median age 64 yrs, treated with primary EBRT (59), brachytherapy (13), penectomy (29); median follow-up 5.2 yrs; 5/10 yr OS 56.5/39%; 5/10 yr CSS 66/57%; 5/10 yr

LC 60/55%; no difference between surgery & RT in LC after salvage; note: 2 attempted suicides after penectomy, 1 successful

RADIATION TECHNIQUES
Simulation and field design
- EBRT
  - Simulate pt supine; apply foley catheter and suspend penis; surround penis by tissue bolus for MV RT. If treating inguinal nodes, pt is treated in the frog-leg position. If treating pelvic nodes, may secure penis cranially into pelvic field
  - Field: cover entire length of penis; cover nodes if clinically involved, consider prophylactic coverage regional nodes
  - Dose: 45–50 Gy in 1.8–2 Gy fx to entire penis, then cone-down boost to GTV of 10–20 Gy for total 65–70 Gy
  - If treating inguinal nodes, techniques may be used to protect the femoral heads
- Plesiobrachytherapy/molds
  - Penis is placed into a cylinder loaded with Ir-192 sources; pt wears mold for calculated amount of time daily; target dose 60 Gy, urethra dose 50 Gy; requires very compliant patient
- Interstitial brachytherapy:
  - Implant requires general or spinal anesthesia, takes 30–45 minutes
  - Catheterize to assist urethra identification to avoid transfixing with it needles/catheters; pts remain catheterized for duration of treatment
  - May use rigid steel needles held in predrilled parallel acrylic templates or parallel flexible nylon catheters, placed 1 to 1.5 cm apart
  - HDR with afterloaded Ir-192
  - Pts wear supporting Styrofoam collar around penis, may need mild analgesia with po meds, DVT prophylaxis if stay in bed

Dose limitations
- Doses >60 Gy increase risk of urethral stenosis & fibrosis
- Sterilization occurs with 2–3 Gy
- For pelvic fields, limit bladder ≤75 Gy and rectum ≤70 Gy

COMPLICATIONS

- Dermatitis, dysuria, urethral stricture (10–40%), urethral fistula, impotence (10–20%), late skin telangiectasia (nearly universal), penile fibrosis, penile necrosis (3–15%, higher with IS), small bowel obstruction (rare)

FOLLOW-UP

- Need close f/u, especially if no prophylactic nodal treatment in clinically N0 patients
- H&P every 1–2 mo for 1 yr, every 3 mo for 2nd yr, every 6 mo for 3rd to 5th yrs, then annually

REFERENCES

Crook J, et al. Interstitial brachytherapy for penile cancer: an alternative to amputation. Jurol 2002; 167:506–511.

Crook J, Jezioranski J, et al. Penile brachytherapy: results for 49 patients. IJROBP 2005; 62:460–467.

Grabstald H, Kelley C. Radiation therapy of penile cancer six to ten year follow-up. Urology 1980;15:575–576.

Krieg R, Luk K. Carcinoma of the penis: review of cases treated by surgery and radiation therapy 1960–70. Urology 1981;18:149–154.

Krieg R, R Hoffman. Current Management of unusual genitourinary cancers part 1: penile cancer. Oncology 1999;13:1347–1352.

Mazeron JJ, Langlois D, et al. Interstitial radiation therapy for carcinoma of the penis using iridium 192 wires: The Henri Mondor experience (1970–79). IJROBP 1984;10:1891–1895.

McLean M, et al. The results of primary radiation therapy in the management of squamous cell carcinoma of the penis. IJROBP 1993;25:623–628.

Sarin R, Norman AR, et al. Treatment results and prognostic factors in 101 men treated for squamous carcinoma of the penis. Int J Radiat Oncol Biol Phys 1997;38:713–722.

Yamada Y. Cancer of the male urethra and penis. In: Leibel SA, Phillips TL, editors. Textbook of Radiation Oncology. 2nd ed. Philadelphia: Saunders; 2004. pp. 1047–1053.

Chapter 27
Testicular Cancer

Brian Missett and Alexander R. Gottschalk

PEARLS

- Spermatogonia → spermatocytes → spermatids → spermatozoa
- LN drainage
  - L testicle: testicular vein → L renal vein → paraaortic LN
  - R testicle: testicular vein → IVC below level of renal vein → paracaval & aortocaval nodes
- Pathology: >95% are germ cell tumors (GCTs) = seminomas & non-seminomatous germ cell tumors (NSGCTs)
- 60% of tumors are mixed & 40% are pure (seminoma most common pure)
- Seminoma is the most common single histology, but together NSGCTs are more common
- Seminoma subtypes: classic (>90% of cases, stains + for PLAP) & spermatocytic (older age, cured by orchiectomy, rarely metastasizes, stains negative for PLAP). Anaplastic no longer considered a subtype
- NSGCTs subtypes: embryonal carcinoma (most common NSGCT), yolk sac tumor (elevated AFP, Schiller Duval bodies), choriocarcinoma (elevated βhCG, rarest pure GCT), teratoma, & mixed GCTs
- Other tumors: Sertoli cell tumors (produce estrogen, present with gynecomastia); Leydig cell tumors (produce androgens & estrogen, present with early puberty, gynecomastia); lymphoma; embryonal rhabdomyosarcoma
- Risk factors: undescended testicle, first-born, pre/perinatal estrogen exposure, polyvinyl chloride exposure, advanced maternal age, Down's syndrome, Klinefelter's syndrome (47XXY), CIS, HIV/AIDS

WORKUP

- H&P, testicular ultrasound, βhCG, AFP, LDH, CBC, chemistries, fertility assessment ± sperm banking, CXR, CT abdomen & pelvis, CT chest if ≥ stage II
- βhCG half-life is 24–36 hrs; AFP half-life is 3.5–6 d
- βhCG is rarely elevated in seminoma, but if AFP elevated, not pure seminoma

STAGING

AJCC Staging	
Primary tumor	**Serum tumor markers nadir after surgery (S)**
Tis: Intratubular germ cell neoplasia (carcinoma in situ)	S0: Marker study levels (LDH, AFP, βhCG) within normal limits
T1: Tumor limited to testis & epididymis without vascular lymphatic invasion; tumor may invade into the tunica albuginea but not tunica vaginalis	S1: LDH <1.5× N* & βhCG (mIu/ml) <5000 & AFP (ng/ml) <1000
	S2: LDH 1.5–10× N* or βhCG 5000–50,000 or AFP 1000–10,000
T2: Tumor limited to testis & epididymis with vascular lymphatic invasion; or tumor extending through the tunica albuginea with involvement of the tunica vaginalis	S3: LDH >10× N* or βhCG >50,000 or AFP>10,000
T3: Tumor invades the spermatic cord with or without vascular /lymphatic invasion	N* indicates the upper limit of normal for the LDH assay
T4: Tumor invades the scrotum with or without vascular/lymphatic invasion	**Stage Grouping** IA = T1N0S0 IB = T2-4N0S0 IS = Any TN0S1-3 IIA = Any TN1 S0-1 IIB = Any TN2 S0-1 IIC = Any TN3 S0-1 IIIA = Any M1a S0-1 IIIB = S2 Any N or M1a IIIC = S3 Any N or M1a, or M1b
Regional lymph nodes N0: No regional lymph node metastasis pN1: Metastasis with a lymph node mass 2 cm or less in greatest dimension and less than or equal to 5	

nodes positive, none more than 2 cm in greatest dimension

pN2: Metastasis with a lymph node mass more than 2 cm but not more than 5 cm in greatest dimension; or more than 5 nodes positive, none more than 5 cm; or evidence of extranodal extension of tumor

pN3: Metastasis with a lymph node mass more than 5 cm in greatest dimension

Metastases

M1a: Nonregional nodal or pulmonary metastases

M1b: Distant metastasis other than to non-regional lymph nodes and lungs

Royal Marsden Staging	**~10 yr Survival (Seminoma)**
I: Limited to testis	I: RFS 96–98%, CSS 99–100%
IIA: Nodes <2 cm	IIA: RFS 92%, CSS 96–100%
IIB: Nodes 2–5 cm	IIB: RFS 86%, CSS 96–100%
IIC: Nodes 5–10 cm	IIC: RFS 70%, OS 90% (RT alone)
IID: Nodes >10 cm	IID: RFS 50% (RT alone) 90% (chemo)
III = Nodes above and below diaphragm	IIIA/B: OS 90%
IV = Extralymphatic mets	IIIC: OS 80%

Used with the permission of the American Joint Committee on Cancer (AJCC), Chicago, Illinois. The original source for this material is the AJCC Cancer Staging Manual, Sixth Edition (2002) published by Springer-Verlag New York, www.springeronline.com.

TREATMENT RECOMMENDATIONS FOR SEMINOMA

Stage	Recommended Treatment
I	Postresection: surveillance (relapse rate 16%) or RT (25.5 Gy to para aortic ± pelvic LN) or carboplatinum × 1–2 cycles
IIA/IIB	RT 25.5 Gy to pelvic & paraaortic LN with boost to gross disease (30 Gy for IIA, 36 Gy for IIB)
IIC/D & III	Chemo (etoposide, cisplatinum, ± bleomycin = BEP or EP) × 3–4 cycles
NSGCT	Treated with inguinial orchiectomy with chemotherapy (BEP) and/or retroperitoneal lymph node dissection for select patients

STUDIES

- MRC (*JCO* 1999). 478 pts w/Stage I seminoma randomized to dog-leg vs paraaortic RT. No difference in 3 yr RFS/OS with dogleg (97/96%) vs paraaortic (99/100%). 3 yr pelvic RFS was 100% with dogleg vs 98% with paraaortic. Para-aortic had decreased nausea & vomiting, lower azospermia (11% vs 35%), & more rapid recovery of sperm count

- Warde (*JCO* 2002). 638 pts with stage I seminoma followed with surveillance with 7 yr follow-up. Increased relapse with tumors >4 cm, LVSI, & rete testis involvement. Relapses: 0 risk factors = 12%, 1 risk factor = 16%, 2 risk factors = 30%. Prior study showed age <34 yrs also increased risk of failure

- Travis (*J Natl Cancer Inst* 1997). >28,000 men with testicular cancer. Risk of 2nd cancer was 16% at 25 yrs & 23% at 30 yr compared to expected 9% & 14% for the general population

- Puc (*JCO* 1996). 104 patients with stage IIC, III or extragonadal primary who underwent surgery & had CR or PR of tumor markers. If a radiographic mass was <3 cm, only 3% of pts had pathologic evidence of failures. For masses >3 cm, 27% of patients had evidence of failure
- De Santis (*JCO* 2004). 51 pts with seminoma treated with chemo with residual masses. Compared pathologic predictive value of PET & CT. PET PPV 100% & NPV 96% for viable tumor. CT (≤3 cm vs >3 cm) PPV 37% & NPV 97%
- MRC (*JCO* 2005). 625 pts with Stage I seminoma randomized to 20 Gy vs 30 Gy. RT in 2 Gy fx. RT was paraaortic (with dogleg for pts with prior inguinal surgery). 5 yr RFS was not different (97% 30 Gy, 96.4% 20 Gy). 20 Gy group had decreased lethargy & inability to carry out normal work 1 mo after treatment
- MRC (ASCO abstr., 2004). 1447 pts with stage I seminoma randomized to carboplatin × 1c vs RT. RT was 20–30 Gy (87% PA, 13% dogleg). 3 yr RFS = RT 97%, carboplatin 95%. Relapse sites: carboplatin = 70% PA, 4% pelvic vs RT = 7% PA, 28% pelvic

RADIATION TECHNIQUES
Simulation and field design
- Prior to simulation, fertility assessment ± sperm bank
- Simulate supine
- Need IVP or CT to block out kidneys & rule-out horseshoe kidney
- Place clamshell on uninvolved testicle. Position penis out of field
- Borders: PA = T10/T11-L5/S1. Dogleg, top of obturator foramen. Lateral = tips of transverse processes of lumbar vertebra or 2 cm margin on all nodes (about 10–12 cm wide). For left-sided tumors, widen field to include left renal hilar nodes
- If prior inguinal surgery, treat contralateral inguinal & iliac regions

Dose prescriptions
- 25.5 Gy at 1.5 Gy/fx
- Boost IIA nodes to 30 Gy & IIB nodes to 36 Gy

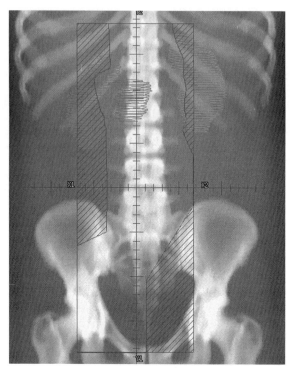

FIGURE 27.1. DRR of a dogleg field used to treat a stage IIB seminoma.

Dose limitations
- 50 cGy causes transient azospermia with recovery at 1 yr, but only 50% of pts reach their baseline
- 80–100 cGy causes total azospermia
- 200 cGy causes sterilization
- Clamshell reduces testicle dose by 2–3× (dogleg without shield ~4 cGy/fx, with shield ~1.5 cGy/fx; paraaortic without shield ~2 cGy/fx, with shield ~0.7 cGy/fx)
- Kidneys: limit at least 70% <20 Gy

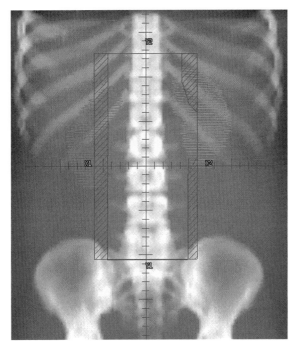

FIGURE 27.2. DRR of a para-aortic field used to treat a stage I seminoma.

COMPLICATIONS

- Acute nausea, vomiting, diarrhea
- Late small bowel obstruction, chronic diarrhea, peptic ulcer disease (<2% with <35 Gy)
- With testicular shielding, most pts will have oligospermia by 4 mo that lasts ~1 yr
- Infertility: 50% of pts have subfertile counts on presentation or after surgery. After RT, 30% able to have children
- BEP causes immediate azospermia, but >50% recover sperm count
- Chemo side effects = alopecia, nausea, myelosuppression, pulmonary fibrosis, ototoxicity
- Second cancers: 5–10% increased risk vs general population after RT

FOLLOW-UP

- After PA RT, H&P, labs, & CXR every 3 mo 1st yr, every 4 mo 2nd yr, every 6 mo 3rd yr, then annually. Also, pelvic CT annually × 3 yrs
- Surveillance = H&P, labs, CT abdomen & pelvis, CXR every 4 mo × 3 yrs, every 6 mo for yrs 4–7, then annually for yrs 8–10

REFERENCES

De Santis M, Becherer A, Bokemeyer C, et al. 2-18fluoro-deoxy-D-glucose positron emission tomography is a reliable predictor for viable tumor in postchemotherapy seminoma: an update of the prospective multicentric SEMPET trial. J Clin Oncol 2004;22:1034–1039.

Fossa SD, Horwich A, Russell JM, et al. Optimal planning target volume for stage I testicular seminoma: A Medical Research Council randomized trial. Medical Research Council Testicular Tumor Working Group. J Clin Oncol 1999;17:1146.

Garwood D. Cancer of the testis. In: Leibel SA, Phillips TL, editors. Textbook of Radiation Oncology. 2nd ed. Philadelphia: Saunders; 2004. pp. 1031–1046.

Hussey D, Meistrich M. The testicle. In: Cox JD, Ang KK, editors. Radiation Oncology: Rationale, Technique, Results. 8th ed. St. Louis: Mosby; 2003. pp. 605–628.

Jones WG, Fossa SD, Mead GM, et al. Randomized trial of 30 versus 20 Gy in the adjuvant treatment of stage I testicular seminoma: a report on Medical Research Council Trial TE18, European Organisation for the Research and Treatment of Cancer Trial 30942 (ISRCTN18525328). J Clin Oncol 2005;23:1200–1208.

Morton G, Thomas G. Testis. In: Perez CA, Brady LW, Halperin EC, et al., editors. Principles and Practice of Radiation Oncology. 4th ed. Philadelphia: Lippincott Williams & Wilkins; 2004. pp. 1763–1784.

National Comprehensive Cancer Network. Clinical Practice Guidelines in Oncology: Testicular Cancer. Available at: http://www.nccn.org/professionals/physician_gls/PDF/testicular.pdf. Accessed on January 19, 2005.

National Cancer Institute. Testicular Cancer (PDQ): Treatment. Available at: http://cancer.gov/cancertopics/pdq/treatment/testicular/healthprofessional/. Accessed on January 19, 2005.

Puc HS, Heelan R, Mazumdar M, et al. Management of residual mass in advanced seminoma: results and recommendations from the Memorial Sloan-Kettering Cancer Center. J Clin Oncol 1996;14:454–460.

Travis LB, Curtis RE, Storm H, et al. Risk of second malignant neoplasms among long-term survivors of testicular cancer. J Natl Cancer Inst 1997;89:1429–1439.

Warde P, Specht L, Horwich A, et al. Prognostic factors for relapse in stage I seminoma managed by surveillance: a pooled analysis. J Clin Oncol 2002;20:4448–4452.

NOTES

Chapter 28
Cervical Cancer

Kim Huang and I-Chow Hsu

PEARLS

- Third most common gynecological cancer in the U.S. (after ovarian and endometrial)
- Screening with Pap smear decreases mortality by 70%. ACS recommends screening for all women who are sexually active or who are >18 yrs old. After 3 normal annual exams, screening may be performed less frequently
- Risk factors = early 1st intercourse, multiple partners, large number of pregnancies, smoking, immunosuppression, prenatal DES (clear cell CA)
- HPV types 16, 18 confer highest risk. HPV 6, 11 associated with benign warts
- Pre-invasive disease = atypical squamous cells of uncertain significance (ASCUS), low-grade (LGSIL) & high-grade (HGSIL) squamous intraepithelial lesion
- ASCUS: 2/3 resolve spontaneously, repeat Pap in 6 mo. If abnormal, perform colposcopy
- LGSIL = mild dysplasia/cervical intraepithelial neoplasia (CIN) 1. Half resolve spontaneously. Repeat Pap in 6 mo. If abnormal, perform colposcopy
- HGSIL = severe dysplasia/CIN 2/3/CIS. One-third resolve spontaneously. All get colposcopy with biopsy
- ~90% of invasive tumors are SCC, 10% are adenocarcinoma, & 1% clear cell

WORKUP

- H&P including bleeding, pain, gynecologic history. Examine abdomen, nodes (SCV, groins). Perform pelvic EUA jointly with the gynecologic oncologist with bimanual palpation. Evaluate cervical os, vaginal vault size, vaginal extension, size & position of uterus, parametrium, adnexa, tumor appearance & bulk
- Pap smear if not bleeding

- Colposcopy with 15× magnification, cold conization if no gross lesion noted and cannot see entire lesion with colposcope. Alternatively, 4 quadrant punch biopsies or D&C for pathology
- For IIB, III, or IVA disease or for symptoms, perform cystoscopy, sigmoidoscopy, &/or barium enema
- Labs: CBC, LFTs, chemistries, BUN/Cr, urinalysis
- Imaging: CT/MRI of abdomen & pelvis. CXR. IVP (if no CT). Consider lymphangiogram
- PET scans are sensitive (~85–90%) & specific (~95–100%)
- If stage IIIB, renal stent should be placed before starting chemo
- Note: FIGO clinical staging does <u>not allow</u> CT, MRI, bone scan, PET, lymphangiography, laparotomy

STAGING

FIGO/AJCC Clinical Staging	
/ TX	Primary tumor cannot be assessed
/ T0	No evidence of primary tumor
0 / Tis	Carcinoma in situ*
I / T1	Cervical carcinoma confined to uterus (extension to corpus should be disregarded)
IA / T1a**	Invasive carcinoma diagnosed only by microscopy. Stromal invasion with a maximum depth of 5.0 mm measured from the base of the epithelium and a horizontal spread of 7.0 mm or less. Vascular space involvement, venous or lymphatic, does not affect classification
IA1 / T1a1	Measured stromal invasion 3 mm or less in depth and 7 mm or less in horizontal spread
IA2 / T1a2	Measured stromal invasion more than 3 mm and not more than 5.0 mm with a horizontal spread 7 mm or less
IB / T1b	Clinically visible lesion confined to the cervix or microscopic lesion greater than IA2 / T1a
IB1 / T1b1	Clinically visible lesion 4.0 cm or less in greatest dimension
IB2 / T1b2	Clinically visible lesion more than 4.0 cm in greatest dimension
II / T2	Cervical carcinoma invades beyond uterus but not to pelvic wall or lower third of vagina
IIA / T2a	Tumor without parametrial invasion

IIB / T2b	Tumor with parametrial invasion
IIIA / T3a	Tumor involves lower third of vagina, no extension to pelvic wall
IIIB / T3b	Tumor extends to pelvic wall and/or causes hydronephrosis or nonfunctioning kidney
IVA / T4	Tumor invades mucosa of bladder, rectum, and/or extends beyond true pelvis (bullous edema is not sufficient to classify a tumor as T4)
/ NX	Regional lymph nodes cannot be assessed
/ N0	No regional lymph node metastasis
/ N1	Regional lymph node metastasis
/ MX	Distant metastasis cannot be assessed
/ M0	Nodistant metastasis
IVB / M1	Distant metastasis

*Bethesda or WHO system is used to further classify

**All macroscopically visible lesions – even with superficial invasion – are T1b/IB

AJCC Stage		~LC		~Survival	
0:	TisN0M0	IA:	95–100%	IA:	95–100%
I:	T1N0M0	IB1:	90–95%	IB1:	85–90%
IA:	T1aN0M0	IB2:	60–80%	IB2:	60–70%
IA1:	T1a1N0M0	IIA:	80–85%	IIA:	75%
IA2:	T1a2N0M0	IIB:	60–80%	IIB:	60–65%
IB:	T1bN0M0	IIIA:	60%	IIIA:	25–50%
IB1:	T1b1N0M0	IIIB:	50–60%	IIIB:	25–50%
IB2:	T1b2N0M0	IVA:	30%	IVA:	15–30%
II:	T2N0M0			IVB:	<10%
IIA:	T2aN0M0				
IIB:	T2bN0M0				
III:	T3N0M0				
IIIA:	T3aN0M0				
IIIB:	T3b any NM0, T1-T3aN1M0				
IVA:	T4 any NM0				
IVB:	Any T any N M1				

Used with the permission of the American Joint Committee on Cancer (AJCC), Chicago, Illinois. The original source for this material is the AJCC Cancer Staging Manual, Sixth Edition (2002) published by Springer-Verlag New York, www.springeronline.com.

TREATMENT
Surgical techniques

- Class I – total abdominal hysterectomy (extrafascial). Removes cervix, cuff (small rim), outside of the pubocervical fascia
- Class II – modified radical hysterectomy (extended). Ureters are unroofed to remove parametrial & paracervical tissue (cardinal, uterosacral) medial to the ureters, & vaginal cuff (1–2 cm)
- Class III – radical abdominal hysterectomy (Wertheim-Miegs). Mobilization of ureters, bladder and rectum to remove parametrial tissue to pelvic sidewall, and pelvic lymphadenectomy, & vaginal cuff (upper 1/3–1/2)
- Class IV – extended radical hysterectomy. Superior vesicular artery, part of ureter and bladder is removed and more vaginal cuff is removed

Indications for post-op RT/chemo-RT

- RT: LVSI, >1/3 stromal invasion, or >4 cm
- Chemo-RT: +margin, +LN, or parametrial or greater extension

Stage	Recommended Treatment
Pre-invasive	Conization or loop electrosurgical excisional procedure (LEEP) or laser or cryotherapy ablation or simple hysterectomy
IA	Total abdominal hysterectomy or cone biopsy with negative margins & close F/U (if fertility preservation desired). For IA2 lesions, radical hysterectomy preferred Alternative is brachytherapy alone (LDR 65–75 Gy or HDR 7 Gy × 5–6 fx). If high risk pathologic features, treat as IB
IB1	Radical hysterectomy with pelvic LN dissection Or definitive RT: EBRT to WP (45 Gy) & brachytherapy (HDR 6 Gy × 5 fx or LDR 15–20 Gy × 2 fx)

Stage	Recommended Treatment
IB2-IIA	Concurrent chemo-RT with cisplatin. EBRT to WP (45 Gy). Brachytherapy = HDR 6 Gy × 5 fx or LDR 15–20 Gy × 2 fx
IIB	Concurrent chemo-RT with cisplatin. EBRT to WP (45–50.4 Gy). Brachytherapy = HDR 6 Gy × 5 fx or LDR 15–20 Gy × 2 fx
IIIA	Concurrent chemo-RT with cisplatin. EBRT to WP & vagina & inguinal LN (45 Gy–50.4 Gy). Brachytherapy = HDR 6 Gy × 5 fx or LDR 17–20 Gy × 2 fx
IIIB-IVA	Concurrent chemo-RT with cisplatin. EBRT to WP (50–54 Gy). Brachytherapy = HDR 6 Gy × 5 or LDR 20 Gy × 2. If LN+, add para-aortic LN IMRT (45–60 Gy)
IVB	Combination chemotherapy

STUDIES
Surgery vs radiation
- Landoni (*Lancet* 1997). 343 pts with IB-IIA randomized to RT vs surgery ± RT. Surgery was radical hysterectomy + pelvic LND with optional adjuvant RT to 50.4 Gy for stage >IIA, <3 mm uninvolved cervix, +margin, or LN+. 45 Gy given to +PAN. 63% of pts in surgery arm received adjuvant RT. RT alone arm was 47 Gy EBRT + LDR to pt A dose 76 Gy. No significant differences in 5 yr OS (83%), DFS (74%), or recurrence (25%). Morbidity worse with surgery ± RT arm (28%) compared to RT alone arm (12%)

LDR vs HDR
- Teshima (*Cancer* 1993). 430 pts randomized to LDR×2 or HDR×4 with EBRT. No differences in CSS or OS except stage I OS was slightly higher with LDR. Gr 2/3 morbidity was also higher with HDR (10% vs 4%)

Extended-field RT (EFRT)
- Rotman RTOG 79-20 (*JAMA* 1995). 337 pts with IIB with no clinical or radiographically involved PAN randomized

to WP 45 Gy or EFRT 45 Gy. EFRT improved 10 yr OS (55% vs 44%), but there was no difference in LRC (65%) or DM (25–30%). Toxicity increased with EFRT (8% vs 4%)

Chemo-RT

- RTOG 90-01 (Morris, *NEJM* 1999; Eifel, *JCO* 2004). 386 pts with surgically staged IIB-IVA, IB-IIA ≥5 cm, or LN+ randomized to EFRT + brachytherapy to 85 Gy point A dose or to WP RT + brachytherapy to 85 Gy pt A dose + cisplatin 75 mg/m² + 5-FU 1000 mg/d × 4 d × 3 cycles. Chemo-RT improved 8 yr OS (67% vs 41%), DFS (61% vs 46%), & decreased LRF (18 vs 35%) & DM (20% vs 35%). Chemo-RT had a non-significant increase in PAN failures (8 vs 4)

- GOG 120 (Rose, *NEJM* 1999). 526 pts with IIB-IVA (surgically staged, paraaortic LN negative) randomized to WP + brachytherapy (to 81 Gy pt A dose) + 3 different chemo regimens: weekly cisplatin 40 mg/m² vs cisplatin/5-FU/hydroxyurea vs hydroxyurea alone. Cisplatin arms improved 4 yr OS (65% vs 47%) & decreased recurrence (34–35% vs 54%). Toxicity was less with cisplatin or hydroxyurea alone.

- NCIC (Pearcey, *JCO* 2002). 353 pts with IA, IIA >5 cm or IIB randomized to WP 45 Gy + LDR 35 Gy ×1 or HDR 8 Gy ×3 vs same RT + weekly cisplatin 40 mg/m² ×6c. No differences in 3/5 yr OS (69/62% vs 66/58%). Study criticized because required only CT staging of nodes & the small # of pts

- GOG 123 (Keys, *NEJM* 1999). 369 pts with IB2 randomized to WP + brachytherapy to pt A dose 75 Gy followed by adjuvant simple hysterectomy vs same RT + weekly cisplatin 40 mg/m² also followed by adjuvant simple hysterectomy. Chemo-RT improved 3 yr OS (83% vs 74%) & decreased LR (21% vs 37%) & increased pCR (52% vs 41%). Authors felt that improved LC led to increased OS due to cisplatin and that adding hysterectomy did not improve OS

Adjuvant hysterectomy after RT

- GOG 71 (Keys, *Cancer J Sci Am* 1997). 282 pts with >4 cm tumors randomized to EBRT + brachytherapy (80 Gy pt A dose) vs same RT but 75 Gy pt A dose followed by adjuvant hysterectomy. No difference in OS (61% vs 64%) but trend for higher LR without adjuvant hysterectomy (26% vs 14%, p = 0.08). No difference in toxicity

Post-op RT

- GOG 92/RTOG 8706 (Rotman, *IJROBP* 2006; Sedlis, *Gynecol Onc* 1999). 277 pts with IB treated with radical hysterectomy with negative margins & LN-, but with ≥2 risk factors (LVSI, >$^1/_3$ stromal invasion, or >4 cm tumors) randomized to observation vs post-op WP RT (46–50.4 Gy). Post-op RT reduced LR (21 → 14%) & DM (9 → 3%), & improved OS (71 → 80%)

Post-op chemo-RT

- GOG 109/SWOG 8797 (Peters, *JCO* 2000, SGO 2004). 243 pts s/p radical hysterectomy with IA2, IB, IIA & LN+ or +margin or +parametria randomized to WP RT (49.3 Gy with 45 Gy to PAN if common iliac LN+) vs WP RT + cisplatin/5-FU every 3 wks × 4c. Post-op chemo-RT improved 4 yr PFS (80% vs 63%), OS (81% vs 71%). Re-analysis demonstrated that chemo-RT decreased LR by 50%, & DM by 30%. ~20% OS benefit from chemo for tumors >2 cm & pts with ≥2 LN+

RADIATION TECHNIQUES

EBRT simulation and field design

- Simulate pt supine. Place 2 radiopaque markers (gold seeds) in cervix and at distal margin of any vaginal disease. Place vaginal & anal markers
- Treat with 4 field or AP/PA technique
- Borders: superior = L4/5; inferior = 3 cm below most inferior vaginal involvement as marked by gold seeds (often at inferior obturator foramen); lateral = 2 cm lateral to pelvic brim; posterior = include entire sacrum; anterior = 1 cm anterior to pubic symphysis. CT planned
- Inguinal fields are treated if stage IIIA (lower 1/3 vagina). Inferior border is vaginal introitus or flash
- If posterior vaginal wall extensively involved, treat perirectal nodes
- If common iliac nodes + raise superior border to have 4 cm margin on known nodes (~L3/4 level)
- EFRT for paraaortic nodes: superior border = T11/12, lateral = encompass tips of transverse processes. CT plan. Block kidneys as determined by CT
- When used, the goal of a midline block is to avoid excess dose adjacent to the implant & to deliver higher dose to potential tumor bearing regions outside the implant. Midline block reduces dose to bladder and rectum, but

may underdose sacrum. Since T&O has 100% dose through Pt A which is ~2 cm from midline, a 4 cm midline block would be at the 100% IDL. If concerned about toxicity, use a wider block (6 cm, ~50% IDL) or if concerned about tumor use a narrower block. Midline blocks narrower than 5 cm may include the ureters which are ~2–2.5 cm from midline. Superior border of midline block = mid-sacroiliac joint

- At many institutions, it is preferred to deliver higher EBRT doses with a midline block for advanced lesions. After 45 Gy to the WP, some institutions drop the superior border to the mid-sacroiliac joint & continue EBRT to 50 Gy. At 50 Gy, the field is further reduced by dropping the superior border to the bottom of the sacro-iliac joint & the EBRT dose is carried to 54 Gy. If parametrial tumor persists after 50–54 Gy, may boost parametria to 60 Gy
- If bulky N+, use 3DCRT or IMRT boost to 60 Gy to involved nodes
- EBRT causes contraction of upper vagina which limits size and packing of vaginal applicators, so try to start brachytherapy 2 wks into EBRT

Brachytherapy

- Proceed when tumor <4 cm (so pt A dose will cover it)
- In general, 1st intracavitary insertion is after 10–20 Gy EBRT unless need more shrinkage. 2nd application is 1–2 wks later. Smitt sleeve may be left in cervical canal between insertions
- If small lesion and narrow vagina, treat with IC RT 1st to optimize brachytherapy before EBRT causes shrinkage and narrowing of vagina
- If large lesion and narrow vagina, use EBRT 1st to shrink the tumor
- If superficial vaginal involvement, use T&O for 1st insertion, then tandem & vaginal cylinder for 2nd insertion (with packing to spare rectum or bladder). Or, use 2 tandem and vaginal cylinder insertions
- For deep vaginal involvement, use IS brachytherapy
- Packing used to push bladder and rectum away. Always soak packing in 40% iodinated contrast (or gauze with imbedded radio-opaque wire). Use Triple-Sulfate soaked gauze for LDR, K-Y Jelly for HDR

- LDR is generally Cs-137 at 0.4–0.8 Gy/hr. Repair of sub-lethal damage with dose rates <0.6–0.8 Gy/hr is similar to fractionated EBRT. 0.4–0.6 Gy/hr has less complications than 0.8–1 Gy/hr
- HDR is generally an Ir-192 high activity (~10 Ci) source with dose rate ~12 Gy/h
- ICRU system: report applicator type, source type, loading, and orthogonal radiographs. Use reference air-kerma strength, volume treated to 60 Gy
- Prescribe to Point A. Point A = 2 cm superior to external cervical os (or vaginal fornices) and 2 cm lateral to central canal/tandem (ideally where uterine vessels cross ureter). Point A dose is very sensitive to the position of the ovoids relative to the tandem
- Point B = 3 cm lateral to Point A, represents parametrial (obturator node). Receives $\sim^1/_3$–$^1/_4$ of dose to Point A
- Pt C = 4 cm lateral to Point A, represents side wall. Receives $\sim^1/_5$ of dose to Pt A
- Point M = 2 cm above ovoids on lateral X-ray
- Bladder point = posterior surface of foley balloon on lateral X-ray & center of balloon on AP film. Foley balloon filled with 7 cc radiopaque fluid & pulled down against urethra
- Rectal point = 5 mm behind posterior vaginal wall between ovoids at inferior point of last intrauterine tandem source, or mid vaginal source
- Vaginal point = lateral edge of ovoid on AP film & mid-ovoid on lateral film
- Tandem placement: Use a looping suture through the cervix for counter-traction. Hegar uterine dilators are used to dilate the os to 6 mm. Tandem inserts usually 6–8 cm (4 cm for postmenopausal women). For tandems >8 cm, use spacer at end to protect small bowel. Tandem should be placed centrally between the ovoids on the AP view & should bisect the ovoids on the lateral view
- Typical tandem loading with Cs-137 = 30–40 mgRaEq with three 10–15 mgRaEq sources (e.g., 15–15–10 cephalad to caudad)
- Ovoids: Cervix should always be marked with 2 gold seeds (usually at 12 & 6 o'clock). Use largest ovoids possible & they should be separated by 0.5–1 cm. Standard loadings for ovoids = 10–15 mgRaEq for 2 cm (small) ovoids or 15–20 mgRaEq for 2.5 cm (medium) ovoids or 5–10 mgRaEq for mini-ovoids

- Pack anteriorly & posteriorly to spare the bladder & rectum
- Films taken in the OR so that the system may be repositioned & re-packed if sub-optimal
- With optimally placed system, LDR dose rate at point A is ~45–55 cGy/hr
- Overall treatment time: prolongation of treatment time increases failure rate by 0.6%/d in IB-IIA and by 0.9%/d in IIB. Try to keep overall treatment time <7 wks

Dose prescriptions

- EBRT: 1.8 Gy/fx. Whole pelvis = 45 Gy. Side wall boost = 50–54 Gy. Persistent or bulky parametrial tumor = 60 Gy. Paraaortic (if treated) = 45 Gy. Bulky LN = 60 Gy
- Brachytherapy
  - LDR = 15–20 Gy × 2 fx
  - HDR = 6 Gy × 5 fx (alternative: 7 Gy × 4 fx)
- Desired cumulative doses
  - Point A: IA = 65–75 Gy, IB1-IIB 75–85 Gy, III-IVA 85–90 Gy
  - Sidewall dose: IB-IIA = 45–50 Gy, IIB = 45–54 Gy, III-IVA = 54–60 Gy

Dose limitations

- Limit bladder & rectal points to <70% of point A dose with HDR. With LDR, limit rectal point <70 Gy & bladder point <75 Gy
- Upper vaginal mucosa tolerance is 120 Gy, mid-vaginal mucosal tolerance is 80–90 Gy, & lower vaginal mucosa tolerance is 60–70 Gy. Vaginal doses >50–60 Gy cause significant vaginal fibrosis & stenosis
- Ovarian failure with 5–10 Gy. Sterilization with 2–3 Gy
- Ureters <75 Gy, femoral heads <50 Gy

COMPLICATIONS

- Acute: pruritis, dry/moist desquamation, hemorrhoids, nausea, colitis (cramping, diarrhea, transient rectal bleeding), cystitis (dysuria, frequency, nocturia), vaginitis or ulceration, vaginal candidiasis
- Procedure-related: uterine perforation (<3%), vaginal laceration (<1%), DVT (<1%)
- Equivalent morbidity after HDR or LDR

- Late: vaginal stenosis, ureteral strictures (1–3%), fistulas (vesicovaginal/rectovaginal <2%), intestinal obstruction or perforation (<5%), femoral neck fracture (<5%)
- Recommend regular vaginal dilation to maintain size of vaginal vault and improve sexual function
- Surgical mortality 1%. Standard post-op complications. Bladder atonia temporarily after surgery

FOLLOW-UP

- H&P every mo for 3 mo, then every 3 mo for 9 mo, then every 4 mo for 1 yr, then every 6 mo for 2 yrs, then annually
- F/U Pap smears controversial due to post-RT change
- CXR annually × 5 yr

REFERENCES

Eifel PJ. The Uterine Cervix. In: Cox JD, Ang KK, editors. Radiation oncology: rationale, technique, results. 8th ed. St. Louis: Mosby; 2003. pp. 681–723.

Eifel PJ, Winter K, Morris M, et al. Pelvic irradiation with concurrent chemotherapy versus pelvic and para-aortic irradiation for high-risk cervical cancer: an update of radiation therapy oncology group trial (RTOG) 90-01. J Clin Oncol 2004;22:872–880.

Greene FL, American Joint Committee on Cancer., American Cancer Society. AJCC cancer staging manual. 6th ed. New York: Springer-Verlag; 2002.

Keys HM, Bundy BN, Stehman FB, et al. Adjuvant hysterectomy after radiation therapy reduces detection of local recurrences in "bulky" stage IB cervical without improving survival: results of a prospective randomized GOG trial. Cancer J Sci Am 1997; 3:117(abstr).

Keys HM, Bundy BN, Stehman FB, et al. Cisplatin, radiation, and adjuvant hysterectomy compared with radiation and adjuvant hysterectomy for bulky stage IB cervical carcinoma. N Engl J Med 1999;340:1154–1161.

Keys HM, Bundy BN, Stehman FB, et al. Radiation therapy with and without extrafascial hysterectomy for bulky stage IB cervical carcinoma: a randomized trial of the Gynecologic Oncology Group. Gynecol Oncol 2003;89:343–353.

Landoni F, Maneo A, Colombo A, et al. Randomised study of radical surgery versus radiotherapy for stage Ib-IIa cervical cancer. Lancet 1997;350:535–540.

Morris M, Eifel PJ, Lu J, et al. Pelvic radiation with concurrent chemotherapy compared with pelvic and para-aortic radiation for high-risk cervical cancer. N Engl J Med 1999;340:1137–1143.

National Comprehensive Cancer Network. Clinical Practice Guidelines in Oncology: Cervical Cancers. Available at: http://www.nccn.org/professionals/physician_gls/PDF/cervical.pdf. Accessed on January 19, 2005.

Pearcey R, Brundage M, Drouin P, et al. Phase III trial comparing radical radiotherapy with and without cisplatin chemotherapy in patients with advanced squamous cell cancer of the cervix. J Clin Oncol 2002;20:966–972.

Perez CA, Kavanagh BD. Uterine cervix. In: Perez CA, Brady LW, Halperin EC, et al., editors. Principles and Practice of Radiation Oncology. 4th ed. Philadelphia: Lippincott Williams & Wilkins; 2004. pp. 1800–1915.

Perez CA, Kavanagh D. Uterine Cervix. In: Perez CA, Brady LW, Halperin EC, et al., editors. Principles and practice of radiation oncology. 4th ed. Philadelphia: Lippincott Williams & Wilkins; 2004. pp. 1800–1915.

Peters WA 3rd, Liu PY, Barrett RJ 2nd, et al. Concurrent chemotherapy and pelvic radiation therapy compared with pelvic radiation therapy alone as adjuvant therapy after radical surgery in high-risk early-stage cancer of the cervix. J Clin Oncol 2000;18:1606–1613.

Rose PG, Bundy BN, Watkins EB, et al. Concurrent cisplatin-based radiotherapy and chemotherapy for locally advanced cervical cancer. N Engl J Med 1999;340:1144–1153.

Rotman M, Pajak TF, Choi K, et al. Prophylactic extended-field irradiation of para-aortic lymph nodes in stages IIB and bulky IB and IIA cervical carcinomas. Ten-year treatment results of RTOG 79-20. JAMA 1995;274:387–393.

Rotman M, Sedlis A, Piedmonte MR, et al. A phase III randomized trial of postoperative pelvic irradiation in stage IB cervical carcinoma with poor prognostic features: follow-up of a gynecologic oncology group study. Int J Radiat Oncol Biol Phys 2006;65:169–176.

Sedlis A, Bundy BN, Rotman MZ, et al. A randomized trial of pelvic radiation therapy versus no further therapy in selected patients with stage IB carcinoma of the cervix after radical hysterectomy and pelvic lymphadenectomy: A Gynecologic Oncology Group Study. Gynecol Oncol 1999;73:177–183.

Swift PS, Hsu IC. Cancer of the Uterine Cervix. In: Leibel SA, Phillips TL, editors. Textbook of Radiation Oncology. 2nd ed. Philadelphia: Saunders; 2004. pp. 1055–1100.

Teshima T, Inoue T, Ikeda H, et al. High-dose rate and low-dose rate intracavitary therapy for carcinoma of the uterine cervix. Final results of Osaka University Hospital. Cancer 1993;72:2409–2414.

NOTES

Chapter 29
Endometrial Cancer

Kim Huang and I-Chow Hsu

PEARLS

- Fourth most common malignancy in women after breast, lung, and colorectal
- Most common gynecological cancer in U.S.
- Second most common cause of gynecological cancer death (after ovarian)
- Risk factors: late menopause, nulliparous, obesity, excess estrogen unopposed with progesterone, tamoxifen (7.5×), oral contraceptives
- Rate of progression to invasive cancer: simple hyperplasia rare (<1%), complex hyperplasia ~3%, atypical simple hyperplasia ~8%, complex hyperplasia ~29%
- 75% of tumors are endometrial adenocarcinomas. Ciliated subtype associated with prior estrogen use and has excellent prognosis
- Grade 1: ≤5% non-squamous or solid growth pattern. Grade 2: 5–50% non-squamous or solid growth pattern. Grade 3: >50% non-squamous or solid growth pattern
- Varying degrees of squamous differentiation: well-differentiated (adenoacanthoma) to poorly differentiated (adenosquamous)
- Most aggressive histologies = papillary serous (UPSC), clear cell, and pure SCC
- Papillary serous has frequent deep invasion, LVSI, & peritoneal spread; most often seen in ovarian & fallopian tube cancer
- Clear cell associated with older women; seen in ovarian, cervical, & vaginal CA
- Most common sarcoma of uterus = carcinosarcoma (mullerian mixed tumor) which contains both malignant epithelial & sarcomatous elements. Generally pts are older than 60 yrs. Next most common = leiomyosarcoma & endometrial stromal sarcomas

■ Primary lymphatic drainage is to pelvic LN (internal & external iliac, obturator, common iliac, presacral, parametrial), but direct spread may occur to paraaortic LN directly (rare in the absence of + pelvic LN). ~1/3 of pts with pelvic LN have + paraaortic LN

■ Risk of LN involvement by depth of invasion & grade was detailed in GOG 33 (Creasman, *Cancer* 1987)

	%Pelvic/Paraaortic LN		
Invasion	**Gr1**	**Gr2**	**Gr3**
Endometrium	0/0	3/3	0/0
Inner 1/3	3/1	5/4	9/4
Middle 1/3	0/5	9/0	4/0
Outer 1/3	11/6	19/14	34/23

■ Other adverse prognostic factors = LVSI, age >60, higher stage, lower uterine segment involvement, anemia, poor KPS

WORKUP

■ H&P. Careful attention to uterine size, cervical & vaginal involvement, ascites, nodes. Pap smear has limited sensitivity (as low as 40%)

■ Endometrial biopsy has 90–98% sensitivity, 85% specificity & therefore obviates need for D&C most of the time. If endometrial biopsy non-diagnostic, then D&C

■ Labs: CBC, blood chemistries, LFTs, CA125 (elevated in 60%), UA

■ Imaging: CXR. For symptoms or advanced disease, CT or MRI of abdomen & pelvis, or transvaginal ultrasound

■ Cystoscopy, sigmoidoscopy for symptoms or advanced lesions

STAGING

AJCC TNM / FIGO Pathologic Staging	~Survival
TX: Primary tumor cannot be assessed	IA: 91%
	IB: 88%
T0: No evidence of primary tumor	IC: 81%
	IIA: 77%
Tis / 0: Carcinoma in situ	IIB: 67%
T1 / I: Tumor confined to corpus uteri	IIIA: 60%
	IIIB: 41%
T1a / IA: Tumor limited to endometrium	IIIC: 32%
	IVA: 5%

T1b / IB:	Tumor invades less than one-half of the myometrium
T1c / IC:	Tumor invades one-half or more of the myometrium
T2 / II:	Tumor invades cervix but does not extend beyond uterus
T2a / IIA:	Tumor limited to glandular epithelium of endocervix. There is no evidence of connective tissue stromal invasion
T2b / IIB:	Invasion of the stromal connective tissue of the cervix
T3 / III:	Local and/or regional spread as defined below
T3a / IIIA:	Tumor involves serosa and/or adnexa (direct extension or metastasis) and/or cancer cells in ascites or peritoneal washings
T3b / IIIB:	Vaginal involvement (direct extension or metastasis)
T4 / IVA:	Tumor invades bladder mucosa and/or bowel mucosa (bullous edema is not sufficient to classify a tumor as T4)
NX:	Regional lymph nodes cannot be assessed
N0:	No regional lymph node metastasis
N1 / IIIC:	Regional lymph node metastasis to pelvic and/or para-aortic nodes
MX:	Distant metastasis cannot be assessed
M0:	No distant metastasis
M1 / IVB:	Distant metastasis (includes metastasis to abdominal lymph nodes other than para-aortic, and/or inguinal lymph nodes; excludes metastasis to vagina, pelvic serosa, or adnexa)

A small number of patients may be treated with primary radiation therapy. In such cases, patients should be staged with the clinical staging system adopted by FIGO in 1971 (*Int J Gynaecol Obstet* 1971;9:172)

TREATMENT RECOMMENDATIONS

Stage	Recommended Treatment
IA G1–2	Surgery [TAH/BSO, peritoneal washings, & pelvic & paraaortic LN sampling (if frozen section >IA or >G1)] → observation
IB G1	If no LVSI & age <60, surgery → observation If LVSI or age >60, consider vaginal cuff brachytherapy (VC)
IA G3, IB G2–3	If no LVSI & age <60, surgery → observation If LVSI or age >60, surgery → VC if complete surgical staging or whole pelvic RT (WP) if incomplete surgical staging
IC G1	If no LVSI & age <60, surgery → VC or observation If LVSI or age >60, surgery → VC (if complete surgical staging) or WP (if incomplete surgical staging)
IC G2	Surgery → VC (if complete surgical staging) or WP (if incomplete surgical staging)
IC G3	If no LVSI & age >60, surgery → WP + VC. Controversial alternative = VC alone if complete surgical staging because several retrospective series have shown only 0–3% pelvic recurrence If LVSI or age >60, surgery → WP + VC. Alternative is WP with increased EBRT dose to vaginal cuff & no brachytherapy

Stage	Recommended Treatment
IIA	If G1–2 with <1/2 myometrial involvement, surgery → WP or VC If G3 with <1/2 myometrial involvement, surgery → WP ± VC If >1/2 myometrial involvement, surgery → WP ± VC (unless G3 = WP + VC)
IIB	Surgery → WP + VC. Or pre-op WP (45 Gy) + T&O (6 Gy ×3)
IIIA (+ peritoneal cytology only)	If + cytology with a IA G1–2 primary tumor, surgery → observation If >IA primary tumor or >G1–2, surgery → WP + VC
IIIA	Surgery → WP + VC. Use extended-field RT (EFRT) for involved paraaortic LN (PAN)
IIIB	Usually no surgery because would require extended radical hysterectomy which combined with RT is very morbid. WP + VC (EFRT for +PAN). Frequently require IS brachytherapy
IIIC	Surgery → WP + VC (if only low pelvic LN+) or EFRT + VC (if high pelvic LN or PAN+)
IVA	EBRT + brachytherapy boost, or chemo (doxorubicin, cisplatin every 3 wks × 7c), or pelvic exenteration
UPSC	For stage I–II, WP + VC. If higher risk, then chemo (carboplatin-paclitaxel × 3–6c) + WP + VC. For stage III–IV, chemo (carboplatin-paclitaxel × 3–6c) with whole-abdominal RT (WART) sometimes sandwiched or at end

Stage	Recommended Treatment
Medically inoperable	WP (50.4 Gy with midline block at 20–40 Gy) + brachytherapy ×2 to deliver 60–80 Gy vaginal surface dose or 54–60 Gy to serosal surface & hotter vaginalsurface dose
Recurrence	If no prior RT → EBRT + IC or IS boost to total dose 60–70 Gy depending on size & normal tolerance
Sarcomas	Surgery. Post-op RT generally used for grade 2–3 to improve LC (but may not have effect on OS)

- Note: intraperitoneal P-32 is effective in reducing subclinical intraperitoneal recurrences but it has significant bowel complications if combined with EBRT, so generally it is not used

STUDIES

- GOG 99 (*Gyn Onc* 2004). 392 pts with IB (60%), IC (30%), & occult II (10%) treated with TAH/BSO, pelvic & PAN sampling, & peritoneal cytology with 6 yr F/U. Pts randomized to observation vs post-op WP RT (50.4 Gy). 1/3 of pts had high-intermediate risk disease (G2–3, outer 1/3 involvement, and LVSI or age >50 + 2 factors, or age >70 + 1 factor). 2/3 pts were low-intermediate risk. WP RT improved LRR (12→3%), mostly among high-intermediate risk pts (26→6%) compared to low-intermediate risk pts (6→2%). No difference in OS (86→92%) but not powered to detect change in OS
- Aalders, Norway (*Ob Gyn* 1980). 500 pts with IB-IC any grade treated with TAH/BSO without LN sampling. Randomized to VC vs VC → WP RT. VC = LDR 60 Gy

to surface. WP = 2/40 Gy with central shielding at 20 Gy. 65% of pts had IB G1–2. Addition of WP RT decreased pelvic & vaginal recurrences (7→2%), but no change in OS (90%) because more DM in WP arm. On subset analysis, most improvement in LRR with IC G3 (20→5%). Poor prognostic factors = IC, G3, LVSI, age >60

- <u>PORTEC</u> (Creutzberg, *Lancet* 2000; Scholten, *IJROBP* 2005). 714 pts with IB G2–3 or IC G1–2 treated with TAH/BSO randomized to observation vs WP RT (46 Gy). No LN dissection (only sampling of suspicious LN). 90% of pts had G1–2 & 40% were IB. WP RT decreased LRR (14 → 4%). 75% of failures were in vaginal vault. No difference in OS (81 vs 85%) or DM (8 vs 7%). With 10 yr f/u & central review of pathology for 80% of pts, WP RT continued to reduce LRR (14 → 5%) without an OS benefit (66 vs 73%) even after excluding IB grade 1 pts

- <u>GOG 122</u> (*JCO* 2005). 396 pts with III/IV disease treated with surgery with maximal residual disease ≤2 cm randomized to whole-abdominal RT (30 Gy + 15 Gy pelvic boost + 15 Gy paraaortic boost if pelvic LN+ or no sampling of pelvic & paraaortic LN) vs chemo (doxorubicin + cisplatin every 3 wks × 7 c). 21% of pts had UPSC in each arm. Chemo improved 5 yr OS (42 → 55%) & DFS (38 → 50%), but increased grade 3–4 hematologic, gastrointestinal, & cardiac toxicity

RADIATION TECHNIQUES
Simulation and field design
- Simulate pt supine with full bladder, bowel contrast, & vaginal marker
- CT planning recommended
- WP borders: superior = L4/5; inferior = lower 1/2 of vagina by marker; lateral = 1.5 cm lateral to pelvic brim; posterior = split sacrum to S3; anterior = pubic symphysis
- EFRT borders: extend superior border to T10/T11 or T11/T12 with CT planning to avoid kidneys
- Brachytherapy boost: place bladder catheter with balloon filled with contrast. 2 marker seeds placed in vaginal cuff at 9 & 3 o'clock. Rectal tube placed. Vaginal cylinder or colpostats can be used. Use largest vaginal cylinder pos-

sible (2.5–3.5 cm). Target upper 2/3 of vaginal cuff unless IIIB when target is whole vaginal cuff. Calculate surface dose and 0.5 cm dose

■ Definitive or pre-op RT may use Heyman capsules or 2 tandems because only looking to cover uterus. Add ovoids to cover cervical extension for stage II. Prescription point is uterine serosa. Dilate using Hegar dilators to 10 mm

■ WART = Use fluoroscopy to determine 1 cm above diaphragm. Need to watch platelets carefully.

Dose prescriptions

■ Post-op
  ■ WP 1.8 Gy/fx to 45 Gy ± VC 6 Gy ×3 (HDR) or 30 Gy (LDR) to vaginal surface. May increase WP dose to 50 Gy if pelvic extension
  ■ If VC used alone, 6 Gy ×6 (HDR) or 60–70 Gy (LDR) to vaginal surface
■ Pre-op: 1.8 Gy/fx to 45 Gy, plus T&O 6 Gy × 3–4 (HDR)
■ Vaginal extension: WP 45–50 Gy plus interstitial implants
■ Paraaortic LN+: EFRT to 45 Gy, plus VC 6 Gy × 3 (HDR)
■ WART: 1.5 Gy/fx to 30 Gy to whole abdomen → cone down to para-aortic LN & WP to 45 Gy. IMRT can improve target coverage and normal tissue sparing
■ Inoperable: WP 40–50 Gy & ICRT 5–6 Gy × 4 (HDR)

Dose limitations

■ Upper vaginal mucosa 150 Gy, lower vaginal mucosa 80–90 Gy
■ Ovarian failure w/ 5–10 Gy. Sterilization w/ 2–3 Gy
■ Rectal point dose <70 Gy, bladder point <75 Gy
■ For WART, use kidney blocks to restrict kidney dose <15 Gy, liver block to shield R lobe of liver after 25 Gy

COMPLICATIONS

■ TAH/BSO mortality <1%
■ Surgical complications = infection, wound dehiscence, fistulas, bleeding
■ Low risk to bowel with <45–50.4 Gy

- Low risk to vagina if total dose <100 Gy
- Vaginal stenosis: use dilators
- Frequency & urgency of urine & stool

FOLLOW-UP

- Every 3 mo × 1 yr, every 4 mo × 1 yr, every 6 mo × 3 yrs, then annually

REFERENCES

Aalders JG, Abeler V, Kolstad P, et al. Postoperative external irradiation and prognostic parameters in satge I endometrial carcinoma: clinical and histopathologic study of 540 patients. Gynecol Oncol 1980;56:419.

Alektiar KM, Nori D. Cancer of the endometrium. In: Leibel SA, Phillips TL, editors. Textbook of radiation oncology. 2nd ed. Philadelphia: Saunders; 2004. pp. 1101–1131.

Creutzberg CL, van Putten WL, Koper PC, et al. Surgery and postoperative radiotherapy versus surgery alone for patients with stage-1 endometrial carcinoma: multicentre randomised trial. PORTEC Study Group. Post Operative Radiation Therapy in Endometrial Carcinoma. Lancet 2000;355:1404–1411.

Glassburn JR, Brady LW, Grigsby PW. Endometrium. In: Perez CA, Brady LW, Halperin EC, et al., editors. Principles and practice of radiation oncology. 4th ed. Philadelphia: Lippincott Williams & Wilkins; 2004. pp. 1916–1933.

Greene FL, American Joint Committee on Cancer., American Cancer Society. AJCC cancer staging manual. 6th ed. New York: Springer-Verlag; 2002.

Jhingran A, Eifel PJ. The Endometrium. In: Cox JD, Ang KK, editors. Radiation oncology: rationale, technique, results. 8th ed. St. Louis: Mosby; 2003. pp. 724–742.

Keys HM, Roberts JA, Brunetto VL, et al. A phase III trial of surgery with or without adjunctive external pelvic radiation therapy in intermediate risk endometrial adenocarcinoma: a Gynecologic Oncology Group study. Gynecol Oncol 2004;92:744–751.

National Comprehensive Cancer Network. Clinical Practice Guidelines in Oncology: Endometrial cancers. Available at: http://www.nccn.org/professionals/physician_gls/PDF/uterine.pdf. Accessed on January 19, 2005.

Randall ME, Filiaci VL, Muss H, et al. Randomized phase III trial of whole-abdominal irradiation versus doxorubicin and cisplatin chemotherapy in advanced endometrial carcinoma: a Gynecologic Oncology Group study. *J Clin Oncol* 2006;24:36–44.

Scholten AN, van Putten WLJ, Beerman H, et al. Postoperative radiotherapy for stage 1 endometrial carcinoma: long-term outcome of the randomized PORTEC trial with central pathology review. *Int J Radiat Oncol Biol Phys* 2005;63:834–838.

Chapter 30
Ovarian Cancer

James Rembert and I-Chow Hsu

PEARLS

- Leading cause of gynecologic cancer death, 2nd most common gynecologic cancer
- Fourth leading cause of cancer death in women
- Highly curable if diagnosed at an early stage, yet no good screening test
- Stage at presentation: I 26%; II 15%; III 42%; IV 17%
- Median age at diagnosis: 63. Peak incidence 8th decade
- Decreased risk: multiple parity, lactation, tubal ligation, oral contraceptive pill use (protection may persist years after stopping)
- Increased risk: nulliparity, ovulation inducing drugs, hormone replacement therapy, 1st parity age >35 yrs, diet (high fat, high lactose, coffee)
- Only 5% of tumors result from a genetic disposition, yet strongest risk factor is a family history of ovarian cancer (1° relatives)
- Lifetime risk: general population 1.6%, One first-degree relative: 5%, two first-degree relatives: 7%
- Familial syndromes
  - BRCA1 – lifetime risk 15–45% (% risk depends on penetrance in family)
  - BRCA2 – lifetime risk 10%
  - Lynch syndrome II – HNPCC and other cancers of Gyn/GU tract
  - Others: Peutz-Jeghers, palmoplantar keratoadenoma, Ollier's syndrome, Maffucci's syndrome
  - Tend to have a more indolent course than sporadic variants

- Pathology: 90% epithelial, stromal 4–8%, germ cell 2–4%
  - Epithelial tumors graded from borderline → undifferentiated
  - Borderline tumors can metastasize, yet have no evidence of stromal invasion
  - Epithelial histologic types: serous 50%, endometrioid 20%, undifferentiated 15%, mucinous 10%, clear cell 4%
- Patterns of spread: exfoliation into peritoneal cavity, angiolymphatic
- Lymphatic spread: mainly pelvic/para-aortic, but inguinals at risk via round ligament
- Patterns of relapse: tend to remain local, only 15% relapses extra-abdominal
- 90% recurrences occur within 5 yrs
- Most patients die from local disease (small bowel obstruction, ascites, etc.)
- Prognostic factors
  - Most important: stage, grade, residual volume of disease
  - Other negative factors: age >65, pre-op ascites, CA125 level > normal after 3c chemo, CA125 nadir >20 U/ml after first-line therapy

WORKUP

- H&P with complete gynecolgic exam and Pap smear
  - Common signs and symptoms: abdominal discomfort/pain, increasing girth, change in bowel habits, early satiety, dyspepsia, nausea, ascites, adnexal mass, pleural effusion (R-sided more common), Sister Mary Joseph's nodule, Blumer's shelf
  - Leser-Trelat sign: sudden appearance of seborrheic keratoses, has been noted to herald ovarian cancer in rare cases
  - Paraneoplastic syndromes: hypercalcemia with clear cell, subacute cerebellar degeneration
- Labs: CBC, LFT, BUN/Cr, serum tumor markers as follows:
  - CA125: most useful, elevated in 85% epithelial ovarian tumors
    - False positives possible, especially in pre-menopausal women due to pregnancy, endometriosis, adenomy-

osis, fibroids, benign cysts, menstruation, PID, peritoneal irritation, cirrhosis, CHF, other cancers (pancreatic, breast, GI cancers, lung, plasma cell dyscrasias, metastatic cervical and endometrial)
- If post-menopausal, CA125 >65 U/ml (normal <35 U/ml) has 97% sensitivity/80% specificity
- CA19-9: low sensitivity but can be positive in GI or mullerian tumors
- CEA: elevated in 58% with Stage III disease
- AFP and ßHCG: measure if <30 yo to help r/o germ cell tumors
- Imaging:
  - Transvaginal US (more useful for adnexal masses than transabdominal)
    - Complex ovarian cyst highly suggestive of cancer, surgery indicated
    - Simple cyst <4 cm can be followed by serial US
    - Ovarian enlargement during reproductive yrs usually benign
  - CT/MRI abd/pelvis: especially helpful pre-operatively if advanced dz
- Cystoscopy, sigmoidoscopy, barium enema as clinically indicated
- Upper GI series or endoscopy indicated in women with anemia & ovarian mass to rule out Krukenberg tumor (metastasis to ovary from a GI primary)
- Endometrial biopsy pre-operatively in women with abnormal vaginal bleeding
- Pre-op percutaneous assessment of ascites/mass NOT recommended – may lead to tumor seeding along tract/peritoneum and delay definitive surgical staging/management
- Surgical exploration: excise intact suspicious adnexal mass, frozen sections → if malignant proceed to complete surgical staging
- Surgical staging: vertical incision, collect ascites/washings, TAH/BSO*, complete abdominal exploration, omentectomy, random peritoneal biopsies (including diaphragm), aortic/pelvic lymph node sampling, optimal debulking

*If proven Stage IA, may preserve fertility with unilateral salpingo-oophrectomy (USO).

STAGING

Primary tumor		
TNM	*FIGO*	
TX		Primary tumor cannot be assessed
T0		No evidence of primary tumor
T1	I	Tumor limited to ovaries (one or both)
1a	IA	Tumor limited to one ovary; capsule intact, no tumor on ovarian surface. No malignant cells in ascites or peritoneal washings[1]
1b	IB	Tumor limited to both ovaries; capsule intact, no tumor on ovarian surface. No malignant cells in ascites or peritoneal washings[1]
1c	IC	Tumor limited to one or both ovaries with any of the following: capsule ruptured, tumor on ovarian surface, malignant cells in ascites or peritoneal washings
T2	II	Tumor involves one or both ovaries with pelvic extension
2a	IIA	Extension and/or implants on uterus and/or tube(s). No malignant cells in ascites or peritoneal washings
2b	IIB	Extension to and/or implants on other pelvic tissues. No malignant cells in ascites or peritoneal washings
2c	IIC	Pelvic extension and/or implants (T2a or T2b) with malignant cells in ascites or peritoneal washings
T3	III	Tumor involves one or both ovaries with microscopically confirmed peritoneal metastasis outside pelvis[2]
3a	IIIA	Microscopic peritoneal metastasis beyond pelvis (no macroscopic tumor)[2]
3b	IIIB	Macroscopic peritoneal metastasis beyond pelvis 2 cm or less in greatest dimension[2]
3c	IIIC	Peritoneal metastasis beyond pelvis more than 2 cm in greatest dimension and/or regional lymph node metastasis[2]

Regional lymph nodes		
NX		No regional lymph node metastasis cannot be assessed
N0		No regional lymph node metastasis
N1:	IIIC	Regional lymph node metastasis

Distant metastasis		
MX		Distant metastasis cannot be assessed
M0		No distant metastasis
M1	IV	Distant metastasis (excludes peritoneal metastasis)

[1]The presence of non-malignant ascites is not classified. The presence of ascites does not affect staging unless malignant cells are present.

[2]Liver capsule metastasis T3/III, liver parencymal metaasatasis M1/Stage IV. Pleural effusion must have positive cytology for M1/Stage IV.

Stage Grouping (AJCC/UICC/FIGO)		5yr OS by Stage: (~40% overall)	
IA/B/C	T1a/b/cN0M0	I:	~80% overall (>90% IA/B)
IIA/B/C	T2a/b/cN0M0	II:	~60% overall
IIIA/B	T3a/bN0M0	III:	~25% overall
IIIC	T3cN0M0 or T1-3N1M0		~30–50% minimal or no
IV	M1		residual ~10% bulky
			residual
		IV	~5–15%

Staging portions of the above table used with the permission of the American Joint Committee on Cancer (AJCC), Chicago, Illinois. The original source for this material is the AJCC Cancer Staging Manual, Sixth Edition (2002) published by Springer-Verlag New York, www.springeronline.com.

TREATMENT RECOMMENDATIONS

Stage	Recommended Treatment
IA/B Gr1 IA/B Gr2	Surgery → observation Surgery → observation OR Surgery → taxane/carboplatin × 3–6c [ICON/GOG157]
IA/B Gr3, IC, II	Surgery → taxane/carboplatin × 3–6c [ICON/GOG157] OR Surgery → WART (if not a chemo candidate & <2cm residual) [Dembo]
III	Surgery → taxane with carboplatin or cisplatin × 6c* [GOG111/158] OR Surgery → WART (if not a chemo candidate & <2cm residual) [Dembo] If CR, observe, clinical trial, consolidative chemo or WART If PR, further chemo, intraperitoneal therapy, or WART If not resectable, chemo first *Intraperitoneal chemo (IP) is an alternative to IV chemo if optimally debulked [GOG 172]

Stage	Recommended Treatment
IV	Manage abdominal disease as for Stage III AND Palliative management of metastatic disease
Abdominal or pelvic recurrence	<6 mo from primary therapy – can retreat with same agents <6 mo from primary therapy – should consider additional agents* AND/OR EBRT for palliation of symptomatic tumor deposits *Other agents: topotecan, liposomal doxorubicin, gemcitabine, vinorelbine, oral altretamine, oral etoposide, tamoxifen, melphalan, oxaliplatin, cyclophosphamide

STUDIES
Adjuvant chemo: early stage
- 4 randomized trials performed using modern chemo (platinum based regimens) vs observation in high-risk early stage patients. The largest (ICON1 and ACTION) individually showed a significant improvement in OS and RFS with immediate adjuvant chemo. Their data was pooled and re-analyzed (see below)
- ICON and ACTION (*J Natl Cancer Inst* 2003). 925 pts, ICON included all stages but mainly stage I–II, ACTION included IA/BG2-3, IC, IIA randomized to observation vs 4–6c immediate adjuvant platinum-based chemo (57% single agent carboplatin, 27% combo cisplatin). Immediate chemo improved 5 yr OS 8% (82% vs 74%; 95% CI 2–12%) and 5 yr RFS 11% (76% vs 65%; 95% CI 5–16%)
- GOG 157 (closed but not published) included IA/BG2–3, IC, II randomized to 3c (considered standard arm) vs 6c adjuvant paclitaxel/carboplatin

Adjuvant chemo-advanced stage
- GOG111 (*NEJM* 1996). 410 pts, stage III/IV with <1 cm residual randomized to cisplatin with either cyclophosphamide or paclitaxel. Paclitaxel improved response rate (73% vs 60%), PFS (18 vs 13 mo), median survival (38 vs

24 mo). Results confirmed in large European/Canadian Intergroup trial (Piccart, *J Natl Cancer Inst* 2000)

- <u>GOG 158</u> (*JCO* 2003). 792 pts, advanced stage with <1 cm residual randomized to paclitaxel with either cisplatin or carboplatin. Carboplatin regimen was less toxic, easier to administer, and no less effective
- <u>GOG 172</u> (*JCO* 2001). 462 pts, stage III <1 cm residual randomized to 2c IV carboplatin followed by 6c IP cisplatin & IV paclitaxel vs 6c IV paclitaxel/cisplatin. LR and OS trend favoring IP over IV, but higher toxicity with IP regimens

Adjuvant WART

- <u>Dembo</u> (*Cancer* 1985). 190 pts with IB, II, asymptomatic III randomized to pelvic RT vs pelvic RT + chlorambucil vs WART. In pts with complete resection, 5 & 10 yr OS improved with WART over pelvic RT +/– chlorambucil (5 yr 78 vs 51%, 10 yr 64% vs 40%), 30% decrease abdominal recurrences with WART

Chemo vs WART for primary adjuvant therapy

- No randomized trial comparing best modern chemo and modern WART techniques has been performed. Smith et al. (*NCI Monograph*, 1975) compared WART vs melphalan in stage II–III pts with <2 cm residual – equivalent 5 yr OS, but less toxicity with chemo; thus most of subsequent focus has been on maximizing chemo. Listed below, one of the randomized trials using now outdated chemo, closed early due to poor accrual, demonstrating equal efficacy of WART. Clearly, WART deserves to be investigated more fully against modern chemo.
- <u>Chiara</u> (*Am J Clin Oncol* 1994). 70 pt with stage I/II randomized to adjuvant cisplatin/cyclophosphamide vs WART (pelvis 43.2 Gy/upper abdomen 30.2 Gy). No difference in 5 yr RFS/OS, yet trend toward poorer outcome with WART

Consolidation after primary chemo with WART

- Some European and small US trials have suggested that addition of WART could improve RFS and possibly OS – needs further prospective evaluation with modern chemo.

RT for local recurrence

■ <u>Cmelak</u> (*Gynecol Oncol* 1997). Retrospective, 41 pts with recurrence treated with WART (median doses: abdomen 28 Gy; pelvis 48 Gy), 10 yr DSS 40% for all Stage I, II, III pts with <1.5 cm residual. 5 yr DSS 0% if residual >1.5 cm

■ <u>Fujiwara</u> (*Int J Gynecol Cancer* 2002). Prospective/non-randomized, 20 pts with local recurrences (<4 cm) after primary therapy given local EBRT (52.3 +/− 8.3 Gy). Regression rates correlated with significantly longer survival, survival best if RT given before symptoms develop and if recurrence limited to LNs. 50% relief of symptoms

RADIATION TECHNIQUES

Simulation and field design

■ Supine, alpha cradle or knee sponge, planning CT scan
■ Must cover entire peritoneal cavity, pelvic RT alone is never adequate as primary adjuvant therapy [Dembo]
■ Open field currently accepted over moving strip technique
■ Treat AP/PA. Borders: superior = above dome of diaphragm; inferior = below obturator foramen; lateral = use CT to set outside peritoneal reflection
■ Plan for shields over kidney at 15 Gy & liver at 25 Gy (UCSF does not use liver block)

Dose prescriptions

■ 30 Gy at 1.2–1.5 Gy/fx whole field; kidney blocks @15 Gy, liver blocks @25 Gy
■ Para-aortic field boosted to 45 Gy
■ Pelvis boosted to 45–55 Gy

Dose limitations (TD 5/5)

■ Kidney <20 Gy
■ Liver <25 Gy
■ Lung: Limit volume receiving ≥20 Gy (V20) <20% to keep risk pneumonitis <10%
■ Spinal cord <45 Gy
■ Bone marrow <30 Gy
■ Stomach <45 Gy
■ Small bowel <45–50 Gy
■ Rectum <60 Gy
■ Bladder <60 Gy

COMPLICATIONS OF WART

- <u>Fyles</u> (*Int J Radiat Oncol Biol Phys* 1992). 598 pts received WART 1971–1985
  - Acute: nausea/vomiting (60%), diarrhea (~70%), leukopenia (11%), thrombocytopenia (11%)
  - 23% required treatment breaks, mainly for hematologic toxicity
  - Late: chronic diarrhea (14%), basal pneumonitis (4%), transient elevation LFT's (44%), serious bowel obstruction (4.2%)

FOLLOW-UP (ADAPTED FROM NCCN 2005 RECOMMENDATIONS

- H&P every 2–4 mo for 2 yrs, then every 6 mo for 3 yrs, then annually
- CA125 each visit if initially elevated
- CBC annually, other labs & imaging as indicated
- US as indicated in patients who underwent USO

REFERENCES

Alektiar K, Fuks Z. Cancer of the ovary. In: Leibel SA, Phiilips TL, editors. Textbook of Radiation Oncology. 2nd ed. Philadelphia: Saunders; 2004. pp. 1131–1156.

Chiara S, Conte P, Franzone P. High-risk early-stage ovarian cancer. Randomized clinical trial comparing cisplatin plus cyclophosphamide versus whole abdominal radiotherapy. Am J Clin Oncol 1994;17(1):72–76.

Cmelak AJ, Kapp DS. Long-term survival with whole abdominopelvic irradiation in platinum-refractory persistent or recurrent ovarian cancer. Gynecol Oncol 1997;65(3):453–460.

Dembo AJ. Abdominopelvic radiotherapy in ovarian cancer. A 10-year experience. Cancer 1985;55(9 Suppl):2285–2290.

Fujiwara K, Suzuki S, Yoden E, et al. Local radiation therapy for localized relapse or refractory ovarian cancer patients with or without symptoms after chemotherapy. Int J Gynecol Cancer 2002; 12(3):250–256.

Fyles AW, Dembo AJ, Bush RS, et al. Analysis of complications in patients treated with abdomino-pelvic radiation therapy for ovarian carcinoma. Int J Radiat Oncol Biol Phys 1992;22(5):847–851.

Greene FL. American Joint Committee on Cancer, American Cancer Society. AJCC Cancer Staging Manual. 6th ed. New York: Springer-Verlag; 2002.

ICON and EORTC-ACTION investigators: International Collaboration on Ovarian Neoplasm Trial 1 and Adjuvant Chemotherapy in Ovarian Neoplasm Trial: Two parallel randomized phase III trials of adjuvant chemotherapy in patients with early stage ovarian cancer. J Natl Cancer Inst 2003;95:105–112.

Markman M, Bundy B, Alberts DS, et al. Phase III trial of standard-dose intravenous cisplatin plus paclitaxel versus moderately high-dose carboplatin followed by intravenous paclitaxel and intraperitoneal cisplatin in small-volume stage III ovarian carcinoma: an Intergroup Study of the Gynecologic Oncology Group, Southwestern Oncology Group, and Eastern Cooperative Group. J Clin Oncol 2001;19:1001–1007.

Martinez A. Ovarian cancer. In: Gunderson L, Tepper J, editors. Clinical Radiation Oncology. 1st ed. Philadelphia: Churchill Livingstone; 2000. pp. 939–957.

McGuire WP, Hosking WJ, Brady MF, et al. Taxol and cisplatin improves outcome in patients with advanced ovarian cancer as compared to Cytoxan/cisplatin. N Engl J Med 1996;334(1):1–6.

National Comprehensive Cancer Network. Clinical Practice Guidelines in Oncology: Ovarian Cancer. Available at: http://www.nccn.org/professionals/physician_gls/PDF/ovarian.pdf. Accessed on December 13, 2004.

Ozols RF, Bundy BN, Greer E, et al. Phase III trials of carboplatin and paxlitaxel compared with cisplatin and paclitaxel in patients with optimally resected stage III ovarian cancer: A Gynecology Oncology Group Study. J Clin Oncol 2003;21:3194–3200.

Piccart M, Bertelsen K, James K, et al. Randomized intergroup trial of cisplatin-paclitaxel versus cisplatin-cyclophosphamide in women with advanced epithelial ovarian cancer: Three-year results. J Natl Cancer Inst 2000;92:699–708.

Rubin SC, Sabbatini P, Alektiar K, Randall M. Ovarian cancer. In: Pazdur R, Coia L, Hoskins W, Wagman L, editors. Cancer Management: A Multidisciplinary Approach. 8th ed. New York: CMP Healthcare Media; 2004. pp. 475–497.

Smith JP, Rutledge FN, Delclos L. Postoperative treatment of early cancer of the ovary: a randomized trial between postoperative irradiation and chemotherapy. Natl Cancer Inst Monogr 1975;42:149–153.

Stambaugh MD. Ovary. In: Perez CA, Brady LW, Halperin EC, et al., editors. Principles and Practice of Radiation Oncology. 4th ed. Philadelphia: Lippincott Williams & Wilkins; 2004. pp. 1934–1957.

Chapter 31
Vaginal Cancer

Eric K. Hansen and Joycelyn L. Speight

PEARLS

- Rare (only 1–2% of all gynecologic malignancies)
- Most commonly presents on the upper posterior 1/3 of the vagina
- Lymph node drainage from the upper 2/3 of the vagina is to the pelvic nodes and from the lower 1/3 of the vagina to the inguinal/femoral nodes
- VAIN (vaginal intraepithelial neoplasia) associated with human papilloma virus (HPV); frequently multifocal, and progresses to invasive disease
- 80–90% of cases are squamous cell carcinomas. Melanoma comprises 5% and is most frequent in the lower 1/3 of the vagina. Adenocarcinoma comprises 5–15% and frequently presents in the Bartholins or Skenes glands. Verrucous carcinomas tend to recur locally but rarely metastasize. Rare histologies include papillary serous adenocarcinoma, small cell carcinoma, botryoid variant of embryonal rhabdomyosarcoma, lymphoma, and clear cell adenocarcinoma (which is associated with *in utero* exposure to DES)
- Risk factors: carcinoma *in situ*, HPV, vaginal irritation, previous abnormal Pap smears, early hysterectomy, and *in utero* exposure to diethylstilbestrol

WORKUP

- H&P with Pap smear. EUA (with the gynecologic oncologist). On speculum exam, rotate the speculum when withdrawing to visualize the posterior wall. Bimanual & rectal exams should be performed
- Colposcopy with Schiller's test & multiple directed biopsies including the cervix & vulva to rule-out primary cervical &/or vulvar cancer
- If suspicious inguinal nodes, FNA or excise

- For ≥ stage II or symptoms, perform cystoscopy & sigmoidoscopy
- Labs: CBC, chemistries, BUN, Cr, LFTs including alkaline phosphatase
- Imaging: CXR & IVP. CT and/or MRI depending on extent (but not to be used for clinical staging)
- Risk of nodes increases with stage: I = 5%, II = 25%, III = 75%, IV = 85%

STAGING

FIGO / AJCC TNM Staging	
TX:	Primary tumor cannot be assessed
T0:	No evidence of primary tumor
0 / Tis:	Carcinoma in situ
I / T1:	Tumor confined to vagina
II / T2:	Tumor invades paravaginal tissues but not to pelvic wall
III / T3:	Tumor extends to pelvic wall (defined as muscle, fascia, neurovascular structures, or skeletal portions of the bony pelvis)
IVA / T4:	Tumor invades mucosa of bladder or rectum and/or extends beyond the true pelvis (bullous edema is not sufficient evidence to classify a tumor as T4)
NX:	Regional lymph nodes cannot be assessed
N0:	No regional lymph node metastasis
IVB / N1:	Pelvic or inguinal lymph node metastasis
MX:	Distant metastasis cannot be assessed
M0:	No distant metastasis
IVB / M1	Distant metastasis

AJCC Stage Groups		~5yr OS by Stage	
0:	TisN0M0	0:	~90%
I:	T1N0M0	I:	70–80%
II:	T2N0M0	II:	40–60%
III:	T3N0M0 or T1-3N1M0	III:	30%
IVA:	T4, any N, M0	IV:	<10%
IVB:	Any T, any N, M1		

| *Note*: Tumors involving the cervix or vulva should be classified as cervical or vulvar tumors, respectively | |

TREATMENT RECOMMENDATIONS

Stage	Recommended Treatment
CIS	CO_2 laser or topical 5-FU or wide local excision. Close follow-up required because of multifocality and frequent progression. For resistant cases, intracavitary (IC) brachytherapy 60–70 Gy to the entire vaginal mucosa
I (<0.5 cm thick, <2 cm, & low grade)	<u>Surgery</u> (wide local excision or total vaginectomy with vaginal reconstruction). Preserves ovarian function. Post-op RT for close/+ margins
	<u>Or, IC ± IS RT</u>. Treat entire vaginal mucosa to surface dose 60–70 Gy. The tumor dose is 60–70 Gy prescribed to 0.5 cm beyond the tumor (corresponding to 80–100 Gy tumor mucosal dose). A 2 cm radial margin is used around the tumor
I (>0.5 cm thick, >2 cm, or high grade)	<u>Surgery</u>: radical vaginectomy & pelvic lymphadenectomy (for upper $^2/_3$) or inguinal lymphadenectomy (for lower $^1/_3$). Post-op RT for close/+ margins

Stage	Recommended Treatment
	<u>Or, RT</u>: EBRT to whole pelvis to 45–50 Gy (consider midline block after 20 Gy). If lower $^1/_3$ involvement, EBRT to inguinal nodes to 45–50 Gy. Treat entire vaginal mucosa with IC RT to surface dose 60–70 Gy → IS boost to tumor (prescribed to 0.5 cm beyond the tumor base) to 70–80 Gy (corresponding to 80–100 Gy tumor mucosal dose). A 2 cm radial margin is used around the tumor
II	EBRT to whole pelvis to 45–50 Gy (consider midline block after 20 Gy). If lower $^1/_3$ involvement, treat inguinal nodes to 45–50 Gy. Treat entire vaginal mucosa to surface dose 60–70 Gy → IS boost to tumor (prescribed to 0.5 cm beyond the tumor base) to 75–85 Gy. A 2 cm radial margin is used around the tumor
III, IV	EBRT to whole pelvis to 50 Gy (with midline block after 40 Gy). If lower $^1/_3$ involvement, treat inguinal nodes to 45–50 Gy. Treat entire vaginal mucosa with IC RT to surface dose 60–70 Gy → IS boost to parametrial and paravaginal extension to 65–70 Gy. Boost the tumor to 75–85 Gy (prescribed to 0.5 cm beyond the tumor). A 2 cm radial margin is used around the tumor. For + nodes, boost additional 15 Gy (to total 60 Gy) with EBRT. Consider concomitant cisplatin-based chemo (based on cervix and vulvar literature).

Stage	Recommended Treatment
	For stage IV, brachytherapy may be avoided due to concern for potential fistula formation. In this case, definitive chemo-RT or exenteration is used
Clear cell adenocarcinoma	Surgery preserves ovarian function, but it is morbid because it includes radical hysterectomy, vaginectomy, pelvic lymphadenectomy, and para- aortic lymph node sampling. If elected, definitive radiation techniques are the same as those described for stages II, III, IV
Mets	Palliative RT ± chemo
Recurrence	Pelvic exenteration (removes vulva, vagina, uterus, anorectum, bladder, urethra, & pelvic and groin lymph node dissections). Pts are left with a permanent colostomy and urinary diversion

STUDIES

- Because of its rarity, most trials are retrospective and have small pt numbers. Data concerning chemotherapy is limited and its use is based on the cervix and vulvar literature
- There are no prospective trials comparing HDR to LDR brachytherapy
- In general, RT is preferred over surgery except for early or posterior stage I lesions, distal lesions, or in the presence of a fistula

RADIATION TECHNIQUES
Simulation and field design

- For EBRT, simulate the patient supine with tumor & introitus markers. Seeds may be placed in the cervix. Bolus on inguinal nodes may be needed. If treating the inguinal nodes, the patient is treated in the frog-leg position

- APPA field borders are as follows: superior = L5/S1; inferior covers entire vagina & 3 cm below lowest extent of disease; lateral = 2 cm lateral to the pelvic brim. If distal 1/3 involvement, lateral borders include the inguinofemoral nodes (superolateral border = anterior superior iliac spine; lateral = greater trochanter; inferior = inguinal crease or 2.5 cm below ischium)
- If treating inguinal nodes, techniques may be used to protect the femoral heads as described for vulvar & anal cancer
- A midline block is optional to decrease the dose to the bladder and rectum. If a midline block is not used, the brachytherapy dose must be reduced
- IC brachytherapy uses largest possible vaginal cylinder to improve the ratio of mucosa to tumor dose
- Dome cylinders are used for homogenous irradiation of the vaginal cuff
- Upper 1/3 lesions may be treated with an intrauterine tandem and vaginal colpostats followed by treatment of the middle and lower 1/3 of the vagina with a vaginal cylinder with a blank source at the top of the cylinder if full dose has already been reached at the apex
- Never carry a source at the level of the ovoids in the tandem or vaginal cylinder to prevent damage to the rectum and bladder

Dose limitations
- Upper vaginal mucosa tolerance is 120 Gy, mid-vaginal mucosal tolerance is 80–90 Gy, & lower vaginal mucosa tolerance is 60–70 Gy. Vaginal doses >50–60 Gy cause significant vaginal fibrosis & stenosis
- Ovarian failure occurs with 5–10 Gy. Sterilization occurs with 2–3 Gy
- Limit bladder ≤65 Gy and rectum ≤60 Gy

COMPLICATIONS
- Complications are dose related and include vaginal dryness & atrophy, pubic hair loss, vaginal stenosis and fibrosis (~50%), cystitis (~50%), proctitis (~40%), rectovaginal or vesicovaginal fistula (<5%), vaginal necrosis (<5–15%), urethral stricture (rare), and small bowel obstruction (rare)
- Vaginal dilators should be used to minimize stenosis

FOLLOW-UP

- H&P (with pelvic exam & pap smear) every 3 mo for 1 yr, every 4 mo for 2nd yr, every 6 mo for 3rd & 4th yrs, then annually. CXR annually for 5 yrs

REFERENCES

Chyle V, Zagars GK, Wheeler JA, et al. Definitive radiotherapy for carcinoma of the vagina: outcome and prognostic factors. Int J Radiat Oncol Biol Phys 1996;35:891–905.

Eifel PJ. The Vulva and Vagina. In: Cox JD, Ang KK, editors. Radiation Oncology: Rationale, Technique, Results. 8th ed. St. Louis: Mosby; 2003. pp. 743–756.

Frank SJ, Jhingran A, Levenback C, et al. Definitive radiation therapy for squamous cell carcinoma of the vagina. Int J Radiat Oncol Biol Phys 2005;62:138–147.

Greene FL. American Joint Committee on Cancer, American Cancer Society. AJCC Cancer Staging Manual. 6th ed. New York: Springer-Verlag; 2002.

Kavanagh B, Segreti E. Vaginal and Vulvar Cancer (#405). Presented at American Society of Therapeutic Radiology and Oncology Annual Meeting, Atlanta, GA, 2004.

Kirkbride P, Fyles A, Rawlings GA, et al. Carcinoma of the vagina – experience at the Princess Margaret Hospital (1974–1989). Gynecol Oncol 1995;56:435–443.

National Cancer Institute. Vaginal Cancer (PDQ): Treatment. Available at: http://cancer.gov/cancertopics/pdq/treatment/vaginal/healthprofessional/. Accessed on January 19, 2005.

Perez CA, Grigsby PW, Garipagaoglu M, et al. Factors affecting long-term outcome of irradiation in carcinoma of the vagina. Int J Radiat Oncol Biol Phys 1999;44:37–45.

Perez CA. Vagina. In: Perez CA, Brady LW, Halperin EC, et al., editors. Principles and Practice of Radiation Oncology. 4th ed. Philadelphia: Lippincott Williams & Wilkins; 2004. pp. 1967–1993.

Stock RG, Green S. Cancer of the vagina. In: Leibel SA, Phillips TL, editors. Textbook of Radiation Oncology. 2nd ed. Philadelphia: Saunders; 2004. pp. 1157–1176.

Thomas GM, Murphy KJ. Vulvar and Vaginal Cancer. In: Gunderson LL, Tepper JE, editors. Clinical Radiation Oncology. 1st ed. Philadelphia: Churchill Livingstone; 2000. pp. 920–938.

Chapter 32
Vulvar Cancer

Brian Missett and Joycelyn Speight

PEARLS

- Anatomy = mons pubis, clitoris, labia majora, labia minora, vaginal vestibule, Bartholin's glands (at posterior labia majora), prepuce over clitoris, posterior forchette, perineal body
- LN spread is to inguino-femoral nodes (superficial & deep). Most superior deep femoral node = Cloquet's node
- Clitoris can theoretically drain directly to pelvic LN, but rare without inguino-femoral LN involvement
- Risk factors = HPV 16, 18, 33 (condyloma acuminatum), vulvar intraepithelial neoplasia (2–5% progress to CA), Bowen's disease, Paget's disease, erythroplasia, chronic irritant vaginitis (e.g., with pessary), leukoplakia, prior GU CA, employment in laundry & cleaning industry, smoking
- Risk of nodes: IA <1 mm deep <5%, 1–3 mm deep 8–10%, 3–5 mm deep 20%, >5 mm deep or >2 cm size 40%, III 30–80%, IV 80–100%. ~20–25% of cN0 pts are pN+. If inguinal LN+, ~30% risk of pelvic LN+

WORKUP

- H&P with EUA. Colposcopic biopsy of primary & FNA or excisional biopsy of inguinal nodes (may be unilateral if well-lateralized). Pap smear of cervix & vagina. Cystoscopy, sigmoidoscopy may be required. CBC, UA. CT or MRI. CXR

STAGING

FIGO / AJCC Primary Tumor	
0 / Tis:	Carcinoma in situ (preinvasive carcinoma)
IA / T1a:	Tumor confined to the vulva or vulva & perineum, 2 cm or less in greatest dimension, and with stromal invasion no greater than 1 mm

IB / T1b: Tumor confined to the vulva or vulva & perineum, 2 cm or less in greatest dimension, and with stromal invasion greater than 1 mm

II / T2:   Tumor confined to the vulva or vulva & perineum, more than 2 cm in greatest dimension

III / T3:   Tumor of any size with contiguous spread to the lower urethra and/or vagina or anus

IVA / T4:   Tumor invades any of the following: upper urethra, bladder mucosa, rectal mucosa, or is fixed to the pubic bone

FIGO / AJCC Regional lymph nodes

III / N1:   Unilateral regional lymph node metastasis (inguinal/femoral LN)

IVA / N2:   Bilateral regionallymph node metastasis (inguinal/femoral LN)

FIGO / AJCC Metastases

IVB / M1 = Distant metastasis (including pelvic LN)

Stage Grouping		~5 yr OS	
IA:	T1aN0	I:	96%
IB:	T1bN0		
II:	T2N0	II:	80%
III:	T3N0 or T1-3N1	III:	50%
IVA:	T4 any N or T1-3N2	IV:	20%
IVB:	Any M1		

Used with the permission of the American Joint Committee on Cancer (AJCC), Chicago, Illinois. The original source for this material is the AJCC Cancer Staging Manual, Sixth Edition (2002) published by Springer-Verlag New York, www.springeronline.com.

TREATMENT RECOMMENDATIONS

Stage	Recommended Treatment
CIS	Local excision or CO_2 laser
IA	Wide local excision (WLE). Post-op RT (50 Gy) to vulva for + margin, margin <8 mm, LVSI, or depth >5 mm. Sample lymph nodes for lesion with >1 mm depth of invasion

Stage	Recommended Treatment
IB/II	WLE with ipsilateral (superficial) LN dissection for lateralized. Bilateral (superficial) LN dissection for central lesions, lesions >5 mm deep, LVSI, or poorly differentiated lesions. If LN+, add deep inguinal dissection. Post-op RT to vulva for + margin, margin <8 mm, LVSI, or lesions >5 mm deep. Post-op RT to inguinal & pelvic nodes for >1 LN+, or nodal ECE. Consider pre-op chemo-RT (50 Gy for cN– or 54 Gy for cN+) → bilateral LN dissection for lesions close to urethra, clitoris, or rectum because margin may be difficult to obtain
III/IVA	If cN0, perform bilateral LN dissection 1st followed by chemo-RT to vulva or vulva & inguinal/pelvic nodes (for ECE, >1 LN) If cN+ fixed or ulcerated, pre-op chemo-RT (45–50 Gy with cisplatin, 5-FU, &/or mitomycin C) provides about 50% CR. Follow with bilateral LN dissection. Surgical salvage for persistent or recurrent disease. If ECE take to 60 Gy; if gross residual take to 65–70 Gy

STUDIES

- **GOG 36** (Homesley, *Obstet Gynecol* 1986). 114 pts treated with radical vulvectomy & bilateral inguinal lymphadenectomy. If inguinal LN+, randomized to pelvic LN dissection vs post-op RT with 45–50 Gy to pelvic & inguinal LN (but not to vulva). RT decreased groin recurrence (5% vs 24%) & improved 2 yr OS (68% vs 54%)

Subset analysis showed benefit only in cN+, pts with >1 pN+ or +LN with ECE. No difference in pelvic recurrence

- GOG 88 (Stehman, *IJROBP* 1992). 121 pts with IB-III cN0 treated with radical vulvectomy randomized to bilateral inguinal RT (50 Gy to D3, without pelvic RT) vs bilateral radical LN dissection. If pLN+, then received RT (50 Gy) to bilateral groin & pelvis. Interim analysis of only 58 pts demonstrated improved 2 yr OS (90% vs 70%) with surgery and decreased inguinal recurrences. Criticisms = RT addressed only inguinal nodes whereas surgery included pelvic LN dissection if inguinal LN+; arms biased because no CT used for staging; poor technique of RT (prescribed to D3, all inguinal recurrences received <prescribed dose); 50 Gy should sterilize microscopic disease as evidenced by Univ of Wisconsin retrospective review with good technique (Petereit, *Int J Radiat Oncol Biol Phys* 1993)

- GOG (Moore, *IJROBP* 1998). Phase II trial of 41 pts with T3 unresectable or T4, any LN status treated with pre-op chemo-RT with 1.7 Gy bid d1–4, 1.7 Gy qd d5–12 to 23.8 Gy w/ cisplatin on d1 & 5-FU on d1–4 → 2 wk break → repeat to total dose 47.6 Gy. For cN0, RT was to vulvar area only & for cN+ included inguinal & pelvic LN. Surgery 4–8 wks after chemo-RT. Pre-op chemo-RT had 47% CR & 55% 4 yr OS (expect 20–50%). 54% of pts had gross residual disease, but only 3% were unresectable

- Dusenbery (*IJROBP* 1994). 27 pts with stage III/IV disease with +LN treated with post-op RT with a midline block s/p resection. 48% central recurrence rate with use of the midline block. Authors recommended discontinuing routine use of the midline block

- Heaps (*Gynecol Oncol* 1990). Review of surgical-patholo-gic factors predictive of LR for 135 pts with vulvar CA. Increased LR with + margin, margin <8 mm pathologi-cally or <1 cm clinically, LVSI, & depth >5 mm

RADIATION TECHNIQUES
Simulation and field design

- Simulate supine, frog-leg position with custom immobilization
- Wire LN, vulva, anus, scars
- Borders: Superior = L5/S1 or mid SI (L4/5 if pelvic N+); inferior = flash vulva & 3 cm inferior to bottom of

ischium; lateral = 2 cm beyond pelvic brim & greater tro-chanter (anterior superior iliac spine) to include inguinal LN
- Energy = 6 MV AP, 18 MV PA. Bolus groins & vulva prn
- CT plan depth of groin nodes
- May need to boost groins with en face electrons

Dose prescriptions
- 1.8 Gy/fx
- 45 Gy to vulva & pelvic LN
- 45–50.4 Gy for cN0 inguinal nodes, & boost to 60 Gy for LN+ or ECE.
- For residual disease, boost to 65–70 Gy (may require brachytherapy)

Dose limitations
- Small bowel <45–55 Gy
- Femoral heads <45 Gy
- Bladder <60 Gy
- Rectum <60 Gy
- Lower vagina <75–80 Gy

COMPLICATIONS
- Acute: epilation of pubic hair, hyperpigmentation, skin reaction. Moist desquamation by 3rd to 5th wk. Treat with Domeboro's solution, loose garments, sitz baths. Also treat candida superinfections, if any. Diarrhea, cystitis
- Late = atrophy of skin and telangiectasia. Gradual short-ening of vagina, vaginal dryness. Femoral neck fracture <5%, associated with osteoporosis and smoking

FOLLOW-UP
- H&P every mo × 3 mo, every 3 mo × 3 mo, every 4 mo × 1 yr, every 6 mo × 2 yrs, then annually
- CXR annually × 5 yr

REFERENCES

Dusenbery KE, Carlson JW, LaPorte RM, et al. Radical vulvectomy with postoperative irradiation for vulvar cancer: therapeutic implications of a central block. Int J Radiat Oncol Biol Phys 1994;29: 989–998.

Eifel P. The vulva and vagina. In: Cox JD, Ang KK, editors. Radiation Oncology: Rationale, Technique, Results. 8th ed. St. Louis: Mosby; 2003. pp. 743–756.

Heaps JM, Fu YS, Montz FJ, et al. Surgical-pathologic variables predictive of local recurrence in squamous cell carcinoma of the vulva. Gynecol Oncol 1990;38:309–314.

Homesley HD, Bundy BN, Sedlis A, et al. Radiation therapy versus pelvic node resection for carcinoma of the vulva with positive groin nodes. Obstet Gynecol 1986;68:733–740.

Montana GS, Kang S. Carcinoma of the vulva. In: Perez CA, Brady LW, Halperin EC, et al., editors. Principles and Practice of Radiation Oncology. 4th ed. Philadelphia: Lippincott Williams & Wilkins; 2004. pp. 2003–2022.

Moore DH, Thomas GM, Montana GS, et al. Preoperative chemoradiation for advanced vulvar cancer: a phase II study of the Gynecologic Oncology Group. Int J Radiat Oncol Biol Phys 1998;42:79–85.

National Cancer Institute. Vulvar Cancer (PDQ): Treatment. Avail-able at: http://cancer.gov/cancertopics/pdq/treatment/vulvar/healthprofessional/. Accessed on January 19, 2005.

Russell A. Cancer of the vulva. In: Leibel SA, Phillips TL, editors. Textbook of Radiation Oncology. 2nd ed. Philadelphia: Saunders; 2004. pp. 1177–1198.

Stehman FB, Bundy BN, Thomas G, et al. Groin dissection versus groin radiation in carcinoma of the vulva: a Gynecologic Oncology Group study. Int J Radiat Oncol Biol Phys 1992;24:389–396.

Chapter 33
Hodgkin's Lymphoma

Hans T. Chung and Alison Bevan

PEARLS

- First-degree relatives of patients have 5-fold increase in risk for Hodgkin's disease
- Hallmark is Reed-Sternberg cells (binucleate CD15+, CD30+), derived from monoclonal B cells
- 80% present with cervical lymphadenopathy
- 50% present with mediastinal disease (most likely NSHL)
- 33% present with B symptoms overall, but only 15–20% of stage I–II have B symptoms
- WHO classification
  - Nodular lymphocyte predominance (NLPHL)
  - Classic (CHL)
    - Nodular sclerosis (NSHL) = 70%
    - Mixed cellularity (MCHL) = 20%
    - Lymphocyte rich (LRCHL) = 10%
    - Lymphocyte depletion (LDHL) = <5%
- NLPHL: CD15–, CD30–, CD45+, CD20+. Occasional late relapse, but best OS. Often stage I–II, B symptoms <10%, more common pts >40 yrs
- NS: Mediastinum often involved. 1/3 have B symptoms
- MC: presents more commonly with advanced disease, often subclinical subdiaphragmatic disease in pts with clinically staged I–II above diaphragm
- LD: rare, mostly advanced with B symptoms in older pts, worst prognosis, associated with HIV

WORKUP

- H&P
- Labs: CBC with differential, LFTs, BUN/Cr, ESR, chemistries, alkaline phosphatase, LDH, albumin. Pregnancy test. HIV test (if risk factors)

- MUGA test & LVEF before ABVD chemo
- Pathology: excisional LN biopsy. Bone marrow biopsy only for pts with B symptoms, stage III–IV, bulky disease, recurrent disease
- Imaging: CXR; CT chest, abdomen & pelvis; PET scan (sensitivity 75–91%). If indicated, gallium, bone scan or MRI
- Consider oophoropexy for women to preserve ovarian function
- Pretreatment dental evaluation if going to treat neck

AJCC / ANN ARBOR STAGING SYSTEM

Stage	Involvement
I	Single lymph node region (1) or one extralymphatic site (1_E)
II	Two or more lymph node regions, same side of the diaphragm (2) or local extralymphatic extension plus one or more lymph node regions same side of the diaphragm (2_E)
III	Lymph node regions on both sides of diaphragm (3) which may be accompanied by local extralymphatic extension (3_E)
IV	Diffuse involvement of one or more extralymphatic organs or sites
B	Unexplained weight loss (>10% in 6 mo prior to diagnosis), unexplained fever >38°C, drenching night sweats
E	Extranodal disease
X	Bulky (>10 cm, or for mediastinal mass >1/3 intrathoracic diameter)

Used with the permission of the American Joint Committee on Cancer (AJCC), Chicago, Illinois. The original source for this material is the AJCC Cancer Staging Manual, Sixth Edition (2002) published by Springer-Verlag New York, www.springeronline.com.

Lymph node groups: Waldeyer's ring; occipital/cervical/preauricular/supraclavicular; infraclavicular; axillary; epitrochlear; mediastinal; right & left hilar (separate); paraaortic; splenic; mesenteric; iliac; inguinal/femoral; popliteal

Prognosis
- B symptoms, bulky mediastinal disease
- Early stage treated with chemo-RT, 5 yr FFF 95% and OS >95%
- Advanced stage (*NEJM* 1998):
  - Poor prognostic factors: male gender, age >45 yr, stage IV, Hgb <10.5, WBC >15k, lymphocyte <0.6 × 10^9/L, albumin <40 g/L
  - If ≤3 factors, 5 yr FFP 70%, whereas >3 factors is 50%

TREATMENT
Chemo agents

- MOPP = mechlorethamine, Oncovin (vincristine), procarbazine, prednisone
- ABVD = Adriamycin (doxorubicin), bleomycin, vinblastine, dacarbazine. (Decreased sterility & second malignancies vs MOPP)
- Stanford V = mechlorethamine, vincristine, prednisone, doxorubicin, bleomycin, vinblastine, etoposide. (Decreased bleomycin & doxorubicin toxicity vs ABVD)

Stage	Recommended Treatment
Favorable IA/IIA (no bulky disease, ≤3 sites, ESR <50)	■ ABVD ×4 then IFRT [30 Gy (subclinical), 36 Gy (clinical)] ■ Alternative chemo = 8 wk Stanford V + IFRT (30 Gy) ■ STLI 40–44 Gy ■ For LP IA, may give IFRT or regional RT alone
Unfavorable IA/IIA (bulky. disease, >3 sites, ESR >50), IB/IIB	■ ABVD × 4–6 then IFRT 30–36 Gy ■ Alternative: 12 wk Stanford V + IFRT 36 Gy (to any node >5 cm)
III IV	■ ABVD ×4 then restage. If CR, ABVD ×2 + IFRT 20–36 Gy to bulky sites (optional). If PR, ABVD × 2–4c, then IFRT 30–36 Gy to bulky sites (optional) ■ Alternative is 12 wk Stanford V chemo ± IFRT 36 Gy for LN >5 cm
Primary refractory disease	■ High-dose chemo + stem cell transplant (30–60% salvage)
Relapse	■ Chemo or chemo-RT salvages ~50–80% of pts initially treated with RT alone. After chemo, may give 15–25 Gy to previously irradiated sites or 30–40 Gy to not previously irradiated sites ■ For pts who relapse after chemo, only 40–60% salvage ■ Most chemo-alone failures occur in sites of initial disease

Stage	Recommended Treatment
	■ If relapse after initial stage III/IV, then autologous bone marrow transplant or autologous peripheral stem cell transplant

STUDIES
Early favorable

- <u>EORTC H6F</u> (*JCO* 1993). 262 pts with clinical stage I–II and favorable factors [1–2 sites, no bulky disease, ESR <50 (or <30 if B symptoms)] randomized to: (1) no laparotomy with STLI; (2) negative laparotomy and NS or LP with mantle 40 Gy or STLI alone if MC or LD; (3) positive laparotomy then chemo-RT. No difference in 6 yr DFS (83% vs 78%) or OS (89% vs 93%) with or without laparotomy. Therefore laparotomy is unnecessary with chemo-RT or STLI

- <u>EORTC H7VF</u> (*ASTRO* 1997). 40 pts with very favorable group (women <40 yrs with IA nonbulky NS or LP with ESR <50) treated with mantle RT alone. Although OS was 96%, RFS was 73%, suggesting that mantle alone is insufficient

- <u>EORTC H7F</u> (*ASTRO* 1997). 333 pts with favorable group randomized to EBVP chemo ×6 and IFRT vs STNI + splenic RT. Chemo-RT improved 5 yr RFS (92% vs 81%) but not OS (98 vs 96%)

- <u>GHSG HD7</u> (*ASH* 2002). 622 pts with favorable clinical stage I–II (no bulky disease, extranodal disease, elevated ESR, >2 LN regions) randomized to EFRT (30 Gy) + boost 10 Gy vs ABVD ×2 and EFRT. Chemo-RT increased 5 yr DFS (90% vs 75%), but no difference in OS (94%)

- <u>SWOG 9133/CALGB 9391</u> (*JCO* 2001). 348 pts with favorable clinical stage I–IIA (no bulky disease, infradiaphragmatic disease, B symptoms) randomized to 3 cycles of doxorubicin and vinblastine and STLI (36–40 Gy) or STLI alone (36–40 Gy). Chemo-RT increased overall response and 3 yr FFS (94% vs 81%), but not OS

- <u>Stanford G4</u> (*ASH* 2004). 87 pts with non-bulky favorable I/IIA received 8 wks of Stanford V followed by IFRT (30 Gy). Median follow-up 5.7 yr. 8 yr FFP and OS were 96% and 98%

- GHSG HD10 (*ESH* 2004, *ASCO* abstr 2005). 1131 pts with favorable I–II with no risk factors randomized to ABVD ×2c vs ×4c, followed by IFRT 20 Gy vs 30 Gy. At medium f/u 2 yrs, no difference between any of the arms (freedom from failure 97%, OS 98.5%)
- EORTC H9F (*ASCO* abstr 2005). 783 pts with favorable IA–IIB randomized to no IFRT, IFRT (20 Gy) or IFRT (36 Gy) after attaining CR with EBVP ×6c (79% of pts had CR & were randomized). Median f/u 33 mo. 4 yr EFS decreased without IFRT (70%) vs 84% (20 Gy) & 87% (36 Gy). No difference in OS (98% all 3 arms)
- Stanford G5. Currently accruing patients with favorable I–IIA to risk-adapted Stanford V-C and low-dose IFRT

Early unfavorable

- EORTC H6U (*JCO* 1993). 316 pts clinical stage I–II and unfavorable factors treated with split course chemo with mantle RT (35 Gy ± boost 5–10 Gy) and no laparotomy were randomized to: MOPP×6 vs ABVD×6. ABVD improved 10 yr DFS (88% vs 77%), but not OS (87% vs 87%). ABVD had higher pulmonary toxicity but less sterility and hematologic complications
- EORTC H7U (*ASTRO* 1997). 316 pts with clinical stage I–II and any unfavorable factor, randomized to MOPP/ABV ×6 vs EBVP ×6, followed by IFRT (36 Gy). MOPP/ABV improved both 6 yr RFS (90% vs 68%), but not OS (89% vs 82%)
- EORTC H8U (*ASH* 2000). 995 pts with unfavorable clinical stage I–II disease randomized to: (1) MOPP/ABV×6 + IFRT; (2) MOPP/ABV×4 + IFRT; (3) MOPP/ABV×4 + STLI. IFRT = 36–40 Gy. No difference in 4 yr FFS and OS
- Milan (*JCO* 2004). Randomized 136 pts with clinical stage IA bulky, IB, IIA or IIA bulky to ABVD ×4 then STLI vs IFRT. Dose 36 Gy for CR, 40 Gy for PR, & 30.6 Gy for STNI prophylactic. No difference in 12 yr FFP (93% vs 94%) or OS (96% vs 94%). 3 pts 2nd CA with STNI vs 0 with IFRT
- GHSG HD8 (*JCO* 2003). 1064 pts with clinical stage I–II and at least 1 unfavorable factor (bulky mediastinal disease, massive splenomegaly, >2 nodal sites, extranodal disease, high ESR) to 4 cycles of COPP/ABVD and EFRT or IFRT (30 Gy + 10 Gy boost). There was no difference in FFS or OS

- Specht meta-analysis (*JCO* 1998). RT alone vs chemo-RT. Chemo-RT decreases 10 yr recurrence by 50% (IA 20 to 10%, IB 30 to 15%). No difference in OS (RT 77%, chemo-RT 79%) or CSS (85–88%)
- NCCTG HD-6/ECOG JHD06 (*JCO* 2005). 399 patients with non-bulky CS I–IIA HD were randomized to STLI ± ABVD×2 or ABVD×4–6. Patients in the STLI arm stratified into favorable and unfavorable risk (MC or LD histology, ≥4 sites, ESR ≥50 or age ≥40). Unfavorable patients received STLI + ABVD × 2. For all patients, STLI improved 5 yr FFP (93% vs 87%), but not EFS and OS. Subgroup analysis of unfavorable risk patients showed improved FFP (95% vs 88%), but not OS. No difference seen in favorable risk patients. 2nd cancers (10 vs 4) and CAD (12 vs 4) were more in STLI arm

Advanced

- CALGB (*NEJM* 1992 & 2002). 361 pts with stage III–IV randomized to MOPP × 6–8c, ABVD × 6–8c, or MOPP-ABVD × 12 mo. No RT. Both ABVD & MOPP-ABVD improved 5 yr FFS, but not OS
- SWOG 7808 (*Ann Int Med* 1994). CS III–IV MOP-BAP × 6 mo. If CR, randomized to observation vs 20 Gy IFRT. Improved FFP for NSHD (60% to 82%), bulky >6 cm (57% to 75%), & patients who actually completed assigned treatment (67% to 85%). No difference in OS
- GHSG HD3 (*Ann Oncol* 1995). IIIB/IV COPP/ABVD × 6 mo. If CR, randomized to 2 mo COPP/ABVD or 20 Gy IFRT. No diff RFS (77%) or OS (90%)
- GELA H89 (*Blood* 2000). 418 pts CS IIIB/IV who achieved CR/PR after 6 cycles of MOPP/ABV or ABVPP were randomized to STLI or 2 more cycles of chemo. 5 yr DFS (79% vs 74%) and OS (88% vs 85%) were not different
- EORTC 20884/GPMC H34 (*NEJM* 2003). CS III/IV MOPP-ABV × 6–8c. If CR, randomized to observation vs consolidative IFRT (24 Gy). IFRT did not improve RFS or OS
- India (*JCO* 2004). 179 (71%) of 251 pts with stage I–IV achieved CR after ABVD ×6, then randomized to no RT or consolidation RT. IFRT was given in 84%. 47% were <15 yrs and 68% had MC histology. RT improved 8 yr EFS (76% vs 88%) and OS (89% vs 100%)
- Stanford G3 (*ASH* 2004). 108 pts with stage III–IV were prospectively treated with 12 wks of Stanford V and IFRT

36 Gy to any sites ≥5 cm. Median F/U was 6.8 yr. 8 yr FFP and OS were 85.9% and 95.2%

- IIL HD9601 Italy (*JCO* 2005). 334 pts with IIB–IV randomized to ABVD ×6 vs MOPPEBVCAD ×6 vs 12 wk modified Stanford V. RT (36–42 Gy) to residual mass or previously bulky disease (>6 cm), and to no more than 2 sites (different than original Stanford V). Median F/U was 61 m. Modified Stanford V had lower CR (89v94v76%), 5 yr FFS (78v81v54%), and FFP (85v94v73%), but no difference in OS (90v89v82%). In ascending order of severity, hematologic toxicity was least in ABVD, Stanford V than MOPPEBVCAD

- ECOG 2496/CALGB 59905. Currently accruing pts with bulky stage I–IIA/B or III–IV disease to either Stanford V with IFRT to bulky disease, or ABVD with IFRT for bulky mediastinal disease

RADIATION TECHNIQUES
Simulation and field design (3DCRT)
- Simulate supine with custom immobilization. Wire nodes
- Consider custom compensator for neck, mediastinal or SCV fields
- Extended RT fields:
    - Mantle: bilateral cervical, SCV, infraclavicular, mediastinal, hilar, & axilla
    - Mini-mantle: mantle without mediastinum, hila
    - Modified mantle: mantle without axilla
    - Inverted Y: paraaortic, bilateral pelvic and inguinofemoral, ± splenic
    - Total lymphoid irradiation (TLI): both mantle & inverted Y-fields
    - Subtotal lymphoid irradiation (STLI): TLI with exclusion of pelvis
- Mantle
    - Simulate with arms-up (to pull axillary LN from chest to allow for more lung blocking) or arms akimbo (to shield humeral heads & minimize tissue in SCV folds). Head extended. Use CT planning
    - Borders: lateral = beyond humeral heads; inferior = bottom of diaphragm (T11/12); superior = inferior mandible
    - Blocks: larynx on AP field. Humeral heads on AP & PA fields. PA cord block (if dose >40 Gy). Lung block at top

of 4th rib to cover infraclavicular LN. If pericardial or mediastinal extension, include entire heart to 15 Gy, then block apex of heart. After 30 Gy, block heart beyond 5 cm inferior to carina (unless residual disease)

■ Margins: pre-chemo cranio-caudad + 2–5 cm; post-chemo lateral + 1.5 cm

■ If plan to treat subdiaphragmatic disease, start 7–10 d after mantle

■ Definition for IFRT (*ASTRO* 2002):

■ IFRT encompasses a region, not an individual LN

■ Major involved-field regions are: neck (unilateral), mediastinum (including bilateral hilum), axilla (including supraclavicular and infraclavicular LN), spleen, PA, inguinal (femoral and iliac nodes)

■ Initially involved pre-chemo sites and volume are treated, except for when the transverse diameter of the

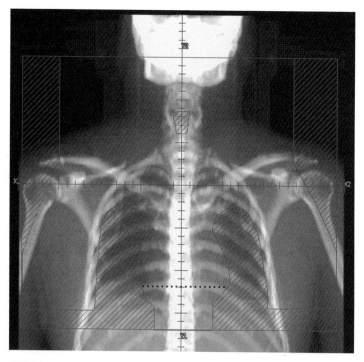

FIGURE 33.1. DRR of an AP mantle field with cardiac block after 30 Gy (black dotted line).

mediastinal and PA LN for which the reduced post-CHT volume is treated
- Neck: include ipsilateral cervical & SCV regions
- Mediastinum: include bilateral hilar regions. If SCV involved, include bilateral SCV & cervical regions
- Axilla: include ipsilateral SCV & infraclavicular regions
- Inguinal: Include external iliac & femoral regions
- Margins: generally 2 cm superior & inferior to pre-chemo volume & 2 cm lateral to post-chemo volume for mediastinal & para-aortic fields
- Shield testes for men & consider oophoropexy for women
- Match fields with half-beam or gap techniques

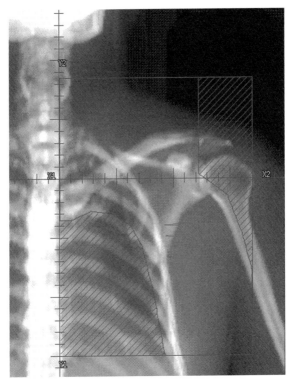

FIGURE 33.2. DRR of IFRT for a stage I axillary Hodgkin's lymphoma.

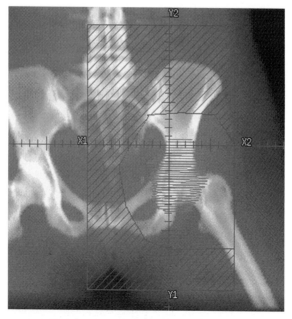

FIGURE 33.3. DRR of IFRT for a stage I inguinal-femoral Hodgkin's lymphoma.

Dose prescriptions
- See treatment algorithm

Dose limitations
- Femoral head: <25 Gy to prevent slipped capital femoral epiphysis; avascular necrosis with steroids or >30–40 Gy
- Mandible dental abnormalities with 20–40 Gy
- Thyroid: <20% to <26 Gy
- Lung blocks
- Entire cardiac silhouette <15 Gy, block at apex, after 30–35 Gy add subcarinal block (5 cm below the carina)
- Renal & liver blocks if necessary

COMPLICATIONS
- Acute: fatigue, dermatitis, esophagitis, nausea, diarrhea
- Subacute: radiation pneumonitis, Lhermitte's syndrome
- Late: coronary artery disease, hypothyroidism, gastric ulcer, pulmonary toxicity, decreased immunity, 2nd malignancies (leukemia RR 22.3×, usually AML peaking at 5–

9 yrs; solid tumors RR 2.8×, usually thyroid, lung, breast, GI occurring >5 yrs after treatment), infertility

FOLLOW-UP

■ Every 3 mo for 2 yr, then every 6 mo for 3 yrs, then annually with H&P, labs, CXR ± CT/PET/gallium. Follow thyroid function if in irradiated field. Annual mammogram for women <30 yrs starting 5–8 yrs after RT

REFERENCES

Aleman BMP, Raemaekers JMM, Tirelli U, et al. Involved-field radiotherapy for advanced Hodgkin's lymphoma. N Engl J Med 2003; 348:2396–2406.

Bonadonna G, Bonfante V, Viviani S, et al. ABVD plus subtotal nodal versus involved-field radiotherapy in early-stage Hodgkin's disease: long-term results. J Clin Oncol 2004;22:2835–2841.

Canellos GP, Anderson JR, Propert KJ, et al. Chemotherapy of advanced Hodgkin's disease with MOPP, ABVD, or MOPP alternating with ABVD. N Engl J Med 1992;327:1478–1484.

Canellos GP, Niedzwiecki D. Long-term follow-up of Hodgkin's disease trial. N Engl J Med 2002;346:1417–1418.

Carde P, Hagenbeek A, Hayat M, et al. Clinical staging versus laparotomy and combined modality with MOPP versus ABVD in early-stage Hodgkin's disease: the H6 twin randomized trials from the European Organization for Research and Treatment of Cancer Lymphoma Cooperative Group. J Clin Oncol 1993;11:2258–2272.

Carde P, Noordijk EM, Hagenbeek A, et al. Superiority of EBVP chemotherapy in combination with involved field irradiation (EBVP/IF) over subtotal nodal irradiation (STNI) in favorable clinical stage (CS) I–II Hodgkin's disease: the EORTC-GPMC H7F randomized trial (Meeting abstract). J Clin Oncol 1997;16:16.

Chisesi T, Federico M, Levis A, et al. ABVD versus stanford V versus MEC in unfavourable Hodgkin's lymphoma: results of a randomised trial. Ann Oncol 2002;13 (Suppl 1):102–106.

Cosset J. MOPP/ABV hybrid and irradiation in unfavourable supradiaphragmatic clinical stages I–II Hodgkin's lymphoma: preliminary results of the EORTC-GELA H8-U randomized trial (#20931) in 995 patients. Leuk Lymphoma 2001;42:12.

Diehl V, Brillant C, Engert A, et al. HD10: Investigating reduction of combined modality treatment intensity in early stage Hodgkin's lymphoma. Interim analysis of a randomized trial of the German Hodgkin Study Group (GHSG). J Clin Oncol (Meeting Abstracts) 2005;23:6506.

Engert A, Schiller P, Josting A, et al. Involved-field radiotherapy is equally effective and less toxic compared with extended-field radiotherapy after four cycles of chemotherapy in patients with early-stage unfavorable Hodgkin's lymphoma: results of the HD8 trial of the German Hodgkin's Lymphoma Study Group. J Clin Oncol 2003;21:3601–3608.

Gobbi PG, Levis A, Chisesi T, et al. ABVD versus modified Stanford V versus MOPPEBVCAD with optional and limited radiotherapy in intermediate- and advanced stage Hodgkin's lymphoma. Final results of a multicenter randomized trial by the Intergruppo Italiano Linfomi. J Clin Oncol 2005;23.

Ferme C, Sebban C, Hennequin C, et al. Comparison of chemotherapy to radiotherapy as consolidation of complete or good partial response after six cycles of chemotherapy for patients with advanced Hodgkin's disease: results of the Groupe d'etudes des Lymphomes de l'Adulte H89 trial. Blood 2000;95:2246–2252.

Hasenclever D, Diehl V, Armitage JO, et al. A prognostic score for advanced Hodgkin's disease. N Engl J Med 1998;339:1506–1514.

Horning SJ, Hoppe RT, Advani R, et al. Efficacy and late effects of Stanford V chemotherapy and radiotherapy in untreated Hodgkin's disease: mature data in early and advanced stage patients. Blood 2004;104:abstr 308.

Laskar S, Gupta T, Vimal S, et al. Consolidation radiation after complete remission in Hodgkin's disease following six cycles of doxorubicin, bleomycin, vinblastine, and dacarbazine chemotherapy: is there a need? J Clin Oncol 2004;22:62–68.

Meyer RM, Gospodarowicz MK, Connors JM, et al. Randomized comparison of ABVD chemotherapy with a strategy that includes radiation therapy in patients with limited-stage Hodgkin's lymphoma: National Cancer Institute of Canada Clinical Trials Group and the Eastern Cooperative Oncology Group. J Clin Oncol 2005;23:4634–4642.

Noordijk E, Carde P, Hagenbeek A. (1997). Combination of radiotherapy and chemotherapy is advisable in all patients with clinical stage I–II Hodgkin's disease. Six-year results of the EORTC-GPMC controlled clinical trials "H7-VF", "H7-F" and "H7-U". Presented at ASTRO,

Noordijk EM, Thomas J, Ferme C, et al. First results of the EORTC-GELA H9 randomized trials: the H9-F trial (comparing 3 radiation dose levels) and H9-U trial (comparing 3 chemotherapy schemes) in patients with favorable or unfavorable early stage Hodgkin's lymphoma (HL). J Clin Oncol (Meeting Abstracts) 2005;23:6506.

Press OW, LeBlanc M, Lichter AS, et al. Phase III randomized intergroup trial of subtotal lymphoid irradiation versus doxorubicin, vinblastine, and subtotal lymphoid irradiation for stage IA to IIA Hodgkin's disease. J Clin Oncol 2001;19:4238–4244.

Sieber M, Franklin J, Tesch H. Two cycles ABVD plus extended field radiotherapy is superior to radiotherapy alone in early stage Hodgkin's disease: results of the German Hodgkin's Lymphoma Study Group (GHSG) Trial HD7. Leuk Lymphoma 2002;43(Suppl 2):52.

Sieber M, Tesch H, Pfistner B, et al. Treatment of advanced Hodgkin's disease with COPP/ABV/IMEP versus COPP/ABVD and consolidating radiotherapy: final results of the German Hodgkin's Lymphoma Study Group HD6 trial. Ann Oncol 2004;15:276–282.

Specht L, Gray RG, Clarke MJ, et al. Influence of more extensive radiotherapy and adjuvant chemotherapy on long-term outcome of early-stage Hodgkin's disease: a meta-analysis of 23 randomized trials involving 3,888 patients. International Hodgkin's Disease Collaborative Group. J Clin Oncol 1998;16:830–843.

Straus DJ, Portlock CS, Qin J, et al. Results of a prospective randomized clinical trial of doxorubicin, bleomycin, vinblastine, and dacarbazine (ABVD) followed by radiation therapy (RT) versus ABVD alone for stages I, II, and IIIA nonbulky Hodgkin disease. Blood 2004; 104:3483–3489.

Chapter 34

Non-Hodgkin's Lymphoma

Hans T. Chung and Alison Bevan

PEARLS

- Rising in incidence; median age 60–65 yrs
- Causative conditions:
  - Immunodeficiency – congenital (SCID, ataxia telangiectasia), acquired (HIV, organ transplant), autoimmune (Sjogren's, Hashimoto's disease, rheumatoid arthritis, systemic lupus erythematosus)
  - Environmental – chemicals (pesticides and solvents)
  - Viral – EBV (Burkitt's lymphoma & NK/T-cell), HTLV-1 (human lymphotrophic virus, type I; adult T-cell leukemia in southern Japan & Caribbean, spread by breast-feeding, sex & blood products), HHV-8 (Kaposi's sarcoma), HCV (extra-nodal B-cell NHL)
  - Bacterial – *H. pylori* (MALT)
  - Radiation – weak association
  - Chemo – alkylating agents
- <u>WHO classification</u>: B cell neoplasms vs T cell & natural killer (NK) cell neoplasms
- B-cell (80%) = DLBCL (31%), follicular (22%), MALT (5%), B-cell CLL (6%) and mantle cell (6%)
- T-cell (13%) = T/NK-cell, peripheral T-cell lymphoma (6%), mycosis fungoides (<1%), anaplastic large cell (2%)
- <u>Low grade</u>: follicular (grade 1–2), CLL, MALT, mycosis fungoides
- <u>Intermediate grade</u>: follicular (grade 3), mantle cell, DLBCL, T/NK-cell, peripheral T-cell lymphoma, anaplastic large cell
- <u>High grade</u>: Burkitt's lymphoma, lymphoblastic
- DLBCL: 30–40% present with stage I–II disease. Extra-nodal disease is common
- Follicular presentation = stage I–II (21%), III (19%), IV (60%). Histologic grade: 1 = follicular small cleaved, 2 = follicular mixed, 3 = follicular large

- MALT (or extranodal marginal zone B-cell lymphoma) commonly involves stomach, ocular adnexae, skin, thyroid, parotid gland, lung, & breast. Most present as stage I–II (65–70%)
- Mantle cell: commonly presents with generalized disease with spleen, bone marrow & gastrointestinal involvement
- Immunophenotyping: see Appendix D
- Cytogenetics: see Appendix D

WORKUP

- H&P. ENT exam if supra-hyoid cervical LN involvement. Ophthalmologic exam for CNS lymphoma
- Excisional LN biopsy with H&E, immunophenotyping, genotyping and molecular profiling with microarrays
- Labs: CBC, LFTs, creatinine, ESR, alkaline phosphatase, uric acid, LDH, HBsAg, HCV Ab, HIV
- Imaging: CXR, CT (chest/abdomen/pelvis ± neck). PET scan or gallium scan. Consider MRI
- Bone marrow biopsy
- CSF cytology if indicated (CNS or epidural lymphoma)

STAGING

- **Ann Arbor staging system** used (See Chapter 33: – Hodgkin's Lymphoma)
- **Limited stage**: stage I–II (≤3 adjacent LN regions), no B symptoms, & non-bulky (<10 cm)
- **Advanced stage**: stage II with >3 contiguous LN regions, stage III–IV, B symptoms, or bulky (≥10 cm)
- Sites that are extranodal, but not extralymphatic (therefore not classified as E): Waldeyer's ring, thymus & spleen

International prognostic index (*N Engl J Med 1993*)

- For intermediate- & high-grade NHL
- Adverse factors: age ≥60 yrs, stage III/IV, elevated LDH, reduced performance status (e.g., ECOG ≥2), & >1 site of extranodal involvement
- 5-year OS by # adverse factors: 0–1 (73%), 2 (51%), 3 (43%), 4–5 (26%)

TREATMENT RECOMMENDATIONS
Low-grade B-cell NHL

Stage	Recommended Treatment
Limited (10% of cases)	IFRT (25–36 Gy at 1.5–1.8 Gy/fx, depending on volume) Median survival 10–15 yr. 10 yr DFS 40–50% Transformation to DLBCL occurs in 10–15%
Advanced (90%)	Asymptomatic – observation Symptomatic – chlorambucil, CVP, fludarabine or RT (8 Gy ×1 for localized disease) Median survival 8–9 yr (among <60 yrs, 10–12 yr)
Relapse	High-dose chemo plus stem cell transplant, or radio-immunotherapy
Transformed disease	Treat as per intermediate-grade disease Rituxan is investigational in maintenance therapy Transplant is also investigational

Intermediate-grade B-cell NHL

Stage	Recommended Treatment
Limited (30% of cases)	Favorable – CHOP-rituximab (R) ×3–4 then IFRT (25–36 Gy) Unfavorable – CHOP-R ×6–8 + IFRT (25–36 Gy)
Advanced (70%)	CHOP-R ×6–8 (rituximab given for DLBCL) IFRT to initially bulky sites is controversial Upfront transplant is investigational
Relapse	High-dose chemo plus stem cell transplant
Palliative	Solitary recurrence – RT Diffuse disease – chemo (rituximab, etoposide, etc.)

High-grade NHL

Stage	Recommended Treatment
All cases	Combination chemo or clinical trial

Gastric MALT

Stage	Recommended Treatment
Stage IAE	4-drug regimen (proton pump inhibitor, bismuth subsalicylate, tetracycline, & metronidazole) for 2 wks CR 97–99%, but median time to CR is 6–8 months
Stage ≥IIAE	Alkylating agent
Recurrent or unresponsive to antibiotics	Suggests *H. pylori*-independent disease IFRT to entire stomach and perigastric nodes (30 Gy/20 fx) Local control >95%

STUDIES
Limited stage low-grade lymphoma

- Stanford (*JCO* 1996). 177 pts with stage I–II follicular lymphoma treated with RT alone. 25% had staging laparotomy. 10 yr RFS and OS was 44% and 64%, respectively. Median survival was 13.8 yr
- Royal Marsden Hospital (*Br J Cancer* 1994). 208 pts with clinical stage I/IE low-grade lymphoma treated with RT alone. 10 yr DFS/CSS were 47%/71%
- Princess Margaret Hospital (*ASCO* 2004). 460 pts with clinical stage I–II follicular lymphoma treated with IFRT alone. Median F/U 12.5 yr. 10 yr DFS, CSS and OS were 41%, 79% and 62%. Late relapses after 10 yrs were infrequent

Advanced stage low-grade lymphoma

- BNLI (*Lancet* 2003). 309 pts with stage III–IVA low-grade lymphoma were randomized to immediate chlorambucil or observation. There was no difference in OS. MS was 5.9 yr (chlorambucil) vs 6.7 yr (observation)
- EORTC 20921 (*JCO* 2006). 381 pts with treatment-naïve, advanced stage, low-grade lymphoma were randomized to CVP or fludarabine. Fludarabine increased overall response rate from 58% to 75%, but had no effect on OS or TTP

Limited stage intermediate-grade lymphoma

- <u>SWOG 8735</u> (*ASH* 2004). 401 pts with intermediate-grade, stage I/IE/II/IIE or bulky stage I lymphoma were randomized to CHOP ×3 + IFRT (40–50 Gy) or CHOP ×8 alone. 5 yr results (*N Engl J Med* 1998) showed improved OS and FFS with CHOP-IFRT. 7- & 10-yr results no longer show any difference in OS or FFS

- <u>ECOG E1484</u> (*JCO* 2004). 352 pts with intermediate-grade, bulky or extranodal stage I, non-bulky stage II/IIE disease received CHOP ×8 then randomized to observation or IFRT (30–40 Gy). IFRT improved 6 yr DFS (73% vs 56%), but no OS difference

- <u>GELA LNH93–1</u> (*NEJM* 2005). 647 pts ≤60 yrs, stage I–II, IPI = 0 intermediate-grade NHL were randomized to ACVBP ×3 followed by consolidation chemo (no RT) or CHOP ×3 + IFRT (40 Gy). ACVBP significantly improved 5 yr EFS and OS, regardless of bulky disease or not

Advanced stage intermediate-grade lymphoma

- <u>SWOG 8516</u> (*NEJM* 1993). 899 pts with bulky stage II, stage III–IV disease randomized to CHOP vs 3 newer and more intensive chemo regimens (m-BACOD, ProMACE-CytaBOM, MACOP-B). No difference in OS, CR or DFS

- <u>GELA LNH98-5</u> (*NEJM* 2002). 399 pts >60 yr with stage II–IV disease randomized to CHOP ×8 or CHOP ×8 plus rituximab. CHOP-R improved CR (76% vs 63%), 2 yr EFS (57% vs 38%) and OS (70% vs 57%)

- <u>MINT</u> (ASCO 2004). 326 pts ≤60 yr with IPI 0-1, stage II–IV or bulky stage I DLBCL randomized to CHOP-like ×6 or CHOP-like + rituximab ×6. CHOP-like + R improved CR, 2 yr time to treatment failure (58% vs 81%) & 2 yr OS (85% vs 95%)

Relapsed intermediate-grade lymphoma

- <u>PARMA</u> (*ASCO* 1998). 109 of 215 pts with relapsed intermediate- or high-grade and responsive to induction DHAP ×2 were randomized to high-dose chemo (BEAC) + autologous bone marrow transplant or DHAP×4. IFRT was indicated in both arms for bulky disease (>5 cm). Median follow-up was 100 months. 8 yr EFS and OS were significantly improved in the BMT arm. Relapses were decreased with the addition of IFRT in the BMT arm (36% vs 55%)

RADIATION TECHNIQUES

Simulation and field design

■ IFRT fields are used. See descriptions in Chapter 33: – Hodgkin's Lymphoma

Dose prescriptions

■ See treatment algorithm

Dose limitations

■ Same as in Chapter 33: – Hodgkin's Lymphoma

COMPLICATIONS

■ Same as in Chapter 33: – Hodgkin's Lymphoma

FOLLOW-UP

■ Same as in Chapter 33: – Hodgkin's Lymphoma

REFERENCES

Ardeshna KM, Smith P, Norton A, et al. Long-term effect of a watch and wait policy versus immediate systemic treatment for asymptomatic advanced-stage non-Hodgkin lymphoma: a randomised controlled trial. Lancet 2003;362:516–522.

Armitage JO. Defining the stages of aggressive non-Hodgkin's lymphoma – a work in progress. N Engl J Med 2005;352:1250–1252.

Coiffier B, Lepage E, Briere J, et al. CHOP chemotherapy plus rituximab compared with CHOP alone in elderly patients with diffuse large-B-cell lymphoma. N Engl J Med 2002;346:235–242.

Fisher RI, Gaynor ER, Dahlberg S, et al. Comparison of a standard regimen (CHOP) with three intensive chemotherapy regimens for advanced non-Hodgkin's lymphoma. N Engl J Med 1993;328:1002–1006.

Hagenbeek A, Eghbali H, Monfardini S, et al. Phase III Intergroup Study of Fludarabine Phosphate Compared With Cyclophospha-mide, Vincristine, and Prednisone Chemotherapy in Newly Diag-nosed Patients With Stage III and IV Low-Grade Malignant Non-Hodgkin's Lymphoma. J Clin Oncol 2006;24:1590–1596.

Horning SJ, Weller E, Kim K, et al. Chemotherapy with or without radiotherapy in limited-stage diffuse aggressive non-Hodgkin's lym-phoma: Eastern Cooperative Oncology Group Study 1484. J Clin Oncol 2004;22:3032–3038.

Mac Manus MP, Hoppe RT. Is radiotherapy curative for stage I and II low-grade follicular lymphoma? Results of a long-term follow-up study of patients treated at Stanford University. J Clin Oncol 1996;14:1282–1290.

Miller TP, Dahlberg S, Cassady JR, et al. Chemotherapy alone compared with chemotherapy plus radiotherapy for localized intermediate-

and high-grade non-Hodgkin's lymphoma. N Engl J Med 1998;339: 21–26.

Petersen PM, Gospodarowicz MK, Tsang RW, et al. Long-term outcome in stage I and II follicular lymphoma following treatment with involved field radiation therapy alone. J Clin Oncol 2004;22:6521.

Pfreundschuh M, Trümper L, Ma D, et al. Randomized intergroup trial of first line treatment for patients <=60 years with diffuse large B-cell non-Hodgkin's lymphoma (DLBCL) with a CHOP-like regimen with or without the anti-CD20 antibody rituximab – early stopping after the first interim analysis. J Clin Oncol 2004;22:6500.

Philip T, Guglielmi C, Hagenbeek A, et al. Autologous bone marrow transplantation as compared with salvage chemotherapy in relapses of chemotherapy-sensitive non-Hodgkin's lymphoma. N Engl J Med 1995;333:1540–1545.

Reyes F, Lepage E, Ganem G, et al. ACVBP versus CHOP plus radiotherapy for localized aggressive lymphoma. N Engl J Med 2005;352:1197–1205.

Spier CM, LeBlanc M, Chase E, et al. Histologic subtypes do not confer unique outcomes in early-stage lymphoma: long-term follow-up of SWOG 8736. Blood 2004;104:abst 3263.

Vaughan Hudson B, Vaughan Hudson G, MacLennan KA, et al. Clinical stage 1 non-Hodgkin's lymphoma: long-term follow-up of patients treated by the British National Lymphoma Investigation with radiotherapy alone as initial therapy. Br J Cancer 1994;69:1088–1093.

NOTES

Chapter 35
Cutaneous Lymphoma

Amy Gillis and Mack Roach III

PEARLS

- Primary cutaneous lymphomas (PCL) include cutaneous B (30%) & T cell (70%) lymphomas
- Overall 1–1.5 new cases per 100,000 per yr
- 2% of new cases of NHL. Most common is cutaneous T cell lymphoma
- Affects older adults (55–60 yrs), 2:1 male predominance, blacks > whites
- Hypothesized links with environmental factors or viral etiology not substantiated
- Presentation: skin lesions, but long natural history. Median time from skin lesion to diagnosis ~5 yrs
- Sezary cells: malignant T cells. Sezary syndrome: erythroderma, lymphadenopathy and sezary cells in peripheral blood
- EORTC and WHO have classification schemes, TNM staging for mycosis fungoides subtype
- Treatment should be tailored to specific subtype of PCL

WORKUP

- H&P. Include LN exam
- Skin biopsies (several often needed to diagnose)
- LN biopsy if clinically indicated
- Laboratory studies: CBC
- For cutaneous T cell lymphoma (CTCL):
  - CXR
  - CT abdomen & pelvis
  - Peripheral blood smear for Sezary cells
  - Bone marrow biopsy

WHO-EORTC CLASSIFICATION WITH SURVIVAL (WILLEMZE, *BLOOD* 2005)*

WHO-EORTC	Frequency (%)	5 yr DS survival (%)
Cutaneous T Cell Lymphomas		
Indolent		
Mycosis fungoides	44	88
Primary cutaneous anaplastic large cell	8	95
Lymphatoid papulosis	12	100
Aggressive		
Sezary Syndrome	3	24
Primary cutaneous T cell, peripheral or aggressive CD8+	~2	16–18
Cutaneous B cell Lymphomas		
Indolent		
Follicle center lymphoma	11	95
Marginal Zone B cell lymphoma	7	99
Intermediate		
Large B cell lymphoma of the leg	4	55
Other diffuse large B cell	<1	50

*Adapted from Willemze R, Jaffe ES, et al. WHO-EORTC classification for cutaneous lymphomas. Blood. 2005; 105(10): 3768–3785 Copyright American Society of Hematology, used with permission. See reference for complete classification.

STAGING: TNM(B) STAGE FOR MYCOSIS FUNGOIDES: T CELL LYMPHOMA

Primary tumor	Blood
T1: Limited patch/plaque (<10% of skin surface involved)	B0: No circulating atypical cells (<1000 Sezary cells [CD4 + CD7–]/ml)
T2: Generalized patch/plaque (>=10% of skin surface involved)	B1: Circulating atypical cells (>=1000 Sezary cells [CD4 + CD7–]/ml)
T3: Cutaneous tumors (one or more)	Stage Grouping
T4: Generalized erythroderma (with or without patches, plaques, or tumors)	IA: T1N0M0 IB: T2N0M0 IIA: T1-2N1M0 IIB: T3N0-1M0

<u>Regional lymph nodes</u>

N0: Lymph nodes clinically uninvolved

N1: Lymph nodes clinically enlarged, histologically uninvolved

N2: Lymph nodes clinically unenlarged, histologically involved

N3: Lymph nodes enlarged and histologically involved

<u>Metastases</u>

M0: No visceral disease

M1: visceral disease present

IIIA: T4N0M0
IIIB: T4N1M0
IVA: T1-4N2-3M0
IVB: T1-4N0-3M1

Used with the permission of the American Joint Committee on Cancer (AJCC), Chicago, Illinois. The original source for this material is the AJCC Cancer Staging Manual, Sixth Edition (2002) published by Springer-Verlag New York, www.springeronline.com.

TREATMENT RECOMMENDATIONS: CTCL (MF)

Stage	Recommended Treatment
IA	Topical treatment: steroids, retinoids, nitrogen mustard Light treatment: UVB or PUVA Local electron beam therapy (EBT)
IB-IIA	Topical nitrogen mustard Light treatment Total skin electron beam therapy (TSEBT)
IIB	Few tumors ■ Local EBT + topical nitrogen mustard ■ PUVA Generalized tumors ■ TSEBT + topical nitrogen mustard ■ PUVA + IFNα ■ PUVA + oral retinoids ■ Other combined modality
IIIA/IIIB	Extracorporeal photopheresis PUVA

Stage	Recommended Treatment
	Oral retinoids IFNα or methotrexate Combined modality
IVA/IVB	Topical therapy + chemotherapy Combined systemic therapy RT for symptomatic lesions Bone marrow transplant

SUBGROUPS
Diffuse large B cell
- Leg presentation thought to have poorer prognosis
- Treat with RT and/or chemotherapy
- MD Anderson experience (Sarris, *JCO* 2001): RT alone has poorer prognosis: OS 25% RT alone vs. 77% with RT + doxorubicin based chemo

Lymphatoid papulosis: T cell
- 14% of PCL, 100% 5 yr survival
- Often generalized, common to have spontaneous remissions
- Relapse common
- Transition to other lymphoma rare
- Often no treatment needed

ALCL (anaplastic large-cell lymphoma): T cell
- Rarely fatal
- Often treated with RT to 40 Gy – usually with good response, CR 90%
- Treat relapse with additional RT

CTCL: Mycosis fungoides (MF) and Sezary syndrome: T cell
- Median duration from lesion onset to diagnosis: 8–10 yrs
- Median survival from diagnosis: 5–10 yrs
- At autopsy: 80% have extracutaneous involvement
- With lymph node involvement: median survival <2 yrs
- Visceral organ involvement: median survival <1 yr
- Quickly responds to RT, & higher doses may decrease recurrence rate

RADIATION TECHNIQUES
Treatment and dose
- Low doses effective, 24–36 Gy

- Palliative: 100–200 kV X-rays or 6–9 MeV electrons, often 15 Gy (3 Gy × 5 fx or 5 Gy × 3 fx)
- Individualize treatment to site of disease. 30–36 Gy (1.5–2 Gy/fx)

Total skin electron beam (TSEB)

- 6 patient postions: Anterior, posterior, 2 posterior obliques and 2 anterior obliques
- Six-dual field technique = 6 pt positions, each with superior and inferior fields
- Patient standing, 3.5 m from electron source
- Lucite plate near patient surface to scatter electrons
- Machine angled at 18 degrees, up/down for homogeneity at pt surface
- Treat 3 patient positions each day, 2 day cycle, 4 days/wk
- 36 Gy in 1.5–2 Gy/fx with 1 week break mid treatment if significant skin erythema occurs
- Thicker or tumorous lesions may require boost

COMPLICATIONS

- Acute complications include erythema & dry desquamation, also hand swelling & lower extremity edema
- Intermediate: alopecia (temporary if scalp dose limited to 25 Gy), hyperpigmentation
- Temporary loss of toe/finger nails, difficulty with sweat production

FOLLOW-UP

- Regular clinic visits with H&P
- With RT, expect continued regression 6–8 weeks post treatment

REFERENCES

Chao KC, Perez CA, Brady LW, editors. Radiation Oncology Management Decisions. 2nd ed. Philadelphia: Lippincott Williams & Wilkins; 2002. pp. 123–128, 598.

Cox JD, Ha CS, Wilder RB. Leukemias and lymphomas. In: Cox JD, Ang KK, editors. Radiation Oncology: Rationale, Technique, Results. 8th ed. St. Louis: Mosby; 2003. pp. 837–855.

Hoppe RT, Kim Y. Mycosis Fungiodes. In: Leibel SA, Phillips TL, editors. Textbook of Radiation Oncology. 2nd ed. Philadelphia: Saunders; 2004. pp. 1417–1431.

Sarris AH, Braunschweig I, et al. Primary cutaneous non-Hodgkin's lymphoma of Ann Arbor stage I: Preferential Cutaneous Relapses but high Cure Rate with Doxorubicin-Based Therapy. *J Clin Oncol.* 2001;19(2):398–405.

Willemze R, Jaffe ES, et al. WHO_EORTC classification for cutaneous lymphomas. *Blood.* 2005; 105(10): 3768–3785.

Yahalom J. Non-Hodgkin's lymphoma. In: Leibel SA, Phillips TL, editors. Textbook of Radiation Oncology. 2nd ed. Philadelphia: Saunders; 2004. pp. 1393–1416.

NOTES

Chapter 36
Multiple Myeloma and Plasmacytoma

Kavita Mishra and Mack Roach III

- Plasma cell tumors are monoclonal tumors of immuno-globulin-secreting cells, derived from B-cell lymphocytes
- Incidence is low overall, ~1–2% of U.S. cancers diagnosed yearly are plasma cell tumors. >90% of these are multiple myeloma (MM); 2–10% are solitary plasmacytoma (SP)
- MM incidence higher in blacks than whites (~2:1). Median age at diagnosis 60 yrs
- SP more common in men than women (4:1). Median age at diagnosis 50–55 yrs
- Etiology is unknown, may involve occupational exposures, RT, solvents
- 20% pts are free of clinical symptoms at diagnosis
- Osseous SP and MM may manifest as bone pain, neurologic symptoms, pathologic fracture, cord compression, anemia, hypercalcemia, renal insufficiency
- ~80% of extraosseous SP occur in upper aerodigestive tract. Common presenting signs include epistaxis, nasal discharge, nasal obstruction
- 50–80% of pts with osseous SP progress to MM at a median ~2–3 yrs after treatment. Factors that predict for conversion are controversial, but may include lesion size ≥5 cm, age >40 yo, presence of M spike, spinal location, persistence of M-protein after RT
- 10–40% of patients with extraosseous SP progress to MM at 10 years

WORKUP

- H&P
- CBC, chemistries, LFTs, albumin, calcium
- SPEP, UPEP. 24 hr urine for Bence-Jones proteins

- Beta-2 microglobulin, LDH, & C-reactive protein reflect tumor burden
- Bone marrow aspirate and biopsy
- Skeletal survey. Bone scan often noncontributory since purely lytic lesions with low isotope uptake
- CXR. Consider MRI or CT imaging of painful weight-bearing areas
- Solitary plasmacytoma: need confirmatory tissue biopsy of single lesion; normal BM biopsy (<10% plasma cells), negative skeletal survey, & no signs or symptoms of systemic disease
- Smoldering Myeloma (Asymptomatic Myeloma): serum M-protein ≥30 g/L *and/or* BM clonal plasma cells ≥10%; no end organ damage (including bone lesions) or symptoms

STAGING

Durie-Salmon Myeloma Staging System[1]		*Measured myeloma cell mass (cells x $10^{12}/m^2$)*
Stage	*Criteria*	

I	All of the following: 1. Hemoglobin value >10 g/ 100 ml 2. Serum calcium value normal (≤12 mg/100 ml) 3. On roentgenogram, normal bone structure or solitary bone plasmacytoma only 4. Low M-component production rates
	  ■ IgG value <5 g/100 ml
	  ■ IgA value <3 g/100 ml
	  ■ Urine light chain M-component on electrophoresis <4 g/24 hours
		<0.6 (Low)

II	Fitting neither Stage I nor III	0.6–1.20 (Intermediate)

III	One or more of the following: 1. Hemoglobin value <8.5 g/100 ml 2. Serum calcium value >12 mg/100 ml 3. Advanced lytic bone lesions 4. High M-component production rates
	  ■ IgG value >7 g/100 ml
	  ■ IgA value >5 g/100 ml
	  ■ Urine light chain M-component on electrophoresis >12 g/24 hours
		>1.20 (High)

Subclassification
A: Relatively normal renal function (serum creatinine value
   <2.0 mg/100 ml)
B: Abnormal renal function (serum creatinine value
   ≥2.0 mg/100 ml)

New International Staging System[2]

Stage	Criteria	MS (months)
I	Serum β2-microglobulin <3.5 mg/L	62
	Serum albumin ≥3.5 g/dL	
II	Not stage I or III	44
III	Serum β2-microglobulin ≥5.5 mg/L	29

1. From: Durie BGM, Salmon SE: A clinical staging system for multiple myeloma. Cancer 36:842–854, 1975, (with permission).
2. From: Greipp PR, San Miguel J, Durie BG, et al. International staging system for multiple myeloma. J Clin Oncol 2005;23:3412–3420. Reprinted with permission from the American Society of Clinical Oncology.

TREATMENT RECOMMENDATIONS

Stage	Recommended Treatment
I or systemic smoldering	Observe
SP – osseous	Involved field RT
SP – extraosseous	Involved field RT alone, surgery alone, or surgery + RT
II or III	Chemo (e.g., melphalan + prednisone) + bisphosphonate. Consider allogeneic or autologous stem cell transplant. Consider RT for palliation of local bone pain, prevention of pathologic fractures, relief of cord compression

STUDIES

- Alexiou (*Cancer* 1999). Review article of 400+ publications with total 869 pts with extraosseous SP treated with RT alone, surgery alone, or combined surgery + RT. In upper aerodigestive (UAD) tract tumors, combined treatment resulted in higher OS; however, in non-UAD located tumors, there was no survival difference between treatment arms. Low risk of lymph node involvement (7.6% in UAD, 2.6% in non-UAD areas)

- Fermand (*Blood* 1998). Randomized 185 pts with MM to early high-dose chemotherapy (HDT) and peripheral blood stem cell autotransplantation (PBSC) vs conventional-dose chemotherapy (CCT) and late HDT + PBSC for nonresponders or recurrence. No difference in OS ~64 mo
- Hu (*Oncology* 2000). Review article of SP literature, including total 338 pts with SP. Pts with osseous SP have LC rate 88–100%, rate of progression to MM 50–80% at 10 yrs, 10 yr OS 45–70%. Pts with extraosseous SP have LC 80–100%, rate of progression to MM 10–40% at 10 yrs, 10 yr OS 40–90%
- IFM 9502 (*Blood* 2002). 282 pts with MM undergoing conditioning regimens before autologous stem cell transplantation randomized to high dose melphalan vs TBI (8 Gy in 4 fx) + lower dose melphalan. TBI arm had greater hematologic toxicity, higher toxic death rate, and decreased 45 mo OS (45.5% vs 66%)
- Myeloma Aredia Study Group (*NEJM* 1996). 377 pts with stage III myeloma and at least 1 lytic lesion randomized to antimyeloma treatment plus either placebo or pamidronate (monthly infusions ×9 cycles). Pamidronate arm had significantly less skeletal events (24% vs 41%) and had decreased bone pain
- Salmon (*JCO* 1990). 180 pts with MM underwent induction chemo and were then randomized to consolidation chemo alone vs double hemibody irradiation (HBI) + chemo. HBI given in 5 daily 1.5 Gy fx, with 6 wk separation between upper and lower HBI. Consolidation chemo arm improved RFS (26 vs 20 mo) and OS (36 vs 28 mo) compared with HBI arm

RADIATION TECHNIQUES
Simulation and field design
- SP: involved field RT including involved bone +2–3 cm margin. Use CT/MRI to delineate tumor extent, especially paravertebral extension. For extraosseous SP, may include primary draining LN
- MM: main indication is for palliation. For symptomatic bony lesions, include entire bone if possible. May limit long bone/pelvis fields to decrease dose to bone marrow. If treating vertebral column, include involved vertebrae + 2 vertebrae above and two below

Dose prescriptions

- SP: 45–50 Gy over 4–5 weeks, 1.8–2 Gy/fx
- MM is very radioresponsive, so lower doses can be given compared with standard palliative RT doses for bony mets from solid tumors
- MM: palliative dose 20–30 Gy in 1.5–2 Gy fractions. May increase dose to 30–36 Gy for cord compression, bulky soft tissue component, and incomplete palliation

Dose limitations

- Varies based on organs within involved field
- Spinal cord <45 Gy at 1.8 Gy/fx

COMPLICATIONS

- Normal tissue toxicity within RT field
- Myelosuppression
- MM: hypercalcemia, anemia, renal insufficiency, infection, skeletal lesions

FOLLOW-UP

- Systemic myeloma: quantitative immunoglobulins + M protein every 3 mo. Follow CBC, serum BUN, Cr, Ca. Bone survey annually or for symptoms. Bone marrow biopsy as indicated
- SP osseous: as above + measure paraprotein every 3–6 mo
- SP extraosseous: paraprotein every 3 mo ×1 yr, then annually. CT/MRI every 6 mo ×1 yr, then as clinically indicated

REFERENCES

Alexiou C, Kau RJ, Dietzfelbinger H, et al. Extramedullary plasmacytoma: tumor occurrence and therapeutic concepts. Cancer 1999;85: 2305–2314.

Fermand J-P, Ravaud P, Chevret S, et al. High-dose therapy and autologous peripheral blood stem cell transplantation in multiple myeloma: up-front or rescue treatment? Results of a multicenter sequential randomized clinical trial. Blood 1998;92:3131–3136.

Hu K, Yahalom J. Radiotherapy in the management of plasma cell tumors. Oncology 2000;14:101–108.

Intergroupe Francophone du Myelome. Comparison of 200 mg/m(2) melphalan and 8 Gy total body irradiation plus 140 mg/m(2) melphalan as conditioning regimens for peripheral blood stem cell transplantation in patients with newly diagnosed multiple myeloma: final analysis of the Intergroupe Francophone du Myelome 9502 randomized trial. Blood 2002;99:731–735.

Kyle, RA, Greipp, PR. Smoldering multiple myeloma. N Engl J Med 1980;302:1347.

Myeloma Aredia Study Group. Efficacy of pamidronate in reducing skeletal events in patients with advanced multiple myeloma. N Engl J Med 1996;334:488–493.

National Comprehensive Cancer Network. Clinical Practice Guidelines in Oncology: Multiple Myeloma. Available at: http://www.nccn.org/professionals/physician_gls/PDF/myeloma.pdf. Accessed on January 21, 2005.

Salmon SE, Tesh D, Crowley J, et al. Chemotherapy is superior to sequential hemibody irradiation for remission consolidation in multiple myeloma: a Southwest Oncology Group study. J Clin Oncol 1990;8:1575–1584.

Schechter NR, Lewis VO. The bone. In: Cox JD, Ang KK, editors. Radiation Oncology: Rationale, Technique, Results. 8th ed. St. Louis: Mosby; 2003. pp. 857–883.

Wasserman TH. Myeloma and plasmacytomas. In: Perez CA, Brady LW, Halperin EC, et al., editors. Principles and Practice of Radiation Oncology. 4th ed. Philadelphia: Lippincott Williams & Wilkins; 2004. pp. 2157–2167.

NOTES

Chapter 37
Bone Tumors

Brian Lee and Jean L. Nakamura

PEARLS

- Diaphysis = shaft; epiphysis = growth plate & end of bone; metaphysis = conical portion between diaphysis & epiphysis
- Prevalence: osteosarcoma > chondrosarcoma > Ewing's > malignant fibrous histiocytoma (MFH)
- 60% cases occur between 10–20 yrs of age (most active age of skeletal growth)
- 80% cases in long bones until epiphyseal closure (then ~even with appendicular skeleton)
- In pts >60 yrs, >50% cases arise from other conditions (i.e., Paget's disease, fibrous dysplasia) → poor chemo response
- Osteosarcoma: malignant osteoid is hallmark (not seen in chondrosarcoma). Most common bone tumor in children. 75% present in metaphyses of long bones with local pain/ swelling. 85% are grade 3–4. Osteosarcoma arising as 2nd malignancy s/p chemo or RT does not necessarily have worse prognosis, but controversial. Associated with Li-Fraumeni syndrome (p53) and retinoblastoma
- Parosteal (juxtacortical) osteosarcomas are usually low-grade, localized with rare DM. Most present in popliteal fossa. 80–90% curable with surgery alone
- Chondrosarcoma: most common in the femur. Frequent local recurrence, DM less common than osteosarcoma. 1/3 are high-grade
- MFH: Very aggressive locally with frequent DM. Often presents with fracture
- Fibrosarcoma: high-grade, behaves like osteosarcoma. Commonly presents with fractures
- Chordoma: physaliferous cell ("bubbly cell") is hallmark. Most often in sacrococcygeal area, base of skull, & spine. Presentation is location specific
- Giant cell tumors = giant multinucleated osteoclast cells. Only 8–15% are malignant. Cyst formation, hemorrhage,

necrosis are important with regards to radiosensitivity. Frequent LR (45–60%)

- Lung metastases common in osteosarcoma, chondrosarcoma, MFH

WORKUP

- H&P
- CBC, chemistries, urinalysis, ESR, alkaline phosphatase
- Plain films (primary region & CXR) – Codman's triangle, perios-teal bone spicules, 1° tumor often seen as cloud-like density
- CT/MRI (primary area & chest) to evaluate soft tissue extensions
- Bone scan – Intramedullary skip metastases. Consider PET scan
- Biopsy lesion after complete radiologic evaluation & avoid incision over area not to be irradiated or re-excised. Biopsy should be performed at institution where treatment will occur

DIFFERENTIATING EWING'S FROM OSTEOSARCOMA

Ewing's	Osteosarcoma
Lytic, destructive lesion	Sclerotic lesion
Diaphysis	Metaphysis
Onion skin effect	Sunburst pattern (periosteal new bone formation)

AJCC STAGING

Primary Tumor		Stage Grouping	
TX:	Primary tumor cannot be assessed	IA:	T1N0M0 G1-2, Low grade
T0:	No evidence of primary tumor	IB:	T2N0M0 G1-2, Low grade
T1:	Tumor ≤8 cm in greatest dimension	IIA:	T1N0M0 G3-4, High grade
T2:	Tumor >8 cm in greatest dimension	IIB:	T2N0M0 G3-4, High grade
T3:	Discontinuous tumors in the primary bone site	III:	T3N0M0 Any G
		IVA:	Any T N0 M1a Any G
Regional LN		IVB:	Any T N1 Any M Any G
NX*:	Regional lymph nodes cannot be assessed		Any T Any N M1b Any G

N0: No regional lymph node metastasis	
N1: Regional lymph node metastasis	~5 yr OS by Histology Osteosarcoma: 60–75% (20% if M1)
*Because of the rarity of lymph node involvement in sarcomas, the desgnation NX may not be appropriate and could be considered N0 if no clinical involvement is evident.	Chondrosarcoma: 50–70% MFH: 15–67% Fibrosarcoma: 25–50% Malignant giant cell tumor: 30%
Distant Metastasis MX: Distant metastasis cannot be assessed M0: No distant metastasis M1 Distant metastasis M1a: Lung M1b: Other distant sites	

Used with the permission of the American Joint Committee on Cancer (AJCC), Chicago, Illinois. The original source for this material is the AJCC Cancer Staging Manual, Sixth Edition (2002) published by Springer-Verlag New York, www.springeronline.com.

TREATMENT RECOMMENDATIONS

- In general, limb sparing strategies are preferred, which may involve a combination of neoadjuvant chemo, RT and surgery
- Input of orthopedic oncologist is essential in determining whether limb sparing is possible. Final limb function may sometimes be better with prosthesis than with partially resected and/or irradiated limb. In children, RT has added implications on growth of limb and future function
- Osteosarcoma: Pre-op chemo → surgery → adjuvant chemo ×4–6 mo
  - Consider clinical trial
  - Inoperable or close/+ margin → RT to 60–75 Gy with shrinking fields
  - Pelvic tumors → Consider intra-arterial chemo (cisplatin/doxorubicin) + RT 60–70 Gy
  - M1a: Surgical resection of lung metastases improves survival
- Chondrosarcoma/MFH/giant cell: surgery = 1° treatment (WLE, amputation). RT for inoperable tumors or close/+ margin

- EBRT = 60–70 Gy. IORT = 15–30 Gy
- Giant Cell: 45–55 Gy
- Chordoma: surgery → RT. RT alone for inoperable cases (66–70 Gy). Consider SRS or proton or charged particle treatment if available

STUDIES
Osteosarcoma
- Randomized trials have established that neoadjuvant and adjuvant chemo help to prevent relapse or recurrence in pts with localized resectable primary tumors (Link, *NEJM* 1986; Eilber, *JCO* 1987)
- Cooperative German/Austrian Osteosarcoma Study Group (*JCO* 2003). Subset analysis of 67 pts with non-metastatic, high-grade pelvic osteosarcomas. RT improved survival for pts with intralesional excision & unresectable tumors
- DeLaney (*IJROBP* 2005). Review of 41 pts with osteosarcoma that were either unresectable or had close or + margins & were treated with RT. No definitive dose-response, although doses >55 Gy had higher LC (p = 0.11). RT more effective for pts with microscopic or minimal residual disease

Chordoma
- Several studies have indicated that charged particle treatment &/or radiosurgery may improve LC

RADIATION TECHNIQUES
Simulation and field design
- Spare 1.5–2 cm strip of skin in extremity XRT if possible to prevent edema
- Include entire surgical bed + scar + 2 cm margin if possible
- Bolus scar for 1st 50 Gy
- CT/MRI data for tx planning
- Try to exclude skin over anterior tibia if possible due to poor vascularity
- Physical therapy instituted as early as possible during treatment to improve functional outcome

Dose limitations
- >20 Gy can prematurely close epiphysis
- >40 Gy will ablate bone marrow

■ ≥50 Gy to bone cortex significantly increases risk of fracture

COMPLICATIONS

■ Abnormal bone & soft tissue growth & development, permanent weakening of affected bone, scoliosis, decreased range of motion due to fibrosis or joint involvement, vascular changes resulting in greater sensitivity to infection, fracture, lymphedema, skin discoloration or telangiectasia, osteoradionecrosis

■ Increased risk of 2° cancers (leukemia, sarcomas)

FOLLOW-UP

■ Intensive physical rehabilitation very important, especially for pediatric cases

■ Regular H&P with functional assessment, CBC, chest imaging, & local imaging every 3 mo for 2 yrs, every 4 mo for 3rd yr, every 6 mo for yrs 4 & 5, then annually

REFERENCES

Bramwell VH, Burgers M, Sneath R, et al. A comparison of two short intensive adjuvant chemotherapy regimens in operable osteosarcoma of limbs in children and young adults: the first study of the European Osteosarcoma Intergroup. J Clin Oncol 1992;10: 1579–1591.

Burgers JM, van Glabbeke M, Busson A, et al. Osteosarcoma of the limbs. Report of the EORTC-SIOP 03 trial 20781 investigating the value of adjuvant treatment with chemotherapy and/or prophylactic lung irradiation. Cancer 1988;61:1024–1031.

DeLaney TF, Park L, Goldberg SI, et al. Radiotherapy for local control of osteosarcoma. Int J Radiat Oncol Biol Phys 2005;61:492–498.

Eilber F, Giuliano A, Eckardt J, et al. Adjuvant chemotherapy for osteosarcoma: a randomized prospective trial. J Clin Oncol 1987;5:21–26.

Link MP, Goorin AM, Miser AW, et al. The effect of adjuvant chemotherapy on relapse-free survival in patients with osteosarcoma of the extremity. N Engl J Med 1986;314:1600–1606.

McNaney D, Lindberg RD, Ayala AG, et al. Fifteen year radiotherapy experience with chondrosarcoma of bone. Int J Radiat Oncol Biol Phys 1982;8:187–190.

Montemaggi P BW, Horowitz SM. Bone. In: Perez CA, Brady LW, Halperin ED, Schmidt-Ullrich RK, editors. Principles and Practice of Radiation Oncology. 4th ed. Philadelphia: Lippincott Williams & Wilkins; 2004. pp. 2168–2184. 2004.

Ozaki T, Flege S, Kevric M, et al. Osteosarcoma of the pelvis: experience of the Cooperative Osteosarcoma Study Group. J Clin Oncol 2003;21:334–341.

Romero J, Cardenes H, la Torre A, et al. Chordoma: results of radiation therapy in eighteen patients. Radiother Oncol 1993;29:27–32.

Schecter NR LV. The bone. In: Cox JD, Ang KK, editors. Radiation Oncology: Rationale, Technique, Results. 8th ed. St. Louis: Mosby; 2003. pp. 857–883. 2003.

Schoenthaler R, Castro JR, Petti PL, et al. Charged particle irradiation of sacral chordomas. Int J Radiat Oncol Biol Phys 1993;26:291–298.

Schupak K. Sarcomas of bone. In: Leibel SA, Phillips TL, editors. Textbook of Radiation Oncology. 2nd ed. Philadelphia: Saunders; 2004. pp. 1363–1374. 2004.

NOTES

Chapter 38
Soft Tissue Sarcoma

Brian Lee and Alexander R. Gottschalk

PEARLS

- ~8700 cases/yr in U.S.
- Median age 40–60 yrs
- Slight male predominance, more frequent among African Americans
- Genetics: NF-1, NF-2, retinoblastoma, Gardner's syndrome, Li-Fraumeni syndrome
- Environmental exposures: herbicides, thorotrast, chlorophenols, vinyl chloride, arsenic
- Lower extremity (45%) > trunk (30%) > upper extremity (15%) > H&N (8%)
- Extremity = liposarcoma, MFH, synovial, fibrosarcoma, myxoid liposarcoma (upper medial thigh)
- Retroperitoneal = liposarcoma (fewer DM) > leiomyosarcoma (increased DM)
- H&N = MFH, usually high-grade (except myxoid MFH = intermediate grade)
- Frequency: MFH (20–30%), liposarcoma (10–20%), leiomyosarcoma (5–10%), fibrosarcoma (5–10%), synovial cell sarcoma (5–10%), rhabdomyosarcoma (5–10%), malignant peripheral nerve sheath tumor/schwannoma (5–10%)
- Synovial sarcoma = usually high-grade, near (but not within) joints in tendon sheaths, bursae, & joint capsules
- Grade based on cellularity, differentiation, pleomorphism, necrosis, #mitoses
- Cytogenetics: See Appendix D

Presentation

- Painless mass. Typically 4–6 mo from symptoms to diagnosis
- Stewart-Treves syndrome = chronic lymphedema of upper extremity → lymphangiosarcoma

- ~20% have metastases at diagnosis. Extremity → lung, retroperitoneal → liver. For low-grade, <10% have metastases vs 50% for high-grade
- Increased risk of LN spread: SCARE = synovial (14%), clear cell (28%), angiosarcoma (11%), rhabdomyosarcoma (15%), epithelioid (20%)

WORKUP

- H&P, CBC, BUN/Cr, ESR, LDH. CT/MRI of primary. Plain X-ray of primary. All pts get CT chest. If myxoid liposarcoma, include CT abdomen because frequently metastasizes to retroperitoneum. MRI brain for alveolar type. Consider PET scan (investigational)
- Always perform imaging prior to biopsy or surgery because cannot fully assess by clinical exam. Perform biopsy at institution where surgery will be performed
- Incisional biopsy or core needle biopsy preferred. Core biopsy predicts type & grade 90% of time. Incisional biopsy should be oriented so can be excised during the definitive excision. Excisional biopsy often contaminates surrounding tissue

PROGNOSIS

- Adverse factors: high grade, increasing size/stage, deep, + margins, >50 yrs age, fibrosarcoma type including desmoid, malignant peripheral nerve sheath tumors, high Ki-67, non-diploid, low level of MDM2 mRNA expression, distal extremity tumors

AJCC STAGING

Primary tumor (T)	
TX:	Primary tumor cannot be assessed
T1:	Tumor ≤5 cm in greatest dimension
	T1a: superficial tumor
	T1b: deep tumor
T2:	Tumor >5 cm in greatest dimension
	T2a: superficial tumor
	T2b: deep tumor

Note: Superficial tumor is located exclusively above the superficial fascia without invasion of the fascia; deep tumor is located either exclusively beneath the superficial fascia, superficial to the fascia with invasion of or through the fascia, or both superficial yet beneath the fascia. Retroperitoneal, mediastinal, and pelvic sarcomas are classified as deep tumors.

Regional lymph nodes (N)
NX: Regional lymph nodes cannot be assessed
N0: No regional lymph node metastasis
N1: Regional lymph node metastasis. *Considered Stg IV

Distant metastasis (M)
MX: Distant metastasis cannot be assessed
M0: No distant metastasis
M1: Distant metastasis

Histologic Grade (G)
GX: Grade cannot be assessed
G1: Well differentiated
G2: Moderated differentiated
G3: Poorly differentitated
G4: Poorly differentiated or undifferentiated (four-tiered systems only)

Stage Grouping					
I:	T1a, 1b, 2a, 2b	N0	M0	G1-2	G1	Low
II:	T1a, 1b, 2a	N0	M0	G3-4	G2-3	High
III:	T2b	N0	M0	Any G	Any G	High or Low
IV:	Any T	N1	M0	Any G	Any G	High or Low
	Any T	N0	M1	Any G	Any G	High or Low

~5 yr OS
I: 90%
II: 81%
III: 56%
IV: <20%, MS 8–12mo

Metastatic relapse: 10% unless isolated lung metastasis (25%)
Retroperitoneal: 40% after gross total resection, 5% after subtotal resection

---

*Not included in AJCC soft tissue sarcoma staging: angiosarcoma, malignant mesenchymoma, desmoid. Included: GI stromal tumors, Ewing's sarcoma/primitive neuroectodermal tumor have been added.
**Used with the permission of the American Joint Committee on Cancer (AJCC), Chicago, Illinois. The original source for this material is the AJCC Cancer Staging Manual, Sixth Edition (2002) published by Springer-Verlag New York, www.springeronline.com.

<u>Not</u> included in AJCC staging: angiosarcoma, dermatofibrosarcoma protuberans, desmoid tumor (fibromatosis)

TREATMENT RECOMMENDATIONS

Stage	Recommended Treatment
I extremity	Surgery alone (unless close/+ margin → post-op RT)
II–III extremity	Surgery + post-op RT or pre-op RT → surgery
IV	For controlled primary, with ≤4 lung lesions &/or extended disease free interval consider surgical resection Otherwise, best supportive care, chemo, &/or palliative surgery or RT
Retroperitoneal	Surgery ± IORT (12–15 Gy) → post-op EBRT 45–50 Gy. Or enroll on trial of pre-op chemo-RT → resection → IORT boost
Desmoid tumors	Surgery. If + margin, post-op RT (50 Gy). If inoperable, RT (56–60 Gy)

Surgery

- Prefer wide en bloc resection with ≥2 cm margin in all directions
- A radical resection removes entire anatomic compartment including neurovascular structures (LC 80–90%)
- Wide excision removes cuff of normal tissue (LC 40–70%)
- Excisional biopsy = marginal excision "shellout" of pseudocapsule only (LC 20%)
- Intralesional biopsy = inside pseudocapsule. Surgical scars should be oriented longitudinally so circumferential RT can be avoided
- Clips should be placed for RT planning

Chemo

- ~50% of pts with high-grade tumors will die of DM despite LC of primary

- Most active single chemo agent = doxorubicin (15–30% response)
- Contradictory results in trials comparing single vs combination chemo. No clear OS benefit to combination chemo
- Post-op chemo controversial. If used, based on meta-analysis (doxo-based) or Italian study (epirubicin/ifosfamide)
- Consider neoadjuvant chemo → surgery for high-grade or unresectable tumors
- Consider checking c-kit level as may respond to Gleevec

STUDIES
Post-op RT

- Pisters (*JCO* 1996). 160 pts with extremity & superficial trunk sarcoma s/p WLE. Randomized to brachytherapy (Ir-192 42–45 Gy over 4–6 d) or observation. RT to tumor + 2 cm margin. Brachytherapy increased LC for high-grade lesions (65→90%) but not for low-grade lesions (~70%). No difference in DSS (80%) & DM
- NCI (Yang, *JCO* 1998). 140 pts with extremity sarcoma treated with WLE. Low-grade randomized to observation vs post-op EBRT. High-grade randomized to post-op chemo vs post-op chemo-RT. RT = large field to 45 Gy → boost to 63 Gy. RT increased LC for low-grade (60→95%) & high-grade (75→100%). No difference in OS (70%) or DMFS (75%)
- NCI (Rosenberg, *Ann Surg* 1982). 43 pts with high-grade STS of extremity randomized to WLE + post-op RT vs amputation alone. RT = 45–50 Gy to compartment with boost to 60–70 Gy. No difference in LC, OS, or DFS. 65 pts also randomized to WLE + post-op RT ± chemo. Chemo decreased LR & increased DFS (60→90%) & OS (75→95%)
- Alektiar (*JCO* 2002). 204 pts with stage IIB treated with limb-sparing surgery with negative margins. 43% got RT & 57% did not get RT. RT was brachytherapy (60%) or EBRT (40%). No difference in 5y LC with or without adjuvant RT (80% vs 84%)

Pre-op or post-op RT

- Pollack (*IJROBP* 1998). Compared pts treated with post-op RT (60–66 Gy) or pre-op RT (50 Gy) before excision or re-excision. No difference in LC between pre vs post-op (81%). For pts presenting with gross disease, best LC with pre-op RT (88% vs 67%). For pts presenting after excision elsewhere, best treated with immediate re-excision & post-op RT (LC 91% vs 72%). More wound healing problems with pre-op (25% vs 5%)

■ NCIC (O'Sullivan, *Lancet* 2002; Davis, *Radiother Oncol*, 2005). 190 pts with extremity STS randomized pre-op RT (50 Gy) vs post-op RT (66 Gy). If +margins, pre-op got 16 Gy boost. No difference in LC (93%), DM (25%), PFS (65%). Initially better OS with pre-op due to deaths other than sarcoma in post-op arm, but on 6 yr F/U, no difference in OS. More wound healing problems with pre-op (35% vs 15%) but increased late fibrosis with post-op RT (48% vs 31%, p = 0.07).

IORT

■ NCI (*Arch Surg* 1993). 35 pts with resectable retroperitoneal STS randomized surgery +/– IORT 20 Gy → post-op 35–40 Gy vs surgery → post-op 50–55 Gy. No difference in 5 yr OS (35%), but non-significant increase in LC (20→ 60%). IORT increased neuropathy if >15 Gy, but lower GI complications

■ Alektiar (*IJROBP* 2000). 32 pts with primary or recurrent retroperitoneal STS treated with surgery + IORT 12–15 Gy → post-op EBRT 45–50 Gy. Results: 5 yr OS 55%, DMFS 80%, LC 62%. 10% neuropathy

Chemo

■ Meta–analysis (Tierney, *Br J Cancer* 1997). 1568 pts treated with WLE ± adjuvant doxorubicin-based chemo. Chemo improved LC (absolute 6%), DMFS (10%), RFS (10%), & OS 4% (non-significant). Largest benefit with high-grade extremity STS

■ No trial of pre-op vs post-op chemo

RADIATION TECHNIQUES
Post-op EBRT

■ Start 10–20 d after surgery for healing
■ 4–6 MV for extremities usually. 2 Gy/fx
■ Bolus scar & drain sites for first 50 Gy unless in tangential beam
■ Field = tumor bed, scar, drainage sites + 5–7 cm longitudinal & 2–3 cm perpendicular margin in initial field. After

50 Gy, reduce field to surgical bed (outlined by clips, scar) + 2 cm margin

- Take negative margins or microscopic residual to 60 Gy, +margins to 66 Gy, gross disease to 75 Gy
- Always spare 1.5–2 cm strip of skin. Try to exclude skin over ant tibia if possible due to poor vascularity
- Never treat whole circumference of extremity to >50 Gy
- Try to spare 1/2 of cross-section of weight-bearing bone, entire or >1/2 of joint cavities, & major tendons (patellar, Achilles)
- Upper inner thigh best treated with frog-leg position
- Buttock/post thigh best treated in prone position
- Nodes: Gross nodes should be resected. No elective nodal radiation
- For distal extremities, pts often have severe reaction with pain, edema, erythema. Usually heals within 1 mo

Pre-op EBRT

- Dose = 2 Gy/fx to 50 Gy
- Field = tumor + 5–7 cm longitudinal margin & 2 cm lateral margin. No cone down
- Surgery 3 wks after RT
- Boost with IORT or brachytherapy: negative margins to 60 Gy, +margins to 65–66 Gy, gross disease to 75 Gy

Post-op brachytherapy

- 45–50 Gy to tumor + 2 cm longitudinal margin + 1–1.5 cm circumferential margin over 4–6 d. Catheters placed in OR 1 cm apart. Load catheters on or after the 6th post-op day to allow time for wound healing
- Do not include scar or drainage site

IORT

- Dose = 12–15 Gy

EBRT alone

- 50 Gy to large field, conedown to 60 Gy, then to 75 Gy
- Consider decreasing RT dose by 10% if doxorubicin given
- Delay RT >3 d from doxorubicin
- Use gonadal shield to preserve fertility
- Physical therapy instituted as early as possible during treatment to improve functional outcome

Dose limitations

- \>20 Gy can prematurely close epiphysis
- ≥40 Gy ablates bone marrow
- ≥50 Gy to bone cortex can cause fracture & healing problems
- Exclude joint space after 40–45 Gy to avoid fibrotic constriction

COMPLICATIONS

- Wound complications 5–15% with post-op RT vs 25–35% with pre-op RT
- Abnormal bone & soft-tissue growth & development
- Limb length discrepancy (2–6 cm managed with shoe lift, otherwise need surgery)
- Permanent weakening of affected bone with highest risk for fracture within 18 mo of RT
- Decreased range of motion secondary to fibrosis
- Lymphedema
- Dermatitis & recall reaction with doxorubicin & dactinomycin
- Skin discoloration, telangiectasia
- 5% pts may develop 2nd malignancy

FOLLOW-UP

- Exam with functional status, MRI of primary, CT chest every 3 mo × 2 yr, every 4 mo in 3rd yr, every 6 mo in 4th & 5th yrs, then annually
- Consider bone scan or PET if clinically indicated

REFERENCES

Alektiar KM, Hu K, Anderson L, et al. High-dose-rate intraoperative radiation therapy (HDR-IORT) for retroperitoneal sarcomas. Int J Radiat Oncol Biol Phys 2000;47:157–163.

Alektiar KM, Leung D, Zelefsky MJ, et al. Adjuvant radiation for stage II-B soft tissue sarcoma of the extremity. J Clin Oncol 2002;20:1643–1650.

Ballo MT ZG. The soft tissue. In: Cox JD, Ang KK, editors. Radiation Oncology: Rationale, Technique, Results. 8th ed. St. Louis: Mosby; 2003. pp. 884–911. 2003.

Davis AM, O'Sullivan B, et al. Late radiation morbidity following randomization to preoperative versus postoperative radiotherapy in extremity soft tissue sarcoma. Radiother Oncol 2005; 75:48–53.

Le Q PT, Leibel SA. Sarcomas of soft tissue. In Leibel SA, Phillips TL, editors. Textbook of Radiation Oncology. 2nd ed. Philadelphia: Saunders; 2004. pp. 1335–1362. 2004.

McGinn C. Soft tissue sarcomas (excluding retroperitoneum). In: Perez CA, Brady LW, Halperin ED, Schmidt-Ullrich RK, editors. Principles and Practice of Radiation Oncology. 4th ed. Philadelphia: Lippincott Williams & Wilkins; 2004. pp. 2185–2205.

O'Sullivan B, Davis AM, Turcotte R, et al. Preoperative versus postoperative radiotherapy in soft-tissue sarcoma of the limbs: a randomised trial. Lancet 2002;359:2235–2241.

Pisters PW, Harrison LB, Leung DH, et al. Long-term results of a prospective randomized trial of adjuvant brachytherapy in soft tissue sarcoma. J Clin Oncol 1996;14:859–868.

Pollack A, Zagars GK, Goswitz MS, et al. Preoperative vs. postoperative radiotherapy in the treatment of soft tissue sarcomas: a matter of presentation. Int J Radiat Oncol Biol Phys 1998;42:563–572.

Rosenberg SA, Tepper J, Glatstein E, et al. The treatment of soft-tissue sarcomas of the extremities: prospective randomized evaluations of (1) limb-sparing surgery plus radiation therapy compared with amputation and (2) the role of adjuvant chemotherapy. Ann Surg 1982;196:305–315.

Sindelar WF, Kinsella TJ, Chen PW, et al. Intraoperative radiotherapy in retroperitoneal sarcomas. Final results of a prospective, randomized, clinical trial. Arch Surg 1993;128:402–410.

Tierney JF, Mosseri V, Stewart LA, et al. Adjuvant chemotherapy for soft-tissue sarcoma: review and meta-analysis of the published results of randomised clinical trials. Br J Cancer 1995;72:469–475.

Yang JC, Chang AE, Baker AR, et al. Randomized prospective study of the benefit of adjuvant radiation therapy in the treatment of soft tissue sarcomas of the extremity. J Clin Oncol 1998;16:197–203.

Chapter 39
Pediatric (Non-CNS) Tumors

Eric K. Hansen and Daphne A. Haas-Kogan

GENERAL PEARLS

- This chapter will discuss **Wilms' tumor, neuroblastoma, rhabdomyosarcoma, Ewing's sarcoma, pediatric Hodgkin's disease, & retinoblastoma**
- The #1 cause of death in children is accidents (44%), followed by cancer (10%), congenital abnormalities (8%), homicide (5%), & heart disease (4%)
- Of childhood cancers, leukemias are the most common (~25–30%, the majority of which are ALL) followed by CNS neoplasms (~17%), lymphomas (~15%, Hodgkin's > NHL > Burkitt's lymphoma), neuroblastoma (~5%), Wilms' tumor (~4%), osteosarcoma (~3%), rhabdomyosarcoma (~3%), non-rhabdomyosarcoma soft-tissue sarcomas (~3%), Ewing's sarcoma (~2%), retinoblastoma (~2%) & others
- Of pediatric CNS neoplasms, gliomas are most common (low-grade astrocytomas ~35–50%, brainstem gliomas ~10–15%, malignant astrocytomas ~10%, optic pathway gliomas ~5%) followed by medulloblastoma (~20%), ependymomas (~5–10%), craniopharyngioma (~5%), & germ cell tumors (<5%). These are discussed in the CNS chapter
- Whenever possible, we recommend that children be enrolled in cooperative group protocols

WILMS' TUMOR

PEARLS

- ~450 cases per year in U.S. 75% of cases present before age 5. Median age at diagnosis is 3–4 yrs, or 2.5 yrs for bilateral tumors (only 4–8% of cases)
- Presents with abdominal mass, pain, hematuria, HTN, fever, &/or malaise

- 90% of cases are favorable histology (FH) = no anaplastic or sarcomatous components, while 10% are unfavorable histology [anaplastic (focal vs diffuse), clear cell sarcoma, or rhabdoid tumor]
- Clear cell sarcoma & rhabdoid tumors may not be true subtypes of Wilms' tumor, but they are included in NWTS trials
- Calcifications are uncommon (~5–15%) in contrast to neuroblastoma (~50–55%)
- Congenital anomalies associated with Wilms' tumor include WAGR syndrome (Wilms', aniridia, genitourinary malformations, retardation due to del 11p13 & WT1 gene), Denys-Drash syndrome (pseudohermaphroditism, renal mesangial sclerosis, renal failure due to WT1 gene mutation), & Beckwith-Wiedemann syndrome (hemihypertrophy, macroglossia, GU abnormalities, gigantism due 11p15 abnormality near WT2 gene)

WORKUP

- H&P, abdominal US, CT or MRI of primary, CXR &/or CT chest, CBC, UA, BUN/Cr, LFTs
- For clear cell variant, add bone scan, MRI brain, & bone marrow biopsy (because propensity for bone & brain mets)
- For rhabdoid variant, add MRI of brain (because 10–15% of pts have PNET of cerebellum or pineal regions).
- Do not biopsy unless unresectable or bilateral

STAGING

NWTS-5 staging system	NWTS 3&4
I: Tumor limited to kidney, completely resected. Renal capsule intact. Tumor not ruptured or biopsied prior to resection. Vessels of renal sinus not involved or <2 mm. Margins negative	10yr OS I FH 97% II FH 93% III FH 90% IV FH 80% V FH 78%
II: Tumor extends beyond kidney but is completely excised. Regional extension (e.g., penetration of renal capsule, or blood vessels involved ≥2 mm); blood vessels outside of renal parenchyma contain tumor. Tumor was biopsied	Anaplastic I–III 49% IV 18%

or tumor spillage confined to the flank. Negative margins	
III: Residual non-hematogenous tumor confined to abdomen: (A) +abdominal nodes; (B) penetration of peritoneal surface or tumor spillage not confined to flank; (C) peritoneal implants; (D) +margins (gross or microscopic); (E) not completely resectable due to extension to other organs	Clear cell sarcoma 77% Rhabdoid tumor I–II 45% III–IV 18%
IV: Hematogenous mets or lymph node mets outside of abdomen or pelvis	
V: Bilateral renal tumors at diagnosis	

TREATMENT RECOMMENDATIONS

Stage	NWTS-5 Treatment
In the U.S., the standard is surgery for all cases (when possible). 90–95% are resectable at diagnosis. Nodes must be sampled, liver & contralateral kidney should be evaluated. If unresectable, biopsy, & give neoadjuvant therapy → resection if possible. Record if tumor spillage is focal in operative cavity or diffuse in peritoneal cavity.	
I & II FH; I anaplasia	Nephrectomy → VCR/AMD pulse intensive (18 wk). No RT
III–IV FH & II–IV focal anaplasia	Nephrectomy → RT by day 9 post-op → VCR/AMD/ADR (24 wk)
II–IV diffuse anaplasia & I–IV clear cell sarcoma	Nephrectomy → RT by day 9 post-op → VCR/ADR/VP-16/CY (24 wk)
I–IV Rhabdoid tumor	Nephrectomy → RT by day 9 post-op → Carboplatin/VP-16/CY (24 wk)

Stage	NWTS-5 Treatment
Bilateral Wilms'	Biopsy & stage each kidney. Give chemo for highest stage. Evaluate response at 5 wks. If possible to resect & leave >2/3 of each kidney, then surgery → re-evaluate at 12 wks. If unresectable after chemo, residual disease, or +margins, give flank RT for stage I/II FH or stage I anaplasia. Also give RT for stage III/IV FH, III/IV anaplasia, & clear cell sarcoma or rhabdoid tumor
Relapsed Wilms'	Chemo + RT to sites of relapse. See RT dose guidelines below

TRIALS

- NWTS 1 (*Cancer* 1976) demonstrated that RT is not needed for group 1 patients <2 yrs if chemo given; there was no radiation dose response seen for 10–40 Gy; RT should be started within 9 days of surgery; VCR/AMD is better than either alone for groups 2 & 3; pre-op chemo was not helpful in group 4

- NWTS 2 (*Cancer* 1981) demonstrated that RT is unnecessary for all group I pts; only 6 months of VCR/AMD are necessary for group 1; adding ADR for groups 2 & 3 improved OS

- NWTS 3 (*Cancer* 1989, 1991) demonstrated that RT was not necessary for stage II when chemo was given; 10 Gy (instead of 20 Gy) was adequate for stage III if ADR used; only 11 wks of chemo were necessary for stage I; ADR is unnecessary for stage II but is necessary for stage III; CY did not benefit stage IV

- NWTS 4 (*JCO* 1998) demonstrated that pulse intensive chemo has less hematologic toxicity & is less expensive that standard chemo and that it should be used in stage I–IV pts with favorable histology

- NWTS 5 (*JCO* 2001; *JCO* 2005) initially randomized stage I FH pts <2 yrs old with tumor <550 g to nephrectomy alone vs nephrectomy → chemo. 69 pts entered, 9 patients relapsed (3 tumor bed, 1 pleural, 4 bilateral lungs, 1 contralateral kidney). Thus, the nephrectomy alone arm closed early. Also found that loss of heterozygosity (LOH) for chromosomes 1p and 16q is associated with increased risk of relapse and death for FH Wilms tumor. Pts with LOH 16q and/or 1p need treatment intensification

RADIATION TECHNIQUES

- Start RT by day 9 post-op (day of surgery = day 0)
- CT plan to contour normal structures
- Fraction size is 1.8 Gy (except for whole abdomen & whole lung = 1.5 Gy)
- Total dose is 10.8 Gy unless gross residual disease. Boost residual disease >3 cm additional 10.8 Gy (to 21.6 Gy)
- The treatment volume is determined by the pre-op CT/MRI and includes the kidney & the tumor + 1 cm margin.
- Pts with stage IV receive flank RT per guidelines for the intra-abdominal tumor stage. For example, flank RT if abdominal tumor is local stage III (but not if stage I–II FH)
- When crossing midline, treat all of the vertebral body to avoid scoliosis
- For para-aortic nodes, treat bilateral paraaortic chains to 10.8 Gy
- For peritoneal seeding, rupture, or diffuse spillage, give whole abdomen RT 1.5/10.5 Gy. Whole abdomen RT borders are the dome of the diaphragm superiorly, the bottom of the obturator foramen inferiorly, & flash laterally. The femoral heads are blocked out
- For lung mets, give whole lung RT 1.5/12 Gy if age >1.5 yrs, or 1.5/9 Gy if age <1.5 yrs. Boost residual disease 1.5/7.5 Gy. If lung mets are only seen on CT, but not on CXR, RT is optional. Whole lung RT borders: flash the supra-clavicular fossa bilaterally, extend 1–4 cm beyond the ribs laterally, and extend below the posterior aspect of the diaphragm inferiorly (usually ~L1). Pts treated with whole lung RT should receive TMP/SMX for PCP prophylaxis
- For liver mets, dose is limited to 19.8 Gy. For focal involvement, may treat involved area + 2 cm. For diffuse involvement, treat whole liver. Lesser volumes may be boosted with an additional 5.4–10.8 Gy
- For brain mets, treat 1.8/30.6 Gy to the whole brain
- For bone mets, treat 1.8/30.6 Gy to lesion + 3 cm margin
- For nodes outside the abdomen or pelvis, treat to 1.8/19.8 Gy with optional 5.4–10.8 Gy boost

- For relapsed disease, dose is 12.6–18 Gy for <1 yr or 21.6 Gy if >1 yr. The cumulative total dose including prior RT should not exceed 30.6 Gy (<3 yr) or 39.5 Gy (>3 yr)

NWTS-5 dose limitations
- Opposite kidney: ≤14.4 Gy
- Liver: 1/2 of uninvolved liver ≤19.8 Gy. With liver mets 75% of liver ≤30.6 Gy
- Bilateral whole lungs: 9 Gy (age <1.5 yrs) or 12 Gy (age >1.5 yrs)

COMPLICATIONS
- Scoliosis, kyphosis, soft tissue hypoplasia, small bowel obstruction, iliac wing hypoplasia, liver/kidney hypoplasia, renal failure, pneumonitis, congestive heart failure (related to doxorubicin), 2nd malignancy

NEUROBLASTOMA

PEARLS
- Neuroblastoma is the most common extracranial solid tumor in children & the most common malignancy in infants <1 yo. The median age at diagnosis is 17 mo
- It arises from primitive neural crest cells of the spinal ganglion, dorsal spinal nerve roots, & adrenal medulla
- It is one of the small round blue cell tumors (along with lymphoma, all – "blastomas", small cell carcinoma of the lung, PNETs/Ewing's sarcoma, & rhabdomyosarcoma)
- Homer-Wright pseudorosettes are found in 15–50% of cases
- Shimada classification divides neuroblastoma into favorable (FH) & unfavorable (UH) histology based on age, amount of Schwann cell stroma, nodular vs diffuse pattern, degree of differentiation, and mitotic index
- Cytogenetic abnormalities associated with poorer prognosis include LOH 1p, N-myc proto-oncogene amplification, diploid tumors (DNA index 1), & increased telomerase activity
- Screening does not change the mortality rate of neuroblastoma due to the high frequency of spontaneous regression in infants as confirmed in international trials
- Neuroblastoma most commonly arises in the adrenal gland, followed by the abdomen & thorax

- 60% of pts <1 year present with localized disease, while 70% of pts >1 year present with metastases
- London (*JCO* 2005) retrospectively analyzed 3666 pts on POG & CCG studies from 1986 to 2001 & demonstrated that the prognostic contribution of age to outcome is continuous in nature. A 460 day cutoff was selected to maximize the outcome difference between younger and older pts
- Classic signs include the blueberry muffin sign (non-tender blue skin nodules), raccoon eyes (orbital mets with proptosis & bruising), & opsoclonus-myoclonus-truncal ataxia (a paraneoplastic syndrome of myoclonic jerking & random eye movements that is associated with early stage and may persist after cure)

WORKUP
- H&P
- Labs include urine catecholamines (epinephrine, norepinephrine, vanillylmandelic acid, & homovanilic acid), CBC, BUN/Cr, LFTs
- Imaging includes CT/MRI of primary, MIBG scan, & CXR. If CXR is +, then order CT chest. The primary is often calcified on X-ray (vs Wilms' which is not)
- Biopsy the primary or involved nodes
- All pts should have a bone marrow biopsy

INSS staging

1: Localized tumor with complete gross excision, negative microscopic margins. Adherent nodes may be + but non-adherent ipsilateral nodes are negative

2A: Localized tumor with incomplete gross excision, & ipsilateral non-adherent nodes negative

2B: Localized tumor with ipsilateral non-adherent nodes +, but contralateral nodes negative

3: Unresectable tumor, tumor extends across midline, or + contralateral nodes, or a midline tumor with bilateral extension

4: Metastases to distant lymph nodes, bone, bone marrow, liver, skin, or other organs

4S: Age <1 yr with an otherwise 1–2B primary tumor with metastases limited to skin, liver, and/or <10% of bone marrow

COG risk groups
Low risk (30% of cases, 3 yr OS 95–100%)
- Any stage I
- Stage 2 <1 yr
- Stage 2 >1 yr without N-myc amplification
- Stage 2 >1 yr with N-myc amplification & FH
- Stage 4S <1 yr without N-myc amplification, with FH & hyperdiploid

Intermediate risk (15% of cases, 3 yr OS 75–98%)
- Stage 3/4 <1 yr without N-myc amplification
- Stage 3 >1 yr without N-myc amplification with FH
- Stage 4S <1 yr without N-myc amplification, with UH or diploid

High risk (55% of cases, 3 yr OS <30%)
- Stage 2 >1 yr with N-myc amplification & UH
- Stage 3/4/4S with N-myc amplification
- Stage 3 >1 yr without N-myc amplification, but with UH
- Stage 4 >1 yr

TREATMENT RECOMMENDATIONS

Risk Group	Recommended Treatment
Low risk	Surgery → observation if GTR. If STR, unresectable, or recurrence after GTR → chemo for 6–12 wks. Chemo regimens consist of carboplatin, VP-16, CY, &/or ADR. However, if pt has severe symptoms from spinal cord compression, respiratory compromise, or GI/GU obstruction, give immediate chemo → surgery. RT (1.5/21 Gy) is used for symptoms that do not respond to chemo or for massive hepatomegaly causing respiratory distress (1.5/4.5 Gy). RT also used for rare local recurrences after chemo & surgery. For clinically-stable stage 4S low-risk pts, observe after biopsy unless massive hepatomegaly causes respiratory distress (then treat

Risk Group	Recommended Treatment
	with chemo ± RT). Biopsy only is necessary as resection does not affect outcome
Intermediate risk	Maximal safe resection with lymphadenectomy → chemo for 12–24 wks depending on biology. Chemo regimens consist of carboplatin, VP-16, CY, &/or ADR. Unresectable tumors may require pre-op chemo to convert them to resectable status If PR to chemo → second look surgery. If viable residual disease present → RT to primary + 2 cm margin (1.5/24 Gy). If stage 4S with respiratory distress → RT to liver (1.5/4.5 Gy). Radiation controversial in intermediate-risk disease.
High risk	High dose chemo (same drugs often with ifosfamide & cisplatin) → attempt maximal safe resection. After surgery → high dose chemo & ABMT (± TBI). All pts then get RT (1.8/21.6 Gy) to the post-chemo pre-surgical extent of tumor +2 cm margin → cis-retinoic acid for 6 mo. If available, IORT may be used at the time of operation, although this is not standard-of-care

STUDIES

Low risk

- <u>POG 8104</u> (Nitschke, *JCO* 1988). Treated 101 pts with POG A (INSS 1) disease with gross total resection → observation, and 2 yr DFS was 89%
- <u>CCG 3881</u> (Perez, *JCO* 2000). Treated 374 pts with Evans I–II (INSS 1-2B) with surgery alone (unless spinal cord compression when RT allowed). For stage I, 4 yr EFS & OS were 93% & 99%, & for stage II, they were 81% & 98%,

respectively. Recurrences were managed successfully with surgery or multimodality therapy. Identified stage 2 pts with N-myc amplification or ≥2 yrs of age with either UH or + lymph nodes as pts at higher risk of death with surgery alone

Intermediate risk

- Castleberry, POG (*JCO* 1991). Randomized 62 pts >1 yr with POG C (INSS 2B-3) to post-op chemo ± concurrent RT → 2nd look surgery → chemo. RT was to the primary & regional nodes (1.5/24 Gy for <2 yrs or 1.5/30 Gy for >2 yrs). Chemo-RT improved DFS (31 → 58%) & CR rate (45 → 67%)
- POG 8742 & 9244 (*Eur J Cancer* 1997). Treated 49 pts >1 yr with INSS 2B–3 with surgery → chemo ×5c → 2nd look surgery → RT for viable residual tumor → chemo. RT was 1.5/24 Gy for age 1–2 yr, 1.5/30 Gy for age >2 yr. 2 yr EFS was 85% after GTR vs 70% after STR, & 92% for FH vs 58% for UH

High risk

- CCG 3891 (*NEJM* 1999, *IJROBP* 2003). Treated 539 high-risk pts with chemo ×5 mo → surgery (+10 Gy RT for gross residual disease), & then randomized them to myeloablative chemo, 10 Gy TBI, & ABMT vs intensive chemo without TBI. If pts were disease-free, they were randomized to observation vs 6 mo of *cis*-retinoic acid. ABMT + TBI improved 3 yr EFS (22 → 34%) & LRC (49 → 67%), & *cis*-retinoic acid improved 3 yr EFS (29 → 46%). For pts with gross residual disease, TBI improved LC (48 → 78%)
- Haas-Kogan (*IJROBP* 2000). Treated 21 high-risk pts with electron beam IORT (mean 10 Gy). If surgery was a GTR, LRC was 89% with IORT, but if surgery was a STR, all pts recurred locally despite IORT

RADIATION TECHNIQUES
Simulation and field design

- CT &/or MRI used for planning 3DCRT or IMRT plans
- Treat the post-chemo pre-surgical tumor extent with a 2 cm margin. If lymph node involvement suspected or proven, cover primary + immediately adjacent nodal drainage areas. Do not give elective nodal RT because of morbidity

- Always cover the full width of vertebrae to avoid scoliosis
- After induction chemo, give RT to metastases if persistent active disease

Dose prescriptions
- Intermediate risk = 1.5/24 Gy (controversial)
- High risk = 1.8/21.6 Gy
- 4S liver involvement = 1.5/4.5 Gy

Dose limitations
- Contralateral kidney: ≥80% of volume <12 Gy
- Liver: ≥50% of volume <9 Gy, ≥2/3 of volume <15 Gy, or ≥75% of volume <18 Gy
- Lung: >2/3 of volume <15 Gy

COMPLICATIONS
- Disturbances of growth, infertility, neuropsychological sequelae, endocrinopathies, cardiac effects, pulmonary effects, bladder dysfunction, 2nd malignancy

---

RHABDOMYOSARCOMA

PEARLS
- Rhabdomyosarcoma accounts for ~3% of childhood cancers
- The most common primary sites are the head & neck [40% = parameningeal (25%), orbit (9%), non-parameningeal sites (6%)], genitourinary tract (30%), extremity (15%), & trunk (15%)
- Primary sites are categorized as favorable or unfavorable (see table below)
- Most cases are sporadic, but predisposing conditions include Li-Fraumeni syndrome (germline p53 mutation), neurofibromatosis type 1, & Beckwith-Wiedemann syndrome (more commonly associated with Wilms' tumor)
- The classic histologic subtypes include embryonal, botyroid & spindle cell subtypes of embryonal, alveolar, & pleomorphic (rare in children)
- The most frequent subtype in children is embryonal (60–70%), & it typically arises in the orbit, head & neck or the genitourinary tract
- Botyroid tumors (10%) arise in the vagina, bladder, nasopharynx, & biliary tract

- Spindle cell tumors are most frequently observed in the paratesticular site
- Alveolar constitutes 20% of cases & is most common in adolescents in the extremity, trunk, or retroperitoneum
- Positive prognostic histologic subtypes include botyroid & spindle cell. Embryonal is an intermediate prognostic subtype. Poor prognostic subtypes include alveolar & undifferentiated
- Embryonal is associated with loss of heterozygosity on 11p15.5
- 70% of alveolar cases are associated with t(2;13) & 20% with t(1;13). The involved genes include FKHR (on chromosome 13), PAX3 (on chromosome 2), & PAX7 (on chromosome 1)

WORKUP

- H&P. EUA may be needed. Cystoscopy should be performed for GU sites
- Labs include CBC, LFTs, BUN/Cr, LDH
- Imaging includes CT/MRI of primary, CT of chest & abdomen, bone scan
- If parameningeal site → lumbar puncture with cytology → if + → neuraxis MRI
- Bone marrow biopsy

STAGING

IRS Pre-operative Staging System (dictates chemo)
Stage 1: Favorable site, any T, N0-1M0
Stage 2: Unfavorable site, T1a/T2a, N0M0
Stage 3: Unfavorable site, T1b/T2b, N0M0, or any T, N1M0
Stage 4: Any M1
<u>Favorable sites</u>: Orbit, non-parameningeal H&N (scalp, parotid, OPX, oral cavity, larynx), GU non-bladder-prostate (paratestes, vagina, vulva, uterus), biliary tract
<u>Unfavorable sites</u>: Parameningeal (NPX, nasal cavity, paranasal sinuses, middle ear, mastoid, pterygopalatine fossa, infratemporal fossa), bladder, prostate, extremity, other (trunk, retroperitoneum)
T1: Tumor is confined to site/organ of origin (a ≤5 cm, b >5 cm)
T2: Tumor extends beyond site/organ of origin (a ≤5 cm, b >5 cm)
N1: Regional lymph node involvement
M1: Distant metastases at diagnosis

IRS Surgical-Pathologic Grouping System (dictates RT)

I: Localized disease, completely resected (~13% of all pts)
  A: Confined to organ or muscle of origin
  B: Infiltration outside organ or muscle of origin

II: Gross total resection (~20% of all pts)
  A: Microscopic residual disease but no regional LN involvement
  B: Resected regional LN
  C: Both microscopic residual disease & resected regional LN

III: Incomplete resection with gross residual disease (~48% of all pts)
  A: Due to biopsy
  B: After major resection (>50%)

IV: Distant metastases at diagnosis (~18% of all pts)

IRS-V Risk Groups

Low risk: Localized embryonal or botyroid histology at favorable sites (Stage 1, Groups I–III) or at unfavorable sites with completely resected or microscopic residual disease (Stages 2–3, Groups I–II)

Intermediate Risk: Embryonal or botyroid histology at unfavorable sites with gross residual disease (Stages 2–3, Group III); pts 2–10 yrs with metastatic embryonal histology (Stage 4); non-metastatic alveolar or undifferentiated histology (Stages 1–3)

High risk: Any Stage 4/Group IV (except for pts 2–10 yrs with embryonal histology)

~3 yr OS by risk group	~5 yr OS by histology	~5 yr OS by site
Low >90–95%	Botyroid 95%	Orbit >90%
Intermed. 55–70%	Spindle cell 88%	Parameningeal 75%
High 30–50%	Embryonal 66–87%	H&N Non-paramen. 80%
	Alveolar 54–71%	Bladder/ prostate 82%
	Undiff. 40–55%	Paratesticular 69–96%
		Gynecologic sites 90–98%
		Extremity 70%

IRS-V TREATMENT

Stage/Group	IRS-V Treatment
All pts require multimodality therapy consisting of surgery (if possible) followed by chemo ± RT. Treatment is based on stage, group, & primary site. Chemotherapy agents include VCR, AMD, CY, topotecan, & irinotecan. VA = VCR/AMD. VAC = VCR/AMD/CY. VTC = VCR/topotecan/CY. VCPT = VCR/irinotecan	
Low risk	
Stage 1–3 group I	Surgery → chemo (VA or VAC). No RT
Stage 1 group II	Surgery → chemo (VA) + RT at wk 3 (36 Gy for N0 or 41.4 Gy for N1)
Stage 1 group III	Surgery (biopsy only for orbit) → chemo (VA) + RT (50.4 Gy except for orbit which is 45 Gy).Most get RT at wk 3, but primary sites at vulva, uterus, biliary tract, & certain non-parameningeal H&N get RT at wk 12 to allow for possible 2nd look surgery. Vaginal primaries get RT at wk 12 (N1) or 28 (N0)
Stage 2 group II	Surgery → chemo (VAC) + RT at wk 3 (36 Gy)
Stage 3 group II	Surgery → chemo (VAC) + RT at wk 3 (36 Gy for N0 or 41.4 Gy for N1)
Intermediate risk Embryonal stages 2–3, group III; embryonal stage 4, age 2–10 yrs; alveolar/undiff stages 1–3	Surgery → chemo (VAC or VAC alternating with VTC). At wk 12, perform 2nd look surgery or definitive RT if unresectable. Definitive RT dose at wk 12 is 50.4 Gy. If 2nd look surgery performed, post-op RT is given at wk 15. Post-op RT doses depend on site, and are 0–36 Gy for complete resection, 36 Gy for microscopic residual & N0, 41.4 Gy for microscopic residual & N1, & 50.4 Gy for gross residual
High risk	Chemo (VCPT → VAC or VAC alternating with VCPT depending on response). RT is

Stage/Group	IRS-V Treatment
	given at wk 15 to primary & metastatic sites, except for pts with intracranial extension, spinal cord compression, or pts requiring emergency RT (day 0). Definitive RT dose is 50.4 Gy except for the orbit which is 45 Gy. If 2nd look surgery is performed, post-op RT doses are 36 Gy for complete resection, 36 Gy for microscopic residual & N0, 41.4 Gy for microscopic residual & N1, & 50.4 Gy for gross residual
Site-specific recommendations	
Orbit	Only a biopsy is required to establish diagnosis → chemo → RT. RT is to the tumor + 2 cm margin. Dose depends on stage & group as above (45 Gy for stage 1 group III). Orbital exenteration is reserved for salvage
Head & neck (non-parameningeal sites)	Follow stage/group guidelines above. For group III, perform 2nd look surgery or definitive RT if unresectable at wk 12. Post-op dose is 36 Gy for complete resection & microscopic residual N0, 41.4 Gy for microscopic residual & N1, & 50.4 Gy for gross residual
Parameningeal sites	If intracranial extension or cranial neuropathy present, RT is given first. Otherwise, RT is given at wk 12 or wk 15 if 2nd look surgery. For focal intracranial extension include a 2 cm margin. If extensive intracranial involvement, treat with whole cranial RT
Biliary tract	Follow stage/group guidelines above. For group III, perform 2nd look surgery or definitive RT if unresectable at wk 12.

Stage/Group	IRS-V Treatment
	Post-op dose is 36 Gy for complete resection & microscopic residual, & 50.4 Gy for gross residual
Extremity	Wide local excision with en bloc removal of a cuff of normal tissue with nodal sampling → chemo → local treatment as described in stage/group guidelines above
Trunk, retroperitoneum, perineum, GI	Follow stage/group guidelines above
Bladder/prostate	Follow stage/group guidelines above. Because one goal is bladder preservation, an initial biopsy is often performed rather than surgery → chemo + RT → surgery for residual disease
Paratesticular	Inguinal orchiectomy with resection of entire spermatic cord & ipsilateral lymph node dissection including high & low infrarenal & bilateral iliac nodes (except group I pts). If scrotal violation, give RT to hemiscrotum. Contralateral testicle can be transposed into thigh prior to RT & later reimplanted. RT dose depends on stage & group as above (50.4 Gy for stage 1 group III)
Uterus, cervix	Follow stage/group guidelines above. For group III, perform 2nd look surgery or definitive RT if unresectable at wk 12. Post-op RT doses are 0 for completely resected N0, 41.4 Gy for completely resected N1, 36 Gy for microscopic residual & N0, 41.4 Gy for microscopic residual & N1, & 50.4 Gy for gross residual
Vulva	Follow stage/group guidelines above. For group III, perform 2nd look surgery or definitive

Stage/Group	IRS-V Treatment
	RT if unresectable at wk 12. Post-op RT doses are 36 Gy for complete resection & microscopic residual N0, 41.4 Gy for microscopic residual & N1, & 50.4 Gy for gross residual
Vagina	Follow stage/group guidelines above, but local treatment is at wk 12 (N1) or 28 (N0) → reassess with biopsy. If biopsy negative, no further local treatment. If + biopsy → resect or RT if unresectable. Definitive RT doses are 36 Gy for group II N0, 41.4 Gy for group II N1, & 50.4 Gy for group III. Post-op RT doses are 0 for complete resection, 36 Gy for microscopic residual & N0, 41.4 Gy for microscopic residual & N1, & 50.4 Gy for gross residual

TRIALS

- IRS-I (*Cancer* 1988). 1972–1978, 686 pts. All pts got chemo for 2 yrs. RT was given initially for groups I & II, & at wk 6 for groups III & IV. RT dose was 40–60 Gy (<3 yrs = 40 Gy; <6 yrs & <5 cm = 50 Gy; >6 yrs or >5 cm = 55 Gy; >6 yrs & >5 cm = 60 Gy). Grp I pts randomized to RT vs no RT & no difference in OS/DFS for embryonal/botyroid. However, there was a benefit of post-op RT for grp I alveolar/undiff histologies. Orbit & GU sites had the best prognosis, & retroperitoneal & alveolar histology had the worst prognosis. DM was much more common than LF.

- IRS-II (*Cancer* 1993). 1978–1984, 990 pts. RT was modified from IRS-I as follows: RT given at wk 0 for grp II, & wk 6 for grps III and IV. RT was to the tumor + 5 cm margin. Pts with CN palsies, base of skull (BOS) involvement, or intracranial disease got whole-brain RT ± intrathecal chemo to prevent meningeal relapse (improved from IRS-I). RT doses were: grp I = 0; grp II = 40–45 Gy; grp III = 40–45 Gy if <6 yrs and <5 cm, 45–50 Gy if >6 yrs or >5 cm, or 50–55 Gy if both. LC for all pts receiving >40 Gy was 93%. LC for grps I&II was 90% vs 80% for grp III. Worse LC & OS for pts with unfavorable histology & tumors >5 cm. Local-regional relapse was more common than distant relapse except for stage IV pts

- <u>IRS-III</u> (*JCO* 1995). 1984–1991, 1062 pts. All pts got postop RT except grp I favorable histology & grp III special pelvic sites in CR after chemo. RT was given at day 0 for CN palsy, BOS erosion, intracranial extension; wk 2 for grp II favorable sites & grp III orbit & H&N; otherwise RT at wk 6. RT was to tumor + 2 cm. RT doses were: grp I unfavorable site or grp II = 41.4 Gy. grp III = 41.4 Gy if <6 yrs & <5 cm, 50.4 Gy if ≥6 yrs & ≥5 cm; 45 Gy for older children or large tumors. 5 yr OS was superior in IRS-III (71%) compared to IRS-II (63%) & IRS-I (55%). LC was 90% for grp I & II pts, but only ~80% for grp III

- <u>IRS-IV</u> (*JCO* 2001, *J Pediatr Hematol Oncol* 2001). 1991–1997, 1000 pts. Pre-treatment staging assigned chemo, & clinical grouping assigned RT. Most pts got surgery → chemo day 0 → RT at wk 9. RT was given at day 0 for CN palsy, BOS erosion, or intracranial extension; at wk 3 for orbit & paratesticular; at wk 18.5 for stage 4. RT was to the pre-surgery, pre-chemo tumor + 2 cm. Whole brain RT omitted for pts with parameningeal primaries except when CSF+. Grp I stages I–II did not get RT. Grp I stage III & all grp II got 41.4 Gy. All grp III got 50.4 Gy in qd fractions vs 1.1 Gy bid to 59.4 Gy. Orbital tumors were usually group III due to biopsy only, so got 50.4 Gy. Prognostic subsets identified (for IRS-V) based on histology, stage, & group

Group/Stage	Treatment	3 yr OS	Findings
I paratesticular	VA	90%	No diff from IRS III
I orbit	VA	100%	No diff from IRS III
II orbit	VA + RT	100%	No diff from IRS III
I, stage 1–2	VAC vs VAI vs VIE; no RT	84–88%	No diff between chemo regimens

Group/Stage	Treatment	3 yr OS	Findings
I stage 3; all II	VAC vs VAI vs VIE + RT	84–88%	No diff between chemo regimens
III	VAC vs VAI vs VIE, + RT(QD vs BID)	72–83% (3 yr FFS)	No diff between chemo regimens. Bid RT did not improve LC (~87%) or OS vs QD RT
IV	VM vs IE → VAC, + RT	27% vs 55%	IE improved FFS, OS vs VM chemo

RADIATION TECHNIQUES
Simulation and field design
- Many pts may require pediatric anesthesia
- Excellent immobilization is required & 3D-CRT &/or IMRT is encouraged to limit doses to normal structures
- In IRS-V RT volumes are to the initial pre-chemo, pre-surgical tumor + 2 cm margin. Involved lymph nodes are included in the RT field, but prophylactic RT is not used. For group III pts requiring 50.4 Gy, the volume is reduced to the pre-chemo, pre-surgical tumor + 0.5 cm margin at 36 Gy for N0 pts or at 41.4 Gy for N1 pts
- The timing of RT is described in the IRS-V treatment summary table above
- Doses are 1.8 Gy/fraction to 36 Gy, 41.4 Gy, or 50.4 Gy
- Dose limitations are as follows: bilateral kidneys <14.4 Gy, whole liver <23.4 Gy, bilateral lungs <15 Gy, optic nerve & chiasm <46.8 Gy, spinal cord <45 Gy, GI tract <45 Gy, whole abdomen 24 Gy in 1.5 Gy fractions, heart <30.6 Gy, lens <14.4 Gy, lacrimal gland & cornea <41.4 Gy
- The ovaries should be shielded, or moved in girls with pelvic primaries
- The normal testicle can be also be transposed prior to RT & later reimplanted

COMPLICATIONS
- Complications are site dependent. Please refer to the chapters on specific anatomic sites

- Chemo complications include nausea, vomiting, mucositis, alopecia, & hematopoietic suppression. Ifosfamide & etoposide can cause renal & electrolyte imbalance. CY can cause hemorrhagic cystitis. ADR can cause cardiomyopathy. Cisplatin can cause hearing impairment. Topoisomerase inhibitors can cause 2nd malignancies, particularly AML
- AMD & ADR can accentuate radiation "recall" reaction if given during or immediately after RT

FOLLOW-UP

- H&P & CXR every 2 mo for 1st yr with repeat imaging studies that were + at diagnosis every 3 mo, then H&P & CXR every 4 mo for 2nd & 3rd yrs, H&P annually for 5–10 yrs, & annual visit or phone contact after 10 yrs

---

EWING'S SARCOMA

PEARLS

- ~200 cases per yr in U.S. Ewing's sarcoma is the 2nd most common bone cancer of children (osteosarcoma is #1). Boys are affected more than girls (1.5–2 : 1). The median age at presentation is 14 yrs (usually 8–25 yrs). Ewing's sarcoma is rare in African Americans & Asians
- Ewing's family of tumors includes Ewing's sarcoma (bone – 87%), extraosseous Ewing's sarcoma (8%), peripheral PNET (5%), & Askin's tumor (PNET of chest wall)
- >90% of pts have t(11;22) [or t(21;22)] involving the EWS gene on chromosome 22. The c-myc protooncogene is frequently expressed in Ewing's (whereas n-myc is often amplified in neuroblastoma)
- Ewing's sarcoma commonly presents in the lower extremity (femur 15–20%, more common than tibia or fibula 5–10%), pelvis (20–30%), upper extremity (humerus 5–10%), ribs (9–13%), & spine (6–8%)
- 75–80% of pts present with localized disease; 20–25% have metastases to lung, bone, or bone marrow. Nearly all pts have micromets at diagnosis, so all need chemo

WORKUP

- H&P. Labs include CBC, LFTs, LDH, & ESR
- X-rays of the primary frequently show a moth-eaten lesion. Lytic lesions are more common than blastic, & "onion-skinning" may be present for subperiosteal lesions

- CT &/or MRI of primary, bone scan, CT chest, ± PET scan
- Biopsy the lesion & obtain a bone marrow biopsy
- Negative prognostic factors include metastases, pelvic or truncal primaries, proximal (vs distal) extremity primaries, large tumors (>8 cm or >100–200 cc), age >17 yrs, high LDH or ESR, poor response to induction chemo, & no surgery

STAGING

- There is no uniform staging system for Ewing's sarcomas. The AJCC staging systems for bone or soft tissue sarcomas may be used. Please refer to the chapters on bone tumors & soft tissue sarcomas for more details on staging
- For localized disease, 5 yr OS is ~60–70%
- For pts with lung/pleural mets only, cure rates are ~30%
- For pts with bone/bone marrow mets, cure rates are ~20–25%
- For pts with both lung & bone/bone marrow mets, cure rates are <15%
- Local treatment alone without chemo cures only ~10%
- Local failure rates after definitive RT for Ewing's sarcoma generally range from ~10–25%, and are correlated with prognostic factors (above) such as site (extremity lesions LF 5–10% vs pelvic lesions LF 15–70%) and size (<8 cm LF 10% vs >8 cm LF 20%)

TREATMENT RECOMMENDATIONS

- Induction chemo (VDC alternating with IE) → local treatment (surgery or RT) at wk 12 → adjuvant chemo
- Chemo agents include vincristine (V), actinomycin-D (A), cyclophosphamide (C), doxorubicin (D), ifosfamide (I), & etoposide (E)
- Limb-salvage surgery is preferred over amputation. Adequate margins for surgery are: >1 cm for bone, >0.5 cm for soft tissue, & >0.2 cm for fascia
- Post-op RT is given for gross residual disease (55.8 Gy) or + microscopic margins (50.4 Gy)
- Consider post-op RT if poor histologic response to induction chemo in resected specimen
- Definitive RT is used for skull, face, vertebra, or pelvic primaries & for unresectable disease. The RT dose is 45 Gy to the pre-chemo GTV + 2 cm margin → boost to

55.8 Gy to the initial bony GTV + the post-chemo soft-tissue extent

- For a rib primary with a +pleural effusion, RT is given to the hemithorax (1.5/15 Gy) → RT to primary to 55.8 Gy as described above
- For lung mets, give whole lung RT (1.5/15 Gy), or consider resection if ≤4 mets
- Adding IE to VDCA does not improve survival for pts with metastatic disease at diagnosis

TRIALS

- IESS-1 (*JCO* 1990). Non-randomized comparison of 342 pts with localized disease treated with VAC+D vs VAC vs VAC + prophylactic bilateral whole lung RT. The 5 yr RFS was best with VAC+D (60%) vs VAC (24%) vs VAC + RT (44%)
- IESS-2 (*JCO* 1991). Randomized 214 pts with localized non-pelvic primaries to high-dose, intermittent VAC+D vs moderate dose continuous VAC+D. Local treatment was surgery ± post-op RT, or RT alone to the whole bone 45 Gy → boost to 55 Gy. High-dose VAC+D improved OS (63 → 77%) & RFS, & there was no difference in OS for local control modalities
- IESS-3 (Grier, *NEJM* 2003). Randomized pts with localized or metastatic disease to VDC vs VDCA alternating with VP-16/ifosfamide. Local treatment was given at wk 9–15 with RT, surgery, or both. Adding VP-16/ifosfamide improved 5 yr OS (61 → 72%) for localized disease, but not for metastatic disease (25%)
- CESS 86 (*JCO* 2001). 177 pts with localized Ewing's treated with chemo → non-randomized local control arms of surgery alone, surgery + 45 Gy, or 60 Gy RT alone (randomized qd vs bid). RT used 5 cm proximal/distal margins & 2 cm lateral & deep margins. The 5 yr OS was 69%. There were no differences in OS or RFS according to local therapy. Local control was 100% for surgery, 95% for surgery + RT, & 86% for RT alone, and there was no difference for qd vs bid RT. 16–26% of pts developed mets
- POG 8346 (*IJROBP* 1998). 178 pts treated with chemo → surgery or RT. For 44 pts, RT volume was randomized to whole bone (39.6 Gy) → boost to initial tumor + 4 cm margin to 55.8 Gy vs involved-field to boost volume alone to 55.8 Gy. The rest were treated with involved-field RT. There was no difference in LC or EFS when RT done

properly. 5 yr EFS was highest for distal extremity & central site (63–65%) vs proximal extremity (46%) & pelvic/sacral (24%)

- <u>CESS 81, CESS 86, EICESS 92</u> (Shuck, *IJROBP* 2003). Reviewed 1058 pts treated on trial for localized disease. After surgery, LF was 7.5% with or without post-op RT, 5.3% after pre-op RT. After definitive RT, LF was 26.3%. RT pts were negatively selected with unfavorable tumor sites. Compared to surgery alone, post-op RT improved LC after intralesional resections and in tumors with wide resection and poor histologic response. After marginal resections, post-op RT had similar LC to surgery alone despite poorer histologic response
- There are no randomized trials that have directly compared RT to surgery for LC of Ewing's

RADIATION TECHNIQUES

- The radiation fields are tailored depending on the primary site
- MRI is recommended for treatment planning in all cases when available
- For definitive RT for bone tumors with no soft-tissue involvement, treat the pre-chemo GTV + 2 cm margin to 55.8 Gy
- For definitive RT for bone tumors with a soft tissue component, treat the pre-chemo GTV + 2 cm margin to 45 Gy → boost to 55.8 Gy to the initial bony GTV + the post-chemo soft-tissue extent
- For post-op RT, treat the pre-op GTV + 2 cm margin to 45 Gy → boost to the post-op residual disease + 2 cm margin (50.4 Gy for microscopic disease, or 55.8 Gy for gross residual disease)
- For N+, resect → 50.4 Gy to nodal bed. If not resected, give 55.8 Gy
- Avoid bladder RT with CY or ifosfamide

Dose limitations

- Depend on primary site
- >20 Gy can prematurely close epiphysis
- For extremity lesions, spare a 1–2 cm strip of skin to prevent lymphedema. 20–30 Gy usually can be given to entire circumference of an extremity, if necessary
- Spinal cord <45 Gy

COMPLICATIONS

■ Dermatitis; recall-reaction may occur with ADR & dactinomycin

■ Abnormal bone & soft-tissue growth & development. Most of leg growth occurs at the distal femur & proximal tibia. Limb length discrepancy of 2–6 cm can be managed with a shoe lift, otherwise surgery is needed

■ Permanent weakening of affected bone. The highest risk for fracture is within 18 mo of RT. Thus, avoid contact & high-impact sports

■ Decreased range of motion secondary to soft-tissue &/or joint fibrosis Spinal cord <45 Gy

■ Skin discoloration

■ Lymphedema

■ Cystitis (especially with CY or ifosfamide)

■ ~5% pts may develop a late 2nd malignancy

FOLLOW-UP

■ H&P + CXR every 3 mo for 2 yrs. X-ray primary every 3 mo (&/or MRI of primary every 6 mo) for 2 yrs. After 2 yrs, may increase follow-up intervals. Obtain CBC annually

PEDIATRIC HODGKIN'S LYMPHOMA

PEARLS

■ Hodgkin's lymphoma constitutes ~6% of childhood cancers. It shares many aspects of biology & natural history with adult Hodgkin's (see the chapter on adult Hodgkin's lymphoma for more details)

■ Due to morbidity from RT, lower-dose RT with chemo is used to treat children

■ Hodgkin's lymphoma is most common among children >10 yrs and rare among children <4 yrs. For children <10 yrs, it is more common among boys than girls (3–4 : 1) but less so for children >10 yrs (1.3 : 1)

■ Nodular sclerosing histology is the most common subtype in all age groups, but is less common among children (44%) than among adolescents & adults (72–77%). Lymphocyte-predominant histology is relatively more common among children <10 yrs (13%) whereas lymphocyte-depleted subtype is rare. Mixed-cellularity histology is more common in children (33%) than in adolescents or adults (11–17%)

- ~80% of children present with cervical lymphadenopathy, ~25–30% have B symptoms, ~20% have bulky mediastinal adenopathy
- ~80–85% of pts present with stage I–III disease, & 15–20% present with stage IV

WORKUP

- History (including B symptoms, pruritis, respiratory symptoms) & physical exam. Labs include CBC, LFTs, BUN/Cr, ESR
- Imaging includes CXR, CT of chest, abdomen, & pelvis, & PET scan. Formerly gallium scan & lymphangiogram (to study nodal architecture) were used. Bone scan is ordered for pts with bone pain or elevated alkaline phosphatase
- Pathologic diagnosis is obtained by excisional biopsy (to study architectural changes). Bone marrow biopsy is obtained for pts with B symptoms or stage III–IV. Histologic assessment is required to diagnose spleen &/or liver involvement
- Adverse prognostic factors include stage IIB, IIIB, IV; bulky disease; B symptoms; male gender; WBC >11,500/mm^3; hemoglobin ≤11 g/dl

STAGING

- **Ann Arbor staging system** used (See Chapter 33: Hodgkin's Lymphoma)
- 10yr OS is ≥90% for stages I–III & 75–80% for stage IV

TREATMENT RECOMMENDATIONS

Stage	Recommended Treatment
Low risk: IA, IIA favorable (no bulky disease, no extranodal disease, ≤3 sites)	Chemo ×2-4c → IFRT 15–25 Gy. Elimination of IFRT for selected low-risk pts controversial
Intermediate risk: stage I or II (not low risk); IIIA	Chemo ×4-6c → IFRT 15–25 Gy
High risk: IIIB, IVA/B, selected IIB with adverse associated features (e.g., bulky disease)	Chemo ×6-8c → IFRT 15–25 Gy
Relapse	For pts with low-risk disease at diagnosis with relapse confined to an area of initial involvement after chemo & no RT, salvage chemo & IFRT is

Stage	Recommended Treatment
	used. For post-pubertal pts, standard dose RT may be used. For all other pts, induction chemo & high-dose chemo with peripheral blood stem cell rescue is used
Chemotherapy	Hybrid regimens that utilize lower cumulative doses of alkylators, doxorubicin, & bleomycin are used [e.g., COPP/ABV, OEPA (males), OPPA (females)]. Drugs include: cyclophosphamide (C), procarbazine (P), vincristine (O) and/or vinblastine (V), prednisone (P) or dexamethasone, doxorubicin (A) or epirubicin, bleomycin (B), dacarbazine (D), etoposide (E), methotrexate (M), & cytosine arabinoside

TRIALS

- CCG 5942 (*JCO* 2002). 501 pts with a CR to risk-adapted combination chemo randomized to IFRT or observation. In an as-treated analysis, 3 yr EFS was increased with IFRT (85 → 93%), but OS was the same (98–99%)
- GPOH-HD 95 (*IJROBP* 2001, ASTRO 2004). 1018 pts were treated with risk-adapted chemo (2–6 cycles) & RT. No RT was given for a CR, 20 Gy for a PR of >75% tumor regression, 30 Gy for PR <75%, or 35 Gy for residual mass >50 ml. DFS was superior for pts given RT after PR (92%) than for pts not given RT after CR (69–77%), but OS was the same (97%). No advantage for RT in low-risk patients, but this result conflicts with CCG-5942

RADIATION TECHNIQUES
Simulation and field design
- Use immobilization for reproducibility & 6 MV photons for better dose distribution
- Involved fields are protocol specific, but generally include the initially involved lymph node region(s)

- Supradiaphragmatic fields may be simulated with the arms up over the head or akimbo. Arms-up pulls the axillary nodes away from the lungs, allowing greater lung shielding, but the nodes are closer to the humeral heads. Attempts should be made to exclude as much lung, humeral head, & breast tissue as possible
- For children <5 yrs, some consider bilateral RT to avoid growth asymmetry. However, with low doses, unilateral fields are usually appropriate
- Treatment of a bulky mediastinal mass generally involves the initial craniocaudad dimension + 2 cm margin & the post-chemo lateral margin + 1.5 cm. The supraclavicular fossa is generally included, but the axilla is not (unless involved)

Dose prescriptions

- In general, the dose is 15–25 Gy (protocol specific). Occasionally a 5 Gy boost is used. Dose may be determined by response to initial chemo

Dose limitations

- Shield femoral head. Doses >25 Gy increase the risk slipped capital femoral epiphysis, & doses >30–40 Gy increase the risk of avascular necrosis
- Dental abnormalities may occur with doses of 20–40 Gy
- Radiation doses <30 Gy & cardiac shielding limit cardiac sequelae
- Thyroid abnormalities are more common with doses >26 Gy
- Pneumonitis is uncommon with doses <20 Gy except when used in combination with bleomycin
- Shield testes to limit oligospermia or infertility
- Consider oophoropexy for girls to preserve ovarian function

COMPLICATIONS

- Chemo complications include bleomycin (pulmonary fibrosis/pneumonitis); doxorubicin (cardiomyopathy); alkylators & etoposide (AML & myelodysplasia); procarbazine (male infertility); prednisone (avascular necrosis)
- Acute side effects of mantle RT include epilation, dermatitis, dysgeusia, xerostomia, odynophagia, esophagitis. Para-aortic RT may cause acute nausea or vomiting

- Subacute & late effects of RT include musculoskeletal hypoplasia, sterility, hypothyroidism, radiation pneumonitis, increased risk for myocardial atherosclerotic heart disease, & increased risk of 2nd malignancy
- The rate of 2nd malignancies is ~8–15% at 20 yrs. Breast cancer is the most common solid 2nd malignancy following treatment

RETINOBLASTOMA

Eric K. Hansen, Alice Wang-Chesebro, and Daphne A. Haas-Kogan

PEARLS

- Retinoblastoma (RB) is the most common intraocular tumor of childhood. 95% of cases occur in children <5 yrs
- The RB1 tumor suppressor gene on chromosome 13 causes RB only when both alleles are "hit"
- 40% of pts have a germline mutation of RB1; 60% of cases are sporadic
- Up to 25–40% of cases are familial in that the affected gene is inherited, but only 10% have a + family history of RB
- 65–80% of cases are unilateral (mostly sporadic) and 20–35% are bilateral (mostly due to germline mutations)
- In the developing world, pts present with proptosis, orbital mass, or mets. In the U.S., the most common presentation is leukocoria, strabismus, painful glaucoma, irritability, failure to eat, & low grade fever
- The 5 patterns of spread are: contiguous spread thru the choroid/sclera/orbit; extension along the optic nerve into the brain; invasion of subarachnoid space/leptomeninges via CSF; hematogenous spread to bone, liver, & spleen; and lymphatic spread from the conjunctiva
- The risk of metastases increases with tumor thickness and size
- Trilateral RB refers to bilateral RB & midline CNS neuroblastic tumors (frequently of the pineal or suprasellar region)
- With germline RB, 15–35% of non-irradiated pts & 50–70% of irradiated pts develop 2nd tumors by 50 yrs after diagnosis, mainly sarcomas or melanomas

■ Genetic counseling should be given to all patients with RB & siblings should be examined

WORKUP

■ H&P includes external ocular examination, slit lamp bimicroscopy, & biocular indirect ophthalmoscopy (often under anesthesia for mapping)
■ Labs: CBC, chemistries, BUN, Cr, LFTs
■ Imaging: Fluorescein angiography, bilateral US (A&B mode), & MRI
■ Bone scan &/or lumbar puncture for symptoms or suspected metastatic disease
■ Risk factors for metastatic disease include optic nerve invasion, uveal invasion, orbital invasion, & choroidal involvement

STAGING

■ The most commonly used system is the Reese-Ellsworth system, which predicts the chance of visual preservation well, but not survival. The Abramson-Grabowski system addresses both intraocular & extraocular Rb. The International Classification ("ABCDE") system for intraocular Rb is under modification and is used in recent clinical protocols. The AJCC TNM system is new as of 2002 and is used less frequently
■ 5yr DFS is >90% for pts with intraocular disease but <10% for pts with extraocular disease

Reese-Ellsworth (R-E)
Group I: Very favorable (refers to chance of salvaging the affected eye)
A: Solitary tumor, less than 4 disc diameters (DD) in size, at or behind the equator
B: Multiple tumors, none over 4DD in size, all at or behind the equator
Group II: Favorable
A: Solitary tumor, 4 to 10DD in size, at or behind the equator
B: Multiple tumors, 4 to 10DD in size, behind the equator
Group III: Doubtful
A: Any lesion anterior to the equator
B: Solitary tumors larger than 10DD behind the equator
Group IV: Unfavorable
A: Multiple tumors, some larger than 10DD
B: Any lesion extending anteriorly to the ora serrata

Group V: Very unfavorable
           A: Massive tumors involving over half the retina
           B: Vitreous seeding

Adapted from Reese AB, Ellsworth RM. The evaluation and current concept of retinoblastoma therapy. Trans Am Acad Ophthalmol Otolaryngol 1963;67:164.

International Classification System for Intraocular Retinoblastoma

Group A
Small intraretinal tumors away from foveola and disc
- All tumors are 3 mm or smaller in greatest dimension, confined to the retina *and*
- All tumors are located further than 3 mm from the foveola **and** 1.5 mm from the optic disc

Group B
All remaining discrete tumors confined to the retina
- All other tumors confined to the retina not in Group A
- Tumor-associated subretinal fluid less than 3 mm from the tumor with no subretinal seeding

Group C
Discrete Local disease with minimal subretinal or vitreous seeding
- Tumor(s) are discrete
- Subretinal fluid, present or past, without seeding involving up to $1/4$ retina
- Local fine vitreous seeding may be present close to discrete tumor
- Local subretinal seeding less than 3 mm (2 DD) from the tumor

Group D
Diffuse disease with significant vitreous or subretinal seeding
- Tumor(s) may be massive or diffuse
- Subretinal fluid present or past without seeding, involving up to total retinal detachment
- Diffuse or massive vitreous disease may include "greasy" seeds or avascular tumor masses
- Diffuse subretinal seeding may include subretinal plaques or tumor nodules

Group E
Presence of any one or more of these poor prognosis features
- Tumor touching the lens
- Tumor anterior to anterior vitreous face involving ciliary body or anterior segment
- Diffuse infiltrating retinoblastoma

■ Neovascular glaucoma
■ Opaque media from hemorrhage
■ Tumor necrosis with aseptic orbital cellulites
■ Phthisis bulbi

From COG Protocol ARET0331 (with permission): Trial of systemic neoadjuvant chemotherapy for Group B Intraocular Retinoblastoma: A Phase III Limited Institution Study. Available at: https://members.childrensoncologygroup.org/ Prot/ARET0331/ARET0331DOC.pdf.

AJCC Clinical Staging

Primary Tumor

TX: Primary tumor cannot be assessed

T0:   No evidence of primary tumor

T1a: Any eye in which the largest tumor is less than or equal to 3 mm in height and no tumor is located closer than 1 DD (1.5 mm) to the optic nerve or fovea

T1b: All other eyes in which the tumor(s) are confined to the retina regardless of location or size (up to half the volume of the eye). No vitreous seeding. No retinal detachment or subretinal fluid >5 mm from the base of the tumor

T2:   Tumor with contiguous spread to adjacent tissues or spaces (vitreous or subretinal space)

    T2a: Minimal tumor spread to vitreous and/or subretinal space. Fine local or diffuse vitreous seeding and/or serous retinal detachment up to total detachment may be present but no clumps, lumps, snowballs, or avascular masses are allowed in the vitreous or subretinal space. Calcium flecks in the vitreous or subretinal space are allowed. The tumor may fill up to $^2/_3$ of the volume of the eye

    T2b: Massive tumor spread to the vitreous and/or subretinal space. Vitreous seeding and/or subretinal implantation may consist of lumps, clumps, snowballs, or avascular tumor masses. Retinal detachment may be total. Tumor may fill up to $^2/_3$ the volume of the eye

    T2c: Unsalvageable intraocular disease. Tumor fills more than $^2/_3$ the eye or there is no possibility of visual rehabilitation or one or more of the following are present: Tumor associated glaucoma, either neovascular or angle closure; anterior segment extension of tumor; ciliary body extension of tumor; hyphema (significant); massive vitreous hemorrhage; tumor in contact with lens; orbital cellulites-like clinical presentation (massive tumor necrosis)

T3:   Invasion of the optic nerve and/or optic coats

T4:   Extraocular tumor

Regional lymph nodes
NX: No regional lymph node metastasis cannot be assessed
N0: No regional lymph node metastasis
N1: Regional lymph node involvement (preauricular, submandibular, or cervical)
N2: Distant lymph node involvement

Distant metastasis
MX: Distant metastasis cannot be assessed
M0: No distant metastasis
M1: Metastasis to central nervous system and/or bone, bone marrow, or other sites

Used with the permission of the American Joint Committee on Cancer (AJCC), Chicago, Illinois. The original source for this material is the AJCC Cancer Staging Manual, Sixth Edition (2002) published by Springer-Verlag New York, www.springeronline.com.

TREATMENT

Stage	Treatment Recommendation
Unilateral intraocular	Chemoreduction ×6c → focal therapy. Chemo agents include vincristine, carboplatin, & etoposide. Focal therapy options include: ■ Enucleation if the tumor is massive or if the eye is unlikely to have useful vision after treatment ■ EBRT (35–46 Gy) for small tumors located within macula, diffuse vitreous seeding, or multifocal tumors ■ Cryotherapy is used in addition to EBRT or in place of photocoagulation for lesions <4 DD in the anterior retina ■ Photocoagulation is used for posteriorly located tumors <4 DD distinct from the optic nerve head & macula. It is occasionally used alone for small tumors, or in addition to EBRT

Stage	Treatment Recommendation
	■ Episcleral plaque brachytherapy is used for either focal unilateral disease or recurrent disease following prior EBRT
Bilateral	Historically, enucleation has been used for the more advanced eye. If there is potential vision preservation in both eyes, bilateral EBRT &/or chemoreduction with close follow-up for focal treatment may be used
Extraocular	Orbital EBRT + chemo for palliation. High-dose chemo with stem cell rescue may also be attempted in select cases. Intrathecal chemo may be given for pts with CNS or meningeal disease

TRIALS
- Eye preservation rates range among series from ~60 to 90% when using EBRT and depend on extent of disease
- Visual preservation rates range among series from ~65 to 100% for R-E groups I–III but are lower for groups IV–V

RADIATION TECHNIQUES
EBRT
- Pediatric anesthesia may be required
- Simulate pt supine with thermoplastic head mask immobilization
- 3DCRT is recommended (or IMRT if at an experienced center) using CT &/or MRI
- 4–6 MV photons are used
- For unilateral RB, 4 anterior oblique non-coplanar fields may be used (superior, inferior, medial, & lateral)
- For bilateral RB when both eyes require treatment, 3DCRT (or IMRT) is used with opposed lateral fields & anterior oblique fields
- Depending on stage & anatomy, 0.5 cm bolus may be required

- At a minimum, the entire retina is treated including 5–8 mm of the optic nerve
- Dose is 42–45 Gy in 1.8–2 Gy fractions
- Critical structures to limit RT dose to include the opposite globe (including lens & retina), lacrimal glands, optic chiasm, pituitary gland, brainstem, posterior mandibular teeth, & upper C-spine

Episcleral plaque brachytherapy

- Refer to the chapter on orbital tumors for details of brachytherapy for orbital melanoma. Many of the techniques for RB are similar to treatment of melanoma
- The treatment volume covers the tumor + radial (~2 mm) & deep (1–2 mm) margin
- The dose to the tumor apex is 40 Gy (while the base receives 100–200 Gy)
- The dose rate is 0.7–1.0 Gy/hr, and ~2–4 days of treatment are required

COMPLICATIONS

- EBRT complications include dermatitis; depigmentation; telangiectasias; ectropion or entropion of the eyelid; loss of cilia of the scalp, eyebrow, or eyelid; facial/temporal bone hypoplasia; decreased tear production due to radiation damage to the lacrimal gland; direct corneal injury; cataracts; vitreous hemorrhage; retinopathy; hypopituitarism; & 2nd tumors in radiation field
- With plaque brachytherapy, the risk of orbital bone hypoplasia is low but long-term retinopathy, cataract, maculopathy, paillopathy, & glaucoma are possible

FOLLOW-UP

- H&P every 3 mo for 1 yr, every 4 mo for 2nd yr, every 6 mo for 3rd & 4th years, then annually. Patients with bilateral or familial RB advised to have screening for CNS midline neuroblastic tumors with biannual CT or MRI of the brain until age five years

REFERENCES
Wilms' tumor

D'Angio GJ, Breslow N, Beckwith JB, et al. Treatment of Wilms' tumor. Results of the Third National Wilms' Tumor Study. Cancer 1989;64: 349–360.

D'Angio GJ, Evans A, Breslow N, et al. The treatment of Wilms' tumor: results of the Second National Wilms' Tumor Study. Cancer 1981;47:2302–2311.

D'Angio GJ, Evans AE, Breslow N, et al. The treatment of Wilms' tumor: Results of the national Wilms' tumor study. Cancer 1976;38:633–646.

Green DM, Breslow NE, Beckwith JB, et al. Comparison between single-dose and divided-dose administration of dactinomycin and doxorubicin for patients with Wilms' tumor: a report from the National Wilms' Tumor Study Group. J Clin Oncol 1998;16:237–245.

Green DM, Breslow NE, Beckwith JB, et al. Treatment with nephrectomy only for small, stage I/favorable histology Wilms' tumor: a report from the National Wilms' Tumor Study Group. J Clin Oncol 2001;19:3719–3724.

Grundy PE, Breslow NE, Li S, et al. Loss of heterozygosity for chromosomes 1p and 16q is an adverse prognostic factor in favorable histology Wilms tumor: a report from the National Wilms Tumor Study Group. J Clin Oncol 2005;23:7312–7321.

Halperin EC. Wilms' tumor. In: Halperin EC, Constine LS, Tarbell NJ, et al., editors. Pediatric Radiation Oncology. 4th ed. Philadelphia, PA: Lippincott Williams & Wilkins; 2005. pp. 379–422.

Kalapurakal JA, Thomas PRM. Wilms' tumor. In: Perez CA, Brady LW, Halperin EC, et al., editors. Principles and Practice of Radiation Oncology. 4th ed. Philadelphia: Lippincott Williams & Wilkins; 2004. pp. 2238–2246.

Kun LE. Childhood cancer. In: Cox JD, Ang KK, editors. Radiation Oncology: Rationale, Technique, Results. 8th ed. St. Louis: Mosby; 2003. pp. 913–938.

Marcus K. Pediatric Tumors (Non-CNS): Wilms' Tumors, Ewings Sarcoma and Neuroblastoma (#107). Presented at American Society of Therapeutic Radiology and Oncology Annual Meeting, Atlanta, GA, 2004.

National Cancer Institute. Wilms' Tumor and Other Childhood Kidney Tumors (PDQ): Treatment. Available at: http://cancer.gov/cancertopics/pdq/treatment/wilms/healthprofessional/. Accessed on January 19, 2005.

National Wilms Tumor Study – 5: Therapeutic Trial and Biology Study. Available at: https://members.childrensoncologygroup.org/Prot/4941/4941DOC.PDF. Accessed on January 19, 2005.

Paulino AC. Role of Radiation Therapy in Wilms' Tumor, Neuroblastoma, and Ewing's Sarcoma. Presented at American Society of Therapeutic Radiology and Oncology Spring Refresher Course, Chicago, IL, 2004.

Spierer M, Tereffe W, Wolden S. Neuroblastoma and Wilms' tumor. In: Leibel SA, Phillips TL, editors. Textbook of Radiation Oncology. 2nd ed. Philadelphia: Saunders; 2004. pp. 1273–1298.

Thomas PRM, D'Angio GJ. WIlms' tumor. In: Gunderson LL, Tepper JE, editors. Clinical Radiation Oncology. 1st ed. Philadelphia: Churchill Livingstone; 2000. pp. 1073–1078.

Neuroblastoma

Bleyer WA. The U.S. pediatric cancer clinical trials programmes: international implications and the way forward. Eur J Cancer 1997;33:1439–1447.

Castleberry RP, Kun LE, Shuster JJ, et al. Radiotherapy improves the outlook for patients older than 1 year with Pediatric Oncology Group stage C neuroblastoma. J Clin Oncol 1991;9:789–795.

Children's Oncology Group P9641: Primary Surgical Therapy for Biologically Defined Low-Risk Neuroblastoma. Available at: https://members.childrensoncologygroup.org/Prot/9641/9641DOC.PDF. Accessed on January 19, 2005.

Haas-Kogan DA, Fisch BM, Wara WM, et al. Intraoperative radiation therapy for high-risk pediatric neuroblastoma. Int J Radiat Oncol Biol Phys 2000;47:985–992.

Haas-Kogan DA, Swift PS, Selch M, et al. Impact of radiotherapy for high-risk neuroblastoma: a Children's Cancer Group study. Int J Radiat Oncol Biol Phys 2003;56:28–39.

Kun LE. Childhood cancer. In: Cox JD, Ang KK, editors. Radiation Oncology: Rationale, Technique, Results. 8th ed. St. Louis: Mosby; 2003. pp. 913–938.

London WB, Castelberry RP, Matthay KK, et al. Evidence for an age cutoff greater than 365 days for Neuroblastoma risk group stratification in the Children's Oncology Group. J Clin Oncol 2005;23:6459–6465.

Marcus K. Pediatric Tumors (Non-CNS): Wilms' Tumors, Ewings Sarcoma and Neuroblastoma (#107). Presented at American Society of Therapeutic Radiology and Oncology Annual Meeting, Atlanta, GA, 2004.

Matthay KK, Haas-Kogan D, Constine LS. Neuroblastoma. In: Halperin EC, Constine LS, Tarbell NJ, et al., editors. Pediatric Radiation Oncology. 4th ed. Philadelphia, PA: Lippincott Williams & Wilkins; 2005. pp. 179–222.

Matthay KK, Villablanca JG, Seeger RC, et al. Treatment of high-risk neuroblastoma with intensive chemotherapy, radiotherapy, autologous bone marrow transplantation, and 13-cis-retinoic acid. Children's Cancer Group. N Engl J Med 1999;341:1165–1173.

Michalski JM. Neuroblastoma. In: Perez CA, Brady LW, Halperin EC, et al., editors. Principles and Practice of Radiation Oncology. 4th ed. Philadelphia: Lippincott Williams & Wilkins; 2004. pp. 2247–2260.

Murray KJ. Neuroblastoma. In: Gunderson LL, Tepper JE, editors. Clinical Radiation Oncology. 1st ed. Philadelphia: Churchill Livingstone; 2000. pp. 1084–1088.

National Cancer Institute. Neuroblastoma (PDQ): Treatment. Available at: http://cancer.gov/cancertopics/pdq/treatment/neuroblastoma/healthprofessional/. Accessed on January 19, 2005.

Nitschke R, Smith EI, Shochat S, et al. Localized neuroblastoma treated by surgery: a Pediatric Oncology Group Study. J Clin Oncol 1988;6:1271–1279.

Paulino AC. Role of Radiation Therapy in Wilms' Tumor, Neuroblastoma, and Ewing's Sarcoma. Presented at American Society of Therapeutic Radiology and Oncology Spring Refresher Course, Chicago, IL, 2004.

Perez CA, Matthay KK, Atkinson JB, et al. Biologic variables in the outcome of stages I and II neuroblastoma treated with surgery as primary therapy: a children's cancer group study. J Clin Oncol 2000;18:18–26.

Spierer M, Tereffe W, Wolden S. Neuroblastoma and Wilms' tumor. In: Leibel SA, Phillips TL, editors. Textbook of Radiation Oncology. 2nd ed. Philadelphia: Saunders; 2004. pp. 1273–1298.

Strother D, van Hoff J, Rao PV, et al. Event-free survival of children with biologically favourable neuroblastoma based on the degree of initial tumour resection: results from the Pediatric Oncology Group. Eur J Cancer 1997;33:2121–2125.

Rhabdomyosarcoma

Blach LE. Pediatric soft tissue sarcomas. In: Gunderson LL, Tepper JE, editors. Clinical Radiation Oncology. 1st ed. Philadelphia: Churchill Livingstone; 2000. pp. 1059–1065.

Breitfeld PP, Lyden E, Raney RB, et al. Ifosfamide and etoposide are superior to vincristine and melphalan for pediatric metastatic rhabdomyosarcoma when administered with irradiation and combination chemotherapy: a report from the Intergroup Rhabdomyosarcoma Study Group. J Pediatr Hematol Oncol 2001;23:225–233.

Breneman JC, Donaldson SS. Rhabdomyosarcoma. In: Perez CA, Brady LW, Halperin EC, et al., editors. Principles and Practice of Radiation Oncology. 4th ed. Philadelphia: Lippincott Williams & Wilkins; 2004. pp. 2261–2276.

Crist W, Gehan EA, Ragab AH, et al. The Third Intergroup Rhabdomyosarcoma Study. J Clin Oncol 1995;13:610–630.

Crist WM, Anderson JR, Meza JL, et al. Intergroup rhabdomyosarcoma study-IV: results for patients with nonmetastatic disease. J Clin Oncol 2001;19:3091–3102.

Friedmann AM, Tarbell NJ, Constine LS. Rhabdomyosarcoma. In: Halperin EC, Constine LS, Tarbell NJ, et al., editors. Pediatric Radiation Oncology. 4th ed. Philadelphia, PA: Lippincott Williams & Wilkins; 2005. pp. 319–346.

IRSG Protocol D9803: Randomized study of vincristine, actinomycin-D, and cyclophosphamide (VAC) versus VAC alternating with vincristine, topotecan and cyclophosphamide for patients with intermediate-risk rhabdomyosarcoma. Available at: https://members. childrensoncologygroup.org/Prot/D9803/D9803DOC.PDF. Accessed on January 19, 2005.

IRSG Protocol D9602: Actinomycin D and vincristine with or without cyclophosphamide and radiation therapy, for newly diagnosed patients with low-risk embryonal/botyroid rhabdomyosarcoma: an IRS-V/STS protocol. Available at: https://members.childrensoncologygroup.org/Prot/D9602/D9602DOC.PDF. Accessed on January 19, 2005.

IRSG Protocol D9802: A phase II "up-front window study" of irinotecan (CPT-11) combined with vincristine followed by multimodal, multiagent, therapy for selected children and adolescents with newly diagnosed stage 4/clinical group IV rhabdomyosarcoma: An IRS-V/STS Study. Available at: https://members.childrensoncologygroup.org/Prot/D9802/D9802DOC.PDF. Accessed on January 19, 2005.

Kun LE. Childhood cancer. In: Cox JD, Ang KK, editors. Radiation Oncology: Rationale, Technique, Results. 8th ed. St. Louis: Mosby; 2003. pp. 913–938.

Maurer HM, Beltangady M, Gehan EA, et al. The Intergroup Rhabdomyosarcoma Study-I. A final report. Cancer 1988;61:209–220.

Maurer HM, Gehan EA, Beltangady M, et al. The Intergroup Rhabdomyosarcoma Study-II. Cancer 1993;71:1904–1922.

National Cancer Institute. Rhabdomyosarcoma (PDQ): Treatment. Available at: http://cancer.gov/cancertopics/pdq/treatment/childrhabdomyosarcoma/healthprofessional/. Accessed on January 19, 2005.

Wharam Jr. MD. Pediatric bone and soft tissue tumors. In: Leibel SA, Phillips TL, editors. Textbook of Radiation Oncology. 2nd ed. Philadelphia: Saunders; 2004. pp. 1251–1272.

Ewing's sarcoma

Blach LE. Pediatric sarcomas of bone. In: Gunderson LL, Tepper JE, editors. Clinical Radiation Oncology. 1st ed. Philadelphia: Churchill Livingstone; 2000. pp. 1066–1072.

Donaldson SS, Torrey M, Link MP, et al. A multidisciplinary study investigating radiotherapy in Ewing's sarcoma: end results of POG #8346. Pediatric Oncology Group. Int J Radiat Oncol Biol Phys 1998;42:125–135.

Dunst J, Jurgens H, Sauer R, et al. Radiation therapy in Ewing's sarcoma: an update of the CESS 86 trial. Int J Radiat Oncol Biol Phys 1995;32:919–930.

Evans RG, Nesbit ME, Gehan EA, et al. Multimodal therapy for the management of localized Ewing's sarcoma of pelvic and sacral bones: a report from the second intergroup study. J Clin Oncol 1991;9:1173–1180.

Grier HE, Krailo MD, Tarbell NJ, et al. Addition of ifosfamide and etoposide to standard chemotherapy for Ewing's sarcoma and primitive neuroectodermal tumor of bone. N Engl J Med 2003;348:694–701.

Marcus Jr. RB. Ewing's sarcoma. In: Perez CA, Brady LW, Halperin EC, et al., editors. Principles and Practice of Radiation Oncology. 4th ed. Philadelphia: Lippincott Williams & Wilkins; 2004. pp. 2277–2284.

Marcus K. Pediatric Tumors (Non-CNS): Wilms' Tumors, Ewings Sarcoma and Neuroblastoma (#107). Presented at American Society of Therapeutic Radiology and Oncology Annual Meeting, Atlanta, GA, 2004.

Marcus KJ, Tarbell NJ. Ewing's sarcoma. In: Halperin EC, Constine LS, Tarbell NJ, et al., editors. Pediatric Radiation Oncology. 4th ed. Philadelphia, PA: Lippincott Williams & Wilkins; 2005. pp. 271–290.

National Cancer Institute. Ewing's Family of Tumors (PDQ): Treatment. Available at: http://cancer.gov/cancertopics/pdq/treatment/ewings/ healthprofessional/. Accessed on January 19, 2005.

Nesbit ME, Jr., Gehan EA, Burgert EO, Jr., et al. Multimodal therapy for the management of primary, nonmetastatic Ewing's sarcoma of bone: a long-term follow-up of the First Intergroup study. J Clin Oncol 1990;8:1664–1674.

Paulino AC. Role of Radiation Therapy in Wilms' Tumor, Neuroblastoma, and Ewing's Sarcoma. Presented at American Society of Therapeutic Radiology and Oncology Spring Refresher Course, Chicago, IL, 2004.

Paulussen M, Ahrens S, Dunst J, et al. Localized Ewing tumor of bone: final results of the cooperative Ewing's Sarcoma Study CESS 86. J Clin Oncol 2001;19:1818–1829.

Schuck A, Ahrens S, Paulussen M, et al. Local therapy in localized Ewing tumors: results of 1058 patients treated in the CESS 81, CESS 86, and EICESS 92 trials. Int J Radiat Oncol Biol Phys 2003;55:168–177.

Wharam Jr. MD. Pediatric bone and soft tissue tumors. In: Leibel SA, Phillips TL, editors. Textbook of Radiation Oncology. 2nd ed. Philadelphia: Saunders; 2004. pp. 1251–1272.

Pediatric Hodgkin's lymphoma

Asselin B, Hudson M, Mandell LR, et al. Pediatric leukemias and lymphomas. In: Leibel SA, Phillips TL, editors. Textbook of Radiation Oncology. 2nd ed. Philadelphia: Saunders; 2004. pp. 1215–1251.

Greene FL, American Joint Committee on Cancer, American Cancer Society. AJCC Cancer Staging Manual. 6th ed. New York: Springer-Verlag; 2002.

Hudson M, Asselin B, Mandell LR, et al. Lymphomas in children. In: Perez CA, Brady LW, Halperin EC, et al., editors. Principles and Practice of Radiation Oncology. 4th ed. Philadelphia: Lippincott Williams & Wilkins; 2004. pp. 2285–2307.

Hudson MM, Constine LS. Hodgkin's disease. In: Halperin EC, Constine LS, Tarbell NJ, et al., editors. Pediatric Radiation Oncology. 4th ed. Philadelphia, PA: Lippincott Williams & Wilkins; 2005. pp. 223–260.

Jenkin D, Danjoux C, Greenberg M. Leukemias and lymphomas in children – Hodgkin's disease. In: Gunderson LL, Tepper JE, editors. Clinical Radiation Oncology. 1st ed. Philadelphia: Churchill Livingstone; 2000. pp. 1098–1103.

Nachman JB, Sposto R, Herzog P, et al. Randomized comparison of low-dose involved-field radiotherapy and no radiotherapy for children with Hodgkin's disease who achieve a complete response to chemotherapy. J Clin Oncol 2002;20:3765–3771.

National Cancer Institute. Childhood Hodgkin's Lymphoma (PDQ): Treatment. Available at: http://cancer.gov/cancertopics/pdq/treatment/childhodgkins/healthprofessional/. Accessed on January 19, 2005.

Ruhl U, Albrecht M, Dieckmann K, et al. Response-adapted radiotherapy in the treatment of pediatric Hodgkin's disease: an interim report at 5 years of the German GPOH-HD 95 trial. Int J Radiat Oncol Biol Phys 2001;51:1209–1218.

Ruhl U, Albrecht M, Lueders H, et al. The German Multinational GPOH-HD 95 Trial: Treatment Results and Analysis of Failures in Pediatric Hodgkins Disease Using Combination Chemotherapy With and Without Radiation. Presented at American Society of Therapeutic Radiology and Oncology 46th Annual Meeting, Atlanta, GA, 2004.

Retinoblastoma

Abramson DA, McCormick B, Schefler AC. Retinoblastoma. In: Leibel SA, Phillips TL, editors. Textbook of Radiation Oncology. 2nd ed. Philadelphia: Saunders; 2004. pp. 1463–1482.

Fontanesi J, Donaldson SS, Pratt CB, et al. Retinoblastoma. In: Gunderson LL, Tepper JE, editors. Clinical Radiation Oncology. 1st ed. Philadelphia: Churchill Livingstone; 2000. pp. 1079–1083.

Freire JE, Brady LW, Shields JA, et al. Eye and orbit. In: Perez CA, Brady LW, Halperin EC, et al., editors. Principles and Practice of Radiation Oncology. 4th ed. Philadelphia: Lippincott Williams & Wilkins; 2004. pp. 876–896.

Halperin EC, Kirkpatrick JP. Retinoblastoma. In: Halperin EC, Constine LS, Tarbell NJ, et al., editors. Pediatric Radiation Oncology. 4th ed. Philadelphia, PA: Lippincott Williams & Wilkins; 2005. pp. 135–178.

Kun LE. Childhood cancer. In: Cox JD, Ang KK, editors. Radiation Oncology: Rationale, Technique, Results. 8th ed. St Louis: Mosby; 2003. pp. 913–938.

National Cancer Institute. Retinoblastoma (PDQ): Treatment. Available at: http://cancer.gov/cancertopics/pdq/treatment/retinoblastoma/healthprofessional/. Accessed on January 19, 2005.

Shields C, Shields J. Diagnosis and management of retinoblastoma. Cancer Control 2004; 11(5):317–327.

Chapter 40
Palliative Care

Laura Millender and William M. Wara

- This chapter will cover brain metastases, bone metastases, spinal cord compression, liver metastases, airway obstruction, superior vena cava obstruction, and gynecologic bleeding

BRAIN METASTASES

PEARLS

- Most common type of intracranial tumor (incidence ~170,000/yr in U.S.)
- "Solitary" = one brain metastasis, only site of disease
- "Single" = one brain metastasis, other sites of disease
- Primary cancers most likely to metastasize to brain are lung, breast, and melanoma
- Hemorrhagic metastases: renal cell CA, choriocarcinoma, and melanoma

WORKUP

- MRI of brain with and without contrast
- If solitary lesion, obtain biopsy

PROGNOSTIC FACTORS

- RTOG recursive partitioning analysis (Gaspar, *IJROBP* 1997)

Class	Characteristics	Survival
I	KPS 70–100 Primary controlled Age <65 Mets to brain only	7.1 mo
II	All Others	4.2 mo
III	KPS <70	2.3 mo

TREATMENT
Steroids

- Improve headache and neurologic function
- No impact on survival
- Start dexamethasone 4 mg q 6 h if patient has neurologic symptoms
- Taper as tolerated
- No role for steroids in asymptomatic patients

Surgery, whole brain RT (WBRT), stereotactic radiosurgery (SRS)

Characteristics	Options
Single lesion RPA class I–II	Surgical resection + WBRT WBRT + SRS SRS alone (with SRS or WBRT for salvage prn) WBRT alone
2–4 lesions RPA class I–II	WBRT alone WBRT + SRS SRS alone (with SRS or WBRT for salvage prn) controversial
>4 lesions RPA class I–II	WBRT alone WBRT + SRS controversial SRS alone (with SRS or WBRT for salvage prn) controversial
RPA class III	WBRT alone

STUDIES
Surgery

- Patchell (*NEJM* 1990). Prospective. Randomized. Pts with solitary brain lesion. Surgical removal of tumor plus WBRT vs needle biopsy plus WBRT. Recurrence at original site, time to recurrence, MS, time to death from neurologic cause, and time with KPS >70 all significantly better in the surgery group. 6/54 pts did not have a pathologic diagnosis of brain met

Post-Op WBRT

- Patchell (*JAMA* 1998). Prospective. Randomized. Pts with solitary brain lesion. All pts treated with surgery then randomly assigned to WBRT or no further therapy. Post-op RT reduced recurrence at the original site and other sites in the brain. Pts in the RT group were less likely to die of neurologic causes. OS and duration of functional independence were not different

SRS boost after WBRT

- Kondziolka (*IJROBP* 1999). Prospective. Randomized. WBRT alone vs WBRT plus SRS. Local failure 100% at 1 yr after WBRT alone, 8% with addition of RS. Non-significant OS benefit in the SRS group (MS 7.5 mo vs 11 mo).
- Andrews (*Lancet* 2004). Prospective. Randomized. Pts with 1–3 brain mets. WBRT plus SRS vs WBRT alone. Survival advantage with addition of SRS in pts with single met (MS 6.5 mo vs 4.9 mo), RPA class I (11.6 mo vs 9.6 mo), lung histology, & tumor size >2 cm. KPS better with addition of SRS

SRS alone or with WBRT

- JROSG 99–1 (*ASCO* abstr. 2004). 132 pts with 1–4 mets randomized to SRS vs WBRT → SRS. No difference in MS (7.9 mo vs 7.6 mo) or neurologic or KPS preservation. WBRT improved freedom from new mets (48% vs 82%), & 1 yr LC (70% vs 86%)
- Sneed (*IJROBP* 1999, 2002). Multi-institutional & UCSF retrospective reviews of SRS vs SRS + WBRT. No difference in OS by RPA class (I = 14–15 mo, II = 7–8 mo, III = 5 mo). Brain FFP worse without WBRT, but brain FFP allowing for 1st salvage not different

Dose and fractionation considerations

- RTOG fractionation papers (Borgelt, *IJROBP* 1980, 1981; Murrary, *IJROBP* 1997). Multiple fractionation regimens evaluated. Most were similar for treatment response, duration of improvement, and OS. Worse outcomes with 10 Gy × 1 and 7.5 Gy × 2
- Shaw (*IJROBP* 2000). Maximum tolerated dose for single fraction radiosurgery: tumor diameter <20 mm, dose 24 Gy; diameter 21–30 mm, dose 18 Gy; diameter 31–40 mm, dose 15 Gy

TECHNIQUES: WBRT

- Opposed laterals, flash anterior/posterior/superior
- Bottom of field at foramen magnum, inferior to C1, or inferior to C2
- Use eye block

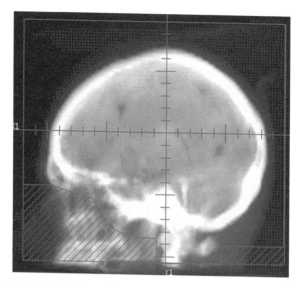

FIGURE 40.1. Lateral DRR of a whole-brain radiation field.

- Acceptable fractionation schemes include 4 Gy × 5, 3 Gy × 10 (most common), 2.5 Gy × 15, and 2 Gy × 20
- Choose fractionation based on performance status and life expectancy

COMPLICATIONS

- Neurocognitive deficits after WBRT in long term survivors
- 5% rate of symptomatic brain necrosis after SRS, generally treated with steroids, sometimes requires surgery for intractable symptoms

FOLLOW-UP

- Brain MRI scan with and without contrast every 3 mo

BONE METASTASES

PEARLS

- Common cause of severe cancer pain
- Pain relief after RT can be expected in 60–90% of pts
- Good pain control may improve OS
- Sites of mets: spine (lumbar > thoracic) > pelvis > ribs > femur > skull

- Primary cancers most likely to metastasize to bone are breast, prostate, thyroid, kidney, and lung

WORKUP
- Bone scan is the primary imaging modality
- Plain films should be used to look for fracture or impending fracture but are not sensitive for diagnosis as cortical involvement occurs late
- MRI is the procedure of choice when evaluating for spinal cord compression or nerve root compromise
- Biopsy and/or PET scan are not routinely needed but should be considered if radiographic studies are equivocal

TREATMENT

Surgery
- Indicated for pathologic fracture
- Mirels (*Clin Orthop* 1989) 12 point scoring system estimates risk of pathologic fracture based on site of disease (upper extremity, lower extremity, peritrochanteric), amount of pain (mild, moderate, functional), type of lesion (blastic, mixed, lytic), and size ($<1/3$, $1/3$–$2/3$, $>2/3$ diameter of bone involved). Scores of 10–12 have 72–100% chance of fracture
- Van der Linden (*J Bone Joint Surg BR* 2004) data shows that axial cortical involvement >30 mm and/or circumferential cortical involvement >50% predict for high rates of fracture

EBRT
- Local field RT for discrete painful lesions
  - Avoid uninvolved sensitive tissues like perineum and joints when possible
  - Dose: 8 Gy × 1, 4 Gy × 5
- Wide-field ("hemibody") RT occasionally used for diffuse bone mets

Radiopharmaceutical therapy
- Best for pts with multiple lesions that show uptake on bone scan

- Should not be used for fractures, spinal cord compression, nerve root compression, or lesions with large extra osseous component
- Pts must have adequate blood counts, no myelosuppressive chemotherapy for 4 weeks before and 6–8 weeks after treatment
- Response rates 40–90%, pain relief at 2–3 weeks, lasts 3–4 months
- Agents: strontium-89, samarium-153 EDTMP

Pharmacologic therapies and supportive care

- Bisphosphonates are used in most patients with multiple bone mets
- Hormone therapy can be very effective in breast and prostate cancer
- Pain management is important (NSAIDs, narcotics, steroids, anticonvulsants, tricyclic antidepressants, electric stimulation, nerve blocks)
- Don't forget braces and walkers

STUDIES
EBRT dose

- Tong (*Cancer* 1982). Various fractionation schemes evaluated. No differences seen in rates of pain relief
- Blitzer (*Cancer* 1985). Reanalysis of RTOG data with conclusion that more fractions with higher total dose was more effective for pain relief
- Bone Pain Trial Working Party (*Radiother Oncol* 1999). 8 Gy in single fx vs 20 Gy in 5 fx or 30 Gy in 10 fx. No difference in pain relief at 12 mo. Re-treatment more frequently needed after 8 Gy
- Hartsell (*ASTRO* abstr. 2003). Pts with breast and prostate cancer randomized to 8 Gy in 1 fraction vs 30 Gy in 10 fractions. Higher acute toxicity with 30 Gy (17% vs 10%). Pain CR/PR rates at 3 mo were equivalent, 15%/50% for 8 Gy and 18%/48% for 30 Gy

Radionuclide therapy

- Porter (*IJROBP* 1993). Randomized local field RT +/– strontium 89 in pts with hormone refractory prostate cancer. Pts in combined arm needed less analgesics, had fewer sites of new pain, had lower PSA and alk phos levels, and had better quality of life

SPINAL CORD COMPRESSION

PEARLS
- Most important prognostic factor is ambulatory status
- Pain precedes neurologic dysfunction and is most common presenting symptom

WORKUP
- MRI scan of entire spine to determine location and extent of disease and to rule out other sites of cord compression
- Biopsy required if metastatic disease has not been previously documented or if patient does not have proven cancer diagnosis

TREATMENT
Steroids
- Start steroids immediately and then taper as tolerated
- Used for symptom relief (improved neurologic function, reduced pain)

Surgery and RT
- Maximum debulking surgery with appropriate spine stabilization followed by post-op RT is treatment of choice for patients with single region of cord compression and life expectancy >3 mo
- Laminectomy is not an alternative to maximal debulking and stabilization (laminectomy plus RT is equivalent to RT alone)
- If pt has multiple levels of compression or is not medically fit for surgery, then give immediate RT

TRIALS
- <u>Patchell</u> (*Lancet* 2005). Prospective randomized trial of surgery with post-op RT to 30 Gy vs RT alone to 30 Gy. Surgery pts regained ability to walk more often (62% vs 19%), retained ability to walk longer (122 days vs 13 days), and required less steroid and pain medication. Improved survival with surgery (126 days vs 100 days)

TECHNIQUES

- PA only is preferred technique at many institutions; however, this technique risks overdosing the spinal cord or under dosing the tumor
  - Example: lumbar spine met, cord depth (7.5 cm), anterior vertebral body depth (12 cm). With 6 MV dosed at 12 cm, cord would receive 128% of the prescription dose. If 18 MV is used, cord would receive 120% of the prescription dose. If the prescription is 3 Gy × 10 fractions, total dose to the cord would be 36–38.4 Gy
- AP/PA gives more homogenous dose distribution and is the preferred technique
- Dose schedules: 4 Gy × 5, 3 Gy × 10 (most common), 8 Gy × 1

LIVER METASTASES

PEARLS

- MS 5–10 mo without intervention
- Colorectal primary is most common with 50,000 cases of colorectal liver mets per year in the USA
- Liver has remarkable ability for regeneration and can grow back after 50% resection in just 3 weeks

WORKUP

- CT is primary imaging modality used for diagnosis and follow-up, special contrast protocols exist to maximize CT yield
- Ultrasound is particularly helpful intra-operatively
- MRI scan is good for distinguishing benign from malignant disease and can provide specific information about involvement of biliary tree

TREATMENT
Surgery

- Surgery with curative intent possible in ~10% of pts
- MS after complete resection is ~30 mo with small number of pts surviving >10 yr
- Contraindications for liver resection
  - Presence of extrahepatic disease (selected pts with limited pulmonary and liver mets are candidates for surgical resection of both sites of disease)

- Complete resection not possible (unacceptable LF rates with + margins)
- Second resections can be performed for liver only failures that meet criteria for surgery. Long term survival after second resection is possible

Chemotherapy

- Systemic chemotherapy for unresectable mets is palliative
- Neoadjuvant chemotherapy can be used to shrink disease, increase resectability
- Adjuvant chemotherapy (including hepatic arterial chemotherapy) can be used to reduce LR rates and possibly improve survival

Radiofrequency ablation, cryoablation, ethanol injection

- Alternative therapies for pts who are not surgical candidates
- See Chapter 20: Hepatobiliary Cancer

EBRT

- Whole liver RT (3 Gy × 7) for symptomatic pts with multiple small lesions who are not candidates for other therapies.
- 3DCRT with concurrent hepatic artery chemo is preferred to whole liver RT for pts with good KPS and limited metastatic disease
- Stereotactic body irradiation & IMRT investigational

PAPERS

- McCarter (*Semin Surg Oncol* 2000). Good review of surgical data
- See Chapter 20: Hepatobiliary Cancer for other papers

RADIATION TECHNIQUES/TOLERANCE/COMPLICATIONS

- See Chapter 20: Hepatobiliary Cancer

FOLLOW-UP

- Liver function tests 2–3 weeks after treatment
- Office visit every 3 months or as needed for symptoms
- CT scan every 3–6 months or sooner for recurrent symptoms

AIRWAY OBSTRUCTION

- Broncoscopy with stent placement
  - If successful, may result in immediate symptom relief
- Intraluminal brachytherapy
  - Use caution in previously treated areas near major vessels
- EBRT
  - Accepted dose and fractionation schedules include: $10\,Gy \times 1$, $8.5\,Gy \times 2$ (one week apart), $4\,Gy \times 5$, $3\,Gy \times 10$
  - Do not exceed spinal cord tolerance when using large fraction sizes
  - If large fields will be necessary, use caution. Do not want to induce radiation pneumonitis in pt needing palliation for shortness of breath

SUPERIOR VENA CAVA SYNDROME

- Most frequently seen in lung cancer pts
- Biopsy required to evaluate for benign conditions and sensitive tumors
- Generally symptoms improve because of collateral circulation
- Treatment includes supportive care, steroids, diuretics, and elevation of the head and torso
- Accepted external beam radiation therapy dose and fractionation schedules include $3\,Gy \times 10$ and $4\,Gy \times 5$

GYNECOLOGIC BLEEDING

- Treatment options
  - Vaginal packing
  - EBRT: $3.7\,Gy$ bid $\times 2$ days, repeat every $2\,wks \times 2\,prn$. Use CT scan to determine field borders
  - Brachytherapy
  - Electron cone

REFERENCES

Andrews DW, Scott CB, Sperduto PW, et al. Whole brain radiation therapy with or without stereotactic radiosurgery boost for patients with one to three brain metastases: phase III results of the RTOG 9508 randomised trial. Lancet 2004;363:1665–1672.

Blitzer PH. Reanalysis of the RTOG study of the palliation of symptomatic osseous metastasis. Cancer 1985;55:1468–1472.

Bone Pain Trial Working Party. 8 Gy single fraction radiotherapy for the treatment of metastatic skeletal pain: randomised comparison with a multifraction schedule over 12 months of patient follow-up. Radiother Oncol 1999;52:111–121.

Borgelt B, Gelber R, Kramer S, et al. The palliation of brain metastases: final results fo the first two studies by the Radiation Therapy Oncology Group. Int J Radiat Oncol Biol Phys 1980;6:1–9.

Borgelt B, Gelber R, Larson M, et al. Ultra-rapid high dose irradiation schedules for the palliation of brain metastases: final results of the first two studies by the Radiation Therapy Oncology Group. Int J Radiat Oncol Biol Phys 1981;7:1633–1638.

Dillehay GL, Ellerbroek NA, Balon H, et al. Practice Guideline for the performance of therapy with unsealed radiopharmaceutical sources. Int J Radiat Oncol Biol Phys 2006;64:1299–1307.

Gaspar L, Scott C, Rotman M, et al. Recursive partitioning analysis (RPA) of prognostic factors in three Radiation Therapy Oncology Group (RTOG) brain metastases trials. Int J Radiat Oncol Biol Phys 1997;37:745–751.

Hartsell WF, Scott C, Bruner DW, et al. Phase III randomized trial of 8 Gy in 1 fraction vs 30 Gy in 10 fractions for palliation of painful bone metastases: preliminary results of RTOG 97-14. ASTRO 2003, abstract.

Janjan NA, Delclos ME, Ballo MT, et al. Palliative care. In: Cox JD, Ang KK, editors. Radiation Oncology: Rationale, Technique, Results. 8th ed. St. Louis: Mosby; 2003. 954–986.

Johnson JD, Young B. Demographics of brain metastasis. Neurosurg Clin North Am 1996;7:337–344.

Kagan RA. Palliation of brain and spinal cord metastases. In: Perez CA, Brady LW, Halperin EC, et al, editors. Principles and Practice of Radiation Oncology. 4th ed. Philadelphia: Lippincott Williams & Wilkins; 2004. 2373–2384.

Kondziolka D, Patel A, Lunsford LD, et al. Stereotactic radiosurgery plus whole brain radiotherapy versus radiotherapy alone for patients with multiple brain metastases. Int J Radiat Oncol Biol Phys 1999;45:427–434.

Leonard GD, Brenner B, Kemeny NE. Neoadjuvant chemotherapy before liver resection for patients with unresectable liver metastases from colorectal carcinoma. J Clin Oncol 2005;23:2038–2048.

McCarter MD, Fong Y. Metastatic liver tumors. Semin Surgl Oncol 2000;19:177–188.

Mirels H. Metastatic disease in long bones. A proposed scoring system for diagnosing impending pathologic fractures. Clin Orthop Relat Res 1989;249:256–264.

Murrary KJ, Scott C, Greenberg HM, et al. A randomized phase III study of accelerated hyperfractionation versus standard in patients with unresected brain metastases: a report of the Radiation Therapy Oncology Group (RTOG) 9104. Int J Radiat Oncol Biol Phys 1997;39:571–574.

Patchell RA, Tibbs PA, Regine WF, et al. Postoperative radiotherapy in the treatment of single metastases to the brain. JAMA 1998; 280:1485–1489.

Patchell RA, Tibbs PA, Regine WF, et al. Direct decompressive surgical resection in the treatment of spinal cord compression caused by metastatic cancer: a randomised trial. Lancet 2005;366: 643–648.

Patchell RA, Tibbs PA, Walsh JW, et al. A randomized trial of surgery in the treatment of single metastases to the brain. N Engl J Med 1990; 322:494–500.

Perez CA, Grigsby PW, Thorstad W. Nonsealed radionuclide therapy. In: Perez CA, Brady LW, Halperin EC, et al, editors. Principles and Practice of Radiation Oncology. 4th ed. Philadelphia: Lippincott Williams & Wilkins; 2004. 636–652.

Porter AT, Benda R, Ben-Josef E. Palliation of Metasteses: Bone and spinal cord. In: Gunderson LL, Tepper JE, editors. Clinical Radiation Oncology. 1st ed. Philadelphia: Churchill Livingstone; 2000. 299–313.

Porter AT, McEwan AJ, Powe JE, et al. Results of a randomized phase III trial to evaluate the efficacy of strontium-89 adjuvant to local field external beam irradiation in the management of endocrine resistant metastatic prostate cancer. Int J Radiat Oncol Biol Phys 1993;25:805–813.

Ratanatharathorn V, Powers WE, Temple HT. Palliation of bone metastases. In: Perez CA, Brady LW, Halperin EC, et al, editors. Principles and Practice of Radiation Oncology. 4th ed. Philadelphia: Lippincott Williams & Wilkins; 2004. 2385–2404.

Shaw E, Scott C, Souhami L, et al. Single dose radiosurgical treatment of recurrent previously irradiated primary brain tumors and brain metastases: final report of RTOG Protocol 90-05. Int J Radiat Oncol Biol Phys 2000;47:291–298.

Sneed PK, Lamborn KR, Forstner JM, et al. Radiosurgery for brain metastases: is whole brain radiotherapy necessary? Int J Radiat Oncol Biol Phys 1999;43:549–558.

Sneed PK, Suh JH, Goetsch SJ, et al. A multi-institutional review of radiosurgery alone vs. radiosurgery with whole brain radiotherapy as the initial management of brain metastases. Int J Radiat Oncol Biol Phys 2002;53:519–526.

Stevens, KR. The liver and biliary system. In: Cox JD, Ang KK, editors. Radiation Oncology: Rationale, Technique, Results. 8th ed. St. Louis: Mosby; 2003. 493–496.

Tong D, Gillick L, Hendrickson FR. The palliation of symptomatic osseous metastases: final results of the study by the Radiation Therapy Oncology Group. Cancer 1982;50:893–899.

Van der Linden YM, Dijkstra PD, Kroon HM, et al. Comparative analysis of risk factors for pathological fracture with femoral metastases. J Bone Joint Surg Br 2004;86:566–573.

NOTES

Abbreviations

3D	3-dimensional
3DCRT	3-dimensional conformal radiotherapy
5-FU	5-fluorouracil
AA	Anaplastic astrocytoma
ABMT	Autologous bone marrow transplant
abstr.	Abstract
ACS	American Cancer Society
ACTH	Adrenocorticotropic hormone
ADR	Doxorubicin
AFP	Alpha fetoprotein
AIDS	Acquired immune deficiency syndrome
Al	Aluminum
AMD	Dactinomycin
AML	Acute myeloid leukemia
AP	Anterior-posterior
APR	Abdominoperineal resection
ASCO	American Society of Clinical Oncology
ASTRO	American Society for Therapeutic Radiology and Oncology
BCC	Basal cell carcinoma
BCG	Bacillus Calmette-Guerin
bPFS	Biochemical progression-free survival
BUN	Blood urea nitrogen
c	Cycles (e.g., ×2c = for two cycles)
ca	Cancer
CALGB	Cancer and Leukemia Group B
CBC	Complete blood count
cCR	Clinical complete response
CESS	German Cooperative Ewing's Sarcoma Study
cGy	CentiGray
Chemo	Chemotherapy
Chemo-RT	Chemo-radiotherapy
CHOP	Cyclophosphamide, doxorubicine, vincristine, & prednisone
CIS	Carcinoma in-situ

cm	centimeter
CN	Cranial nerve (e.g., CN X)
COG	Children's Oncology Group
CR	Complete response
Cr	Creatinine
CR	Complete response
CSF	Cerebrospinal fluid
CSI	Craniospinal irradiation
CSS	Cause-specific survival
CT	Computed tomography
CTV1	Clinical target volume 1
CTV2	Clinical target volume 2
Cu	Copper
CXR	Chest X-ray
CY	Cyclophosphamide
d	Day
D&C	Dilation & curettage
DCIS	Ductal carcinoma *in situ*
DES	Diethylstibestrol
DFS	Disease-free survival
DLBCL	Diffuse large B-cell lymphoma
DLCO	Diffusing capacity
DM	Distant metastases
Dmax	Maximum dose
DRE	Digital rectal exam
DRR	Digitally-reconstructed radiograph
DSS	Disease specific survival
DVH	Dose-volume histogram
EBCTCG	Early Breast Cancer Trialists' Collaborative Group
EBRT	External beam radiation therapy
EBV	Epstein-Barr virus
ECE	Extracapsular extension
ECOG	Eastern Cooperative Oncology Group
EFRT	Extended field radiotherapy
EFS	Event free survival
EGD	Esophogastroduodenoscopy
EORTC	European Organisation for Research and Treatment of Cancer
EPID	Electronic portal imaging device
ERCP	Endoscopic retrograde cholangiopancreatography
ESR	Erythrocyte sedimentation rate
EtOH	Alcohol
EUA	Exam under anesthesia

EUS	Endoscopic ultrasound
F/U	Follow-up
FEV1	Forced expiratory volume in 1 second
FFF	Freedom from failure
FFP	Freedom from progression
FFS	Failure-free survival
FH	Family history
FOBT	Fecal occult blood test
fx	Fraction(s)
GBM	Glioblastoma multiforme
GERD	Gastroesophageal reflux disease
GHSG	German Hodgkin's Study Group
GS	Gleason score
GTR	Gross total resection
GTV	Gross tumor volume
GU	Genitourinary
Gy	Gray
H&N	Head and neck
H&P	History & physical exam
hCG	Human chorionic gonadotropin
HCV	Hepatitis C virus
HDR	High dose rate
HIV	Human immunodeficiency virus
HNPCC	Hereditary non-polyposis colon cancer
HPV	Human papilloma virus
hr	Hour
HTN	Hypertension
HVL	Half-value layer
Hx	History
IC	Intracavitary
IDL	Isodose line
IESS	Intergroup Ewing's Sarcoma Study
IE	Ifosfamide & etoposide (VP-16)
IFN	Interferon
IFRT	Involved-field radiation therapy
IJROBP	International Journal of Radiation Oncology*Biology*Physics
IMRT	Intensity modulated radiotherapy
INSS	International Neuroblastoma Staging System
Int	Intergroup
IORT	Intraoperative radiation therapy
IS	Interstitial
IVC	Inferior vena cava
IVP	Intravenous pyelogram

JCO	Journal of Clinical Oncology
JPA	Juvenile pilocytic astrocytoma
LAR	Low anterior resection
LC	Local control
LCSG	Lung Cancer Study Group
LDH	Lactate dehydrogenase
LDR	Low dose rate
LF	Local failure
LFTs	Liver function tests
LN	Lymph node(s)
LND	Lymph node dissection
LR	Local recurrence/relapse
LRC	Local-regional control
LRF	Local-regional failure
LVEF	Left ventricular ejection fraction
LVSI	Lymphovascular space invasion
MALT	Mucosa associated lymphoid tissue
MFH	Malignant fibrous histiosarcoma
mm	millimeter
mo	Month
MRC	Medical Research Council
MRI	Magnetic resonance imaging
MRSI	Magnetic resonance spectroscopy imaging
MS	Median survival
MUGA	Multiple gated acquisition scan
N0	Node negative
N+	Node positive
NCI	National Cancer Institute
NCIC	National Cancer Institute of Canada
NED	No evidence of disease
NEJM	New England Journal of Medicine
NHL	Non-Hodgkin's lymphoma
NPX	Nasopharynx
NPV	Negative predictive value
NSABP	National Surgical Adjuvant Breast and Bowel Project
NSCLC	Non-small cell lung cancer
NSGCT	Non-seminomatous germ cell tumor
NWTS	National Wilms' Tumor Study
OS	Overall survival
OPX	Oropharynx
PA	Posterior-anterior
Pb	Lead
pCR	Pathologic complete response

PET	Positron emission tomography
PLAP	Placental alkaline phosphatase
PNET	Primitive neuroectodermal tumor
PNI	Perineural invasion
Post-op	Post-operative
PPV	Positive predictive value
PR	Partial response
Pre-op	Pre-operative
PS	Performance status
PSA	Prostate specific antigen
pt	Patient
pts	Patients
PTV	Planning target volume
PUVA	Psoralen & ultraviolet light A
QOL	Quality of life
RAI	Radioactive iodine
RBE	Relative biological effectiveness
RCC	Renal cell carcinoma
RFS	Relapse-free survival
RT	Radiation therapy
RTOG	Radiation Therapy Oncology Group
S/P	Status post
SCC	Squamous cell carcinoma
SCID	Severe combined immunodeficiency
SCLC	Small cell lung cancer
SCV	Supraclavicular
SI	Sacroiliac
SIADH	Syndrome of inappropriate antidiuretic hormone
SPEP	Serum protein electrophoreses
SRS	Stereotactic radiosurgery
STD	Sexually transmitted disease
STLI	Subtotal lymphoid irradiation
STR	Subtotal resection
SWOG	Southwest Oncology Group
T&O	Tandem & Ovoid
TAH/BSO	Total abdominal hysterectomy/bilateral salpingo-oophorectomy
TBI	Total body irradiation
TCC	Transitional cell carcinoma
TMP/SMX	Trimethoprim/sulfamethoxazole
TNM	Tumor Node Metastasis
TRUS	Transrectal ultrasound
TSH	Thyroid stimulating hormone
TURBT	Transurethral resection of bladder tumor

U.S.	United States of America
UA	Urinalysis
UCSF	University of California, San Francisco
UPEP	Urine protein electrophoreses
US	Ultrasound
USO	Unilateral salpingo-oophorectomy
UVB	Ultraviolet light B
VAC	Vincristine, actinomycin-D, & cyclophosphamide
VDC	Vincristine, doxorubicin, cyclophosphamide
VDCA	Vincristine, doxorubicin, cyclophosphamide, & actinomycin-D
VCR	Vincristine
VP-16	Etoposide
VM	Vincristine & melphalan
vs	Versus
wk	Week
WHO	World Health Organization
WLE	Wide local excision
yo	Years old
yr	Year

Appendixes

A: PERFORMANCE STATUS SCALES

KARNOFSKY PERFORMANCE STATUS

100	Normal; no complaints; no evidence of disease
90	Able to carry on normal activity; minor signs or symptoms of disease
80	Normal activity with effort; some signs or symptoms of disease
70	Cares for self; unable to carry on normal activity or to do active work
60	Requires occasional assistance, but is able to care for most of his/her personal needs
50	Requires considerable assistance and frequent medical care
40	Disabled; requires special care and assistance
30	Severely disabled; hospital admission is indicated although death not imminent
20	Very sick; hospital admission necessary; active support treatment necessary
10	Moribund; fatal processes progressing rapidly
0	Dead

From: Karnofsky D, Abelman W, Craver L, Burchenal J. The use of nitrogen mustards in the palliative treatment of carcinoma. Cancer 1948;1:634–656, with permission.

ECOG PERFORMANCE STATUS

0	Fully active, able to carry on all pre-disease performance without restriction
1	Restricted in physically strenuous activity but ambulatory and able to carry out work of a light or sedentary nature (e.g., light house work, office work)
2	Ambulatory and capable of all self-care but unable to carry out any work activities. Up and about more than 50% of waking hours
3	Capable of only limited self-care, confined to bed or chair more than 50% of waking hours
4	Completely disabled. Cannot carry on any self-care. Totally confined to bed or chair
5	Dead

From: Oken MM, Creech RH, Tormey DC, et al. Toxicity And Response Criteria Of The Eastern Cooperative Oncology Group. Am J Clin Oncol 1982;5:649–655, with permission.

B: RADIONUCLEOTIDES USED IN BRACHYTHERAPY

Radionuclide	Photon Energy (MeV)	Half-Life	Exposure Rate Constant (Rcm²/mCi-hr)	Half-value Layer (mm of Lead)
Au-198	0.412	2.7 d	2.38	2.5
Co-60	1.25 avg	5.26 yr	13.07	11
Cs-137	0.662	30 yr	3.26	5.5
I-125	0.028 avg	60 d	1.46	0.025
Ir-192	0.38 avg	74 d	4.69	2.5
Pd-103	0.021 avg	17 d	1.48	0.008
Ra-226	0.83 avg	1622 yr	8.25*	12
Rn-222	0.83 avg	3.83 d	10.15*	12

*Exposure rate constant per mg instead of mCi.

C: RADIATION SAFETY

Release of patients administered radioactive materials falls under the NRC Regulatory Guide 8.39

RELEASE CRITERIA FOR PATIENTS TREATED WITH BRACHYTHERAPY

Isotope	Activity at or below which pts may be released <u>with</u> instructions	Dose rate at 1 meter at or below which pts may be released <u>with</u> instructions
I-125	9 mCi	0.01 mSv/hr (1 mrem/hr)
Pd-103	40 mCi	0.03 mSv/hr (3 mrem/hr)
I-131	33 mCi	0.07 mSv/hr (7 mrem/hr)

Isotope	Activity at or below pts may be released <u>without</u> instructions	Dose rate at 1 meter at or below which pts may be released <u>without</u> instructions
I-125	2 mCi	0.002 mSv/hr (0.2 mrem/hr)
Pd-103	8 mCi	0.007 mSv/hr (0.7 mrem/hr)

Release criteria can be based on either of these measures. For patients who exceed these levels, they can still be released with instructions if a calculation can be provided which proves no member of family or general public could receive more than 5 mSv (0.5 rem) as a result of exposure from the patient, or that lead shielding is provided (e.g., lead cap for brain patients) to reduced the dose rate level at 1 meter.

ANNUAL DOSE LIMITS

Occupational effective dose equivalent (EDE) for whole body	50 mSv (5 rem)/yr
Occupational EDE for lens of eye	150 mSV (15 rem)/yr
Occupational EDE for skin, hands, feet	500 mSv (50 rem)/yr
Occupational EDE for declared pregnant workers (fetus)	0.5 mSv (0.05 rem)/mo
General public EDE, frequent/continuous exposure	1 mSv (0.1 rem)/yr
General public EDE, infrequent exposure	5 mSv (0.5 rem)/yr

Note: 1 rem = 0.01 Sv.

LD-50 is defined as the dose of any agent or material that causes a mortality of 50% in the experimental group. For acute whole body human radiation exposure, the LD-50 in 30–60 days is ~3–4 Gy without medical intervention. The hematopoietic syndrome results from exposure of 3–8 Gy. With appropriate nursing care, antibiotics, &/or transfusions some patients may be saved. Bone marrow transplants are useful after whole-body exposure of 8–10 Gy. The gastrointestinal syndrome results from 5–12 Gy with death in 3–10 days. The cerebrovascular syndrome results from ~100 Gy exposure with death in ~1–3 days

Background radiation in the San Francisco Bay Area is in the range 2–2.5 mSv per year. Dose equivalent flying from San Francisco to New York round trip is <0.06 mSv

D: TUMOR MARKERS, IMMUNOPHENOTYPING, AND CYTOGENETICS

Tumor Marker	Primary Tumor	Other Tumors	Benign Conditions
AFP	Hepatocellular carcinoma, non-seminomatous germ cell tumors (yolk sac tumorsand embryonal cell carcinoma)	Gastric, biliary, and pancreatic	Cirrhosis, viral hepatitis, pregnancy
β-2 microglobulin	Multiple myeloma	Other B cell neoplasms, lung, hepatoma, breast	Ankylosing spondylitis, Reiters syndrome
CA125	Ovarian	Endometrial, fallopian tube, breast, lung, esophageal, gastric, hepatic, and pancreatic	Menstruation, pregnancy, fibroids, ovarian cysts, pelvic inflammation, cirrhosis, ascites, pleural and pericardial effusions, endometriosis
CA15-3	Breast	Ovary, lung, prostate	Benign breast or ovarian disease, endometriosis, pelvic inflammatory disease, hepatitis, pregnancy, lactation

Tumor Marker	Primary Tumor	Other Tumors	Benign Conditions
CA19-9	Pancreatic, biliary tract	Colon, esophageal, hepatic	Pancreatitis, biliary disease, cirrhosis
CA27.29	Breast	Colon, gastric, hepatic, lung, pancreatic, ovarian, prostate	Breast, liver, & kidney disorders, ovarian cysts
Calcitonin	Medullary thyroid	Metastatic breast, lung, pancreas, hepatoma, renal cell, carcinoid	Zollinger-Ellison syndrome, pernicious anemia, chronic renal failure, cirrhosis, Paget's disease, pregnancy, benign breast or ovarian disease
CEA	Colorectal	Breast, lung, gastric, pancreatic, bladder, medullary thyroid, head and neck, cervical, hepatic, lymphoma, melanoma	Cigarette smoking, peptic ulcer disease, inflammatory bowel disease, pancreatitis, hypothyroidism, cirrhosis, biliary obstruction
Gamma globulin	Multiple myeloma, macroglobulinemia	Leukemia	Chronic infections, hepatic disease, autoimmune diseases, collagen diseases
Neuron-specific enolase	Neuroblastoma, small cell lung cancer	Wilms' tumor, melanoma, thyroid, kidney, testicle, pancreas	

Tumor Marker	Primary Tumor	Other Tumors	Benign Conditions
Prostatic acid phosphatase	Prostate	Testicular, leukemia, non-Hodgkin's lymphoma	Paget's disease, osteoporsis, cirrhosis, pulmonary embolism, hyperparathyroidism
PSA	Prostate	None	Prostatitis, BPH, prostate trauma, after ejaculation
Thyroglobulin	Differentiated thyroid cancer (not medullary)		Hyperthyroidism, subacute thyroiditis, benign adenoma
β-HCG	Non-seminomatous germ cell tumors (embryonal cell carcinoma, choriocarcinoma), gestational trophoblastic disease	Rarely, gastrointestinal tumors, seminoma (occasional minimal)	Hypogonadal states, marijuana use

IMMUNOPHENOTYPING

- All lymphoid cells = CD45+
- B-cells = CD19+, CD20+, CD22+
- T-cells = CD2+, CD3+, CD5+, CD7+. CD4+ = helper cells, CD8+ = cytotoxic cells
- Natural-killer cells = CD16+, CD56+, CD57+
- Follicular cell lymphoma = CD5−, CD10+, CD43−
- Mantle cell lymphoma = CD5+, CD23−, CD43+
- MALT lymphoma = CD5−, CD10−, CD23−
- Hodgkin's disease = CD15+, CD30+

CYTOGENETICS

- t(2:13) and t(1:13) = Alveolar rhabdomyosarcoma
- t(8:14) and t(8:22) = Burkitt's lymphoma and B-cell ALL (c-myc gene)
- t(11:14) = Mantle cell lymphoma (bcl-1 gene, cyclin D1 over expression)

- t(11:22) = Ewing's sarcoma & PPNET
- t(12:22) = Clear cell sarcoma
- t(14:18) = Follicular lymphoma and diffuse large B-cell lymphoma (BCL-2 gene)
- t(14:19) = Chronic lymphocytic leukemia (BCL-3 gene)
- t(X:18) = Synovial cell sarcoma

E: COMMONLY PRESCRIBED DRUGS

SKIN

Name	Use	Dose	Comments
Aquaphor (OTC)	Dry desquamation	Apply bid–tid	Original ointment (14 oz jar) or Healing ointment (1.75 oz tube or 3.5 oz jar)
Eucerin (OTC)	Dry desquamation	Apply prn	Lotion 4–16 oz, Cream 2–16 oz
Hydrocortisone (OTC)	Dry desquamation	Apply qid	0.5–1%
Dermoplast (OTC) topical anesthetic	Dry desquamation	Apply tid	Spray (2 and 2.75 oz) or lotion (3 oz)
Desonide (Tridesilon)	Dry-moist desquamation	Apply bid–tid	0.05% cream
Domeboro soaks (OTC)	Moist desquamation	Moist soak 20 min tid–qid	Dissolve 1 tablet or packet in 1 pint water
Aquaphor/ Xylocaine 5% ointment	Moist desquamation	Apply tid	Pharmacist mix 1:1
Neosporin (neomycin, polymixin B, bacitracin; OTC)	Moist desquamation	Apply bid–qid	Cream (7.5 g)
Bacitracin	Moist desquamation	Apply bid–tid	Ointment (30 g)

Note: Drug selection, method and duration of administration, and dosage should be verified by the reader with the most current product information provided by the manufacturer.

Name	Use	Dose	Comments
Silvadene creme 1%	Moist desquamation	Apply tid	Tube (20 or 85 g) or jar (50, 400, & 1000 g)
Telfa (OTC non-adhesive pads)	Moist desquamation	Apply prn	
Hydrogel wound dressings (e.g., Vigilon, Radicare, Geliperm)	Moist desquamation	Apply prn	
Pentoxifylline (Trental)	Ulceration	400 mg po tid	Avoid if recent cerebral bleed or retinal hemorrhage. If GI or CNS side effects, decrease to 400 mg bid; if they persist, discontinue
Ketoconazole 2%	Yeast infection	Apply bid	15, 30, or 60 g
Fluconazole	Yeast infection	200 mg po × 1, then 100 mg po qd × 14 d	
Acyclovir	Herpes	200 mg po 5x/d × 10 d for herpes infections. For zoster, 800 mg po 5x/d × 7–10 d	
Valacyclovir	Herpes	500 mg po bid × 3 d (recurrent)	
Diphenhydramine (Benadryl; OTC)	Pruritis	25–50 mg po q 6 h	

Note: Drug selection, method and duration of administration, and dosage should be verified by the reader with the most current product information provided by the manufacturer.

Name	Use	Dose	Comments
Hydroxyzine (Vistaril)	Pruritis	25 mg po tid–qid	

HEAD AND NECK

Name	Use	Dose	Comments
Cortisporin ophthalmic	Conjunctivitis or keratitis	Apply ointment or 1–2 gtts suspension q 3–4 hrs	Contraindicated for viral infections or ulcerative keratitis & after foreign body removal. Do not use for more than 5–10 d. Caution if glaucoma
Lacrilube (OTC)	Dry eye	Apply qhs	
Saline solutions (OTC)	Dry eye	Apply prn	
Proparacaine hydrochloride 5%	Topical anesthetic for conjunctiva	2 gtts	Use care when manipulating eye because abrasions will not be felt
Auralgan (benzocaine/ antipyrine otic)	Otic analgesic	2–4 gtt OTIC qid prn	Contraindicated if perforated TM
Cortisporin otic suspension	External otitis	4 gtts OTIC q 6h × 7–10 d	
Diphenhydramine (Benadryl; OTC)	Antihistamine, sedating	25–50 mg po q 4–6 h	
Loratadine (OTC; Claritin)	Antihistamine, non-sedating	10 mg po qd	
Pseudoephedrine (OTC)	Decongestant	30–60 mg po q 4–6 h prn	Max 240 mg/d

Note: Drug selection, method and duration of administration, and dosage should be verified by the reader with the most current product information provided by the manufacturer.

Name	Use	Dose	Comments
Dextromethorphan/ Guaifenesin	Antitussive/ Expectorant	1–2 tab po bid or 10 ml po q 4 h	Tabs 30/600 or solution 10/100/5 ml. Max 4 tab/d or 60 ml/d
Ibuprofen (OTC)	Parotitis	600 mg po tid	Should resolve rapidly after first several treatments
Ulcerease (OTC)	Apthous ulcers, mucositis	Rinse or gargle prn. Do not swallow	6 oz bottle
"Triple mix" or "Pink Passion" (Benadryl elixir, Maalox, viscous lidocaine 2%)	Mucositis	2 tsp po 10 min ac &qhs. Swish& spit prn	Pharmacist mix 1 : 1 : 1 in 600 ml bottle. Swallow no more than 8 tsp/d
Sucralfate	Mucositis	2 tsp swish & swallow qid	Suspension 1 g/ 10 cc. Do not use within 30 min of lidocaine (interferes with binding)
Fluconazole	Candidiasis	200 mg po × 1, then 100 mg po qd × 14 d	
Nystatin suspension	Candidiasis	10 cc swish & swallow qid	Continue 2 d post symptom resolution
Amifostine (Ethylol)	Xerostomia	200 mg/m^2 IV qd over 3 min, 15–30 min before RT	Monitor BP
Artificial saliva (OTC)	Xerostomia	Apply prn	e.g., Salivart, Xerolube, Saliva substitute

Note: Drug selection, method and duration of administration, and dosage should be verified by the reader with the most current product information provided by the manufacturer.

Name	Use	Dose	Comments
Baking soda mouthwash (OTC)	Xerostomia	1–3 tsp swish & spit prn	Mix 1 tsp baking soda, 1 tsp salt, 1 quart water
Flouride carriers	Xerostomia		Arrange via dental consultation
Pilocarpine (Salagen)	Xerostomia	5–10 mg po tid	Requires some salivary function. Max 30 mg/d. Caution if asthma, glaucoma, liver dysfunction, cardiovascular disease, COPD
Cevimeline (Evoxac)	Xerostomia	30 mg po tid	Max: 90 mg/d. Similar cautions as Pilocarpine

LUNG

Name	Use	Dose	Comments
Albuterol	Asthma	2 puffs q 4 h prn	
Dextromethorphan/ guaifenesin (OTC)	Antitussive/ expectorant	1–2 tab po bid or 10 ml po q 4 h	Tabs 30/600 or solution 10/100/5 ml. Max 4 tab/d or 60 ml/d
Benzonatate (Tessalon Perles)	Cough	100–200 mg po tid	Max 600 mg/d
Tylenol with codeine (300/30)	Cough	1–2 tabs po q 4 h prn	Max 12 tabs/d
Ibuprofen (OTC)	Mild radiation pneumonitis	600–800 mg po q 6–8 h	
Prednisone	Radiation pneumonitis	1 mg/kg at diagnosis with slow taper over weeks	

Note: Drug selection, method and duration of administration, and dosage should be verified by the reader with the most current product information provided by the manufacturer.

Name	Use	Dose	Comments
Beclomethasone	Radiation pneumonitis	2 puffs qid or 4 puffs bid	May help reduce systemic steroid dose
Methylprednisolone (Solu-Medrol)	Status asthmaticus	0.5–1 mg/kg IV q 6 h	Start 2 mg/kg

BREAST

Name	Use	Dose	Comments
Tamoxifen (Nolvadex)	Breast cancer	10 mg po bid or 20 mg qd	Binds to estrogen receptors, producing estrogenic & anti-estrogenic effects
Raloxifene (Evista)	Breast cancer	60 mg po qd	Selective estrogen receptor modulator
Anastrozole (Arimidex)	Breast cancer, postmenopausal	1 mg po qd	Aromatase inhibitor, non-steroidal
Letrozole (Femara)	Breast cancer, postmenopausal	2.5 mg po qd	Aromatase inhibitor, non-steroidal
Exemestane (Aromasin)	Breast cancer, postmenopausal	25 mg po qd	Aromatase inhibitor, steroidal
Fulvestrant (Faslodex)	Breast cancer, Metastatic	250 mg IM q mo	Binds to estrogen receptors (ER), down-regulates ER protein, producing anti-estrogenic effects
Megestrol (Megace)	Breast cancer, palliative	40 mg po qid	Progestin

Note: Drug selection, method and duration of administration, and dosage should be verified by the reader with the most current product information provided by the manufacturer.

Name	Use	Dose	Comments
Clonidine	Hot flashes	0.1 mg po bid	Anti-hypertensive, watch for rebound hypertension
Venlafaxine (Effexor)	Hot flashes	50–75 mg po qhs	
Paroxetine (Paxil)	Hot flashes	20 mg po qd	

GASTROINTESTINAL

Name	Use	Dose	Comments
Triple mix (Benadryl elixir, Maalox, viscous lidocaine 2%)	Esophagitis	2 tsp po 10 min ac & qhs. Swish & spit prn	Pharmacist mix 1:1:1 in 600 ml bottle. Swallow no more than 8 tsp/d
Miracle Mouthwash	Esophagitis	Mix 60 cc tetracycline oral suspension (125 mg/5 cc), 30 cc mycostatin oral suspension (100,000 u/cc), 30 cc hydrocortisone oral suspension (10 mg/5 cc), and 240 cc benadryl solution (12.5 mg/5 cc)	
Sucralfate	Esophagitis	2 tsp swish & swallow qid	Suspension 1 g/10 cc. Do not use within 30 min of lidocaine (interferes with binding)
Fluconazole	Candidiasis	200 mg po × 1, then 100 mg po qd × 14 d	

Note: Drug selection, method and duration of administration, and dosage should be verified by the reader with the most current product information provided by the manufacturer.

Name	Use	Dose	Comments
Mylanta (aluminum, magnesium, & simethicone; OTC)	Dyspepsia, flatulence	15–30 ml po qid prn	200/200/20 per 5 ml susp (1 bottle = 355 or 710 ml)
Famotidine (Pepcid; OTC)	GERD	20 mg po bid	
Omeprazole (Prilosec; OTC)	GERD	20–40 mg po qd	
Amitriptyline	Appetite stimulant	10–25 mg po qhs to q 8 h	
Megestrol (Megace) suspension	Appetite stimulant	400–800 mg po qd	
Dronabinol (Marinol)	Appetite stimulant	2.5 mg po bid	
Chlorpromazine (Thorazine)	Hiccups	25–50 mg po tid–qid	
Metoclopramide (Reglan)	Gastroparesis N/V	10 mg po qac, qhs 5–10 mg po/IV q 6–8 h prn	Give 30 min before meals
Prochlorperazine (Compazine)	N/V	5–10 mg po q 6–8 h	
Promethazine (Phenergan)	N/V	12.5–25 mg po/pr/IV q 4–6 h	
Ondansetron (Zofran)	N/V	8 mg po tid	First dose 1–2 h before RT
Lorazepam (Ativan)	N/V	Anticipitory: 1–2 mg po 45 min before treatment. Adjunct: 0.5–1 mg po tid	
Simethicone	Flatulence	80–120 mg po qac & qhs	Max 480 mg/d. Chew tabs before swallowing

Note: Drug selection, method and duration of administration, and dosage should be verified by the reader with the most current product information provided by the manufacturer.

Name	Use	Dose	Comments
Loperamide (Imodium; OTC)	Diarrhea	4 mg × 1, then 2 mg po after each unformed stool	Max 16 mg/d
Atropine/ diphenoxylate (Lomotil)	Diarrhea	1–2 tabs po tid–qid prnv	Max 8 tabs/d
Bismuth subsalicylate (Pepto-Bismol; OTC)	Diarrhea	2 tab po q 1 h prn	Max 4200 mg/d
Metamucil	Constipation	1–3 tsp in juice qd with meals	Bulking agent
Colace	Constipation	100 mg po bid	Stool softener
Bisacodyl (Dulcolax)	Constipation	10 mg po or pr	Laxative
Senna	Constipation	2–4 tabs po qd–bid	Stool softener and laxative
Fleet Enema	Constipation	1–2 as directed pr prn	
Anusol HC (Hydrocortisone)	Perianal pain / Proctitis	1–2.5%, apply qid / 25 mg supp pr bid–tid	
Hydrocortisone enema	Proctitis	1 prn qhs, retain for 1 h	
Proctofoam HC 2.5%	Proctitis	Apply prn tid–qid	

GENITOURINARY

Name	Use	Dose	Comments
Phenazopyridine (Pyridium)	Dysuria	200 mg po tid–qid	Urine turns orange
Tolterodine (Detrol)	Bladder spasm	2 mg po bid	Anticholinergic
Flavoxate (Urispas)	Bladder spasm	100–200 mg po tid–qid	Anticholinergic
Oxybutynin (Ditropan)	Bladder spasm	5 mg po bid–tid	Anticholinergic

Note: Drug selection, method and duration of administration, and dosage should be verified by the reader with the most current product information provided by the manufacturer.

Name	Use	Dose	Comments
Finasteride (Proscar)	BPH	5 mg po qd	Type-2 alpha reductase inhibitor
Dutasteride (Avodart)	BPH	0.5 mg po qd	Type-1 & -2 alpha reductase inhibitor
Doxazocin (Cardura)	Bladder outlet obstruction	1–8 mg po qd (start 1)	Alpha-1 blocker
Terazosin (Hytrin)	Bladder outlet obstruction	1–10 mg po qhs (start 1)	Alpha-1 blocker
Tamsulosin (Flomax)	Bladder outlet obstruction	0.4–0.8 mg po qd	Selective alpha-1a blocker
Alfuzosin (Uroxatral)	Bladder outlet obstruction	10 mg po qd	Selective alpha-1a blocker
Trimethoprim/ sulfamethoxazole	Urinary tract infection	1 DS tab po bid × 5–7 d	
Ciprofloxacin	Urinary tract infection	250 mg po bid × 3–7 d	
Sildenafil (Viagra)	Erectile dysfunction	25–50 mg po × 1	Max 100 mg. Contraindicated with nitrates. Caution if HTN, cardiovascular disease
Tadalafil (Cialis)	Erectile dysfunction	10 mg po × 1	Lasts up to 36 h, max 20 mg. Contraindicated with nitrates, alpha-blockers. Caution if HTN, cardiovascular disease

Note: Drug selection, method and duration of administration, and dosage should be verified by the reader with the most current product information provided by the manufacturer.

Name	Use	Dose	Comments
Vardenafil (Levitra)	Erectile dysfunction	5–10 mg po × 1	Max 20 mg. Contraindicated with nitrates, alpha-blockers. Caution if HTN, cardiovascular disease
Bicalutamide (Casodex)	Prostate cancer	50 mg po qd	Antiandrogen. Monitor LFTs at baseline, every mo × 4.
Flutamide (Eulixen)	Prostate cancer	250 mg po q 8 h	Antiandrogen. Monitor LFTs every mo × 4.
Leuprolide (Lupron)	Prostate cancer	Depot (1 mo = 7.5 mg, 3 mo = 22.5 mg, 4 mo = 30 mg)	Gonadotropin-releasing hormone analogue, inhibits gonadotropin release
Goserelin (Zoladex)	Prostate cancer	Depot (1 mo = 3.6 mg, 3 mo = 10.8 mg)	Gonadotropin-releasing hormone analogue, inhibits gonadotropin release
Pentoxifylline (Trental)	Chronic hematuria or radiation cystitis	400 mg po tid	Avoid if recent cerebral bleed or retinal hemorrhage. If GI or CNS side effects, decrease to 400 mg bid; if they persist, discontinue
Vitamin E (tocopherol)	Chronic hematuria or radiation cystitis	1000 IU po qd	

Note: Drug selection, method and duration of administration, and dosage should be verified by the reader with the most current product information provided by the manufacturer.

GYNECOLOGIC

Name	Use	Dose	Comments
Replens vaginal moisturizer (OTC)	Vaginitis	One applicator full q 2–3 d prn	
Premarin vaginal cream	Atrophic vaginitis	1/2–2 g PV 1–3x/wk	Conjugated estrogens
Metronidazole	Bacterial vaginitis	500 mg po bid × 7 d	
Fluconazole	Candidiasis	150 mg po × 1; if refractory, 100 mg po qd × 14 d	
Miconazole	Candidiasis	1 supp qhs × 3 or cream qhs × 7 d	

NERVOUS SYSTEM

Name	Use	Dose	Comments
Dexamethasone (Decadron)	Brain or tumor edema	RT induced: 2–6 mg po q 8 h; tumor induced: 16–25 mg IV × 1, then 4–10 mg po/IV q 6 h; impending herniation: 100 mg IV × 1, then 25 mg IV q 6 h	
Meclizine	Vertigo	25–50 mg po qd	
Scopolamine patch	Vertigo	Apply behind ear, 1 patch q 3 d	
Phenytoin (Dilantin)	Seizure	300–400 mg po div qd–tid	Monitor therapeutic levels
Carbamazepine (Tegretol)	Seizure / Trigeminal neuralgia	800–1200 mg po div bid–qid. Start 200 mg bid. 200–400 mg po bid	Monitor therapeutic levels
Phenobarbital	Seizure	60 mg po bid–tid	Monitor therapeutic levels
Gabapentin (Neurontin)	Seizure, neuropathic pain	300–1200 mg po tid Start 300 mg qd	

Note: Drug selection, method and duration of administration, and dosage should be verified by the reader with the most current product information provided by the manufacturer.

PSYCHIATRIC

Name	Use	Dose	Comments
Lorazepam (Ativan)	Anxiety	0.5–2 mg po/IV q 6–8 h prn	
Haldol (Haloperidol)	Agitation, psychosis	0.5–5 mg po/IM q 1–4 h	
Temazepam (Restoril)	Insomnia	7.5–30 mg po qhs	Short-term treatment
Ambien (Zolpidem)	Insomnia	5–10 mg po qhs	Short-term treatment

PAIN

Name	Use	Dose	Comments
Acetominophen (OTC)	Mild-mod	325–1000 mg po q 4–6 h prn	Max 1 g/dose, 4 g/d
Aspirin (OTC)	Mild-mod	325–650 mg po q 4 h prn	Max 4 g/d
Ibuprofen (Motrin; OTC)	Mild-mod	200–800 mg po q 4–6 h prn	Max 3200 mg/d
Naproxen (Naprosyn)	Mild-mod	250–500 mg po bid	Max 1500 mg/d
Celecoxib (Celebrex)	Mild-mod	200 mg po qd	
Codeine	Mild-mod	15–60 mg po qd	Max 60 mg/dose, 360 mg/d
Acetaminophen/ codeine (Tylenol #2,#3, #4)	Mild-mod	1–2 tabs po q 4–6 h prn	300 mg/15, 30, or 60 mg
Hydrocodone/ acetaminophen (Vicodin, Lortab elixir)	Mod-severe	1–2 tabs po q 4–6 h prn 5–15 ml po q 4–6 h prn	5/500 mg or ES 7.5/750 mg 7.5/500 mg per 15 ml
Oxycodone	Mod-severe	5–30 mg po q 4 h prn	5, 15, 30 mg tabs

Note: Drug selection, method and duration of administration, and dosage should be verified by the reader with the most current product information provided by the manufacturer.

Name	Use	Dose	Comments
Oxycodone/ acetaminophen (Percocet)	Mod-severe	1–2 tabs po q 4–6 h prn	2.5/325, 5/325, 7.5/325, 10/325, 7.5/500, or 10/650 mg
Oxycontin	Mod-severe	10–160 mg po bid prn	10, 20, 40, 80 mg tabs. Start 10 mg bid
Morphine	Mod-severe	10–30 mg po q 3–4 h prn 2.5–10 mg IV q 2–6 h prn	10, 15, 30 mg tabs
MS contin	Mod-severe	15–30 mg po q 8–12 h prn	15, 30, 60, 100, 200 mg tabs
Morphine elixir (Roxanol)	Mod-severe	10–30 mg po q 4 h	20 mg/ml solution
Fentanyl transdermal (Duragesic)	Mod-severe	25–100 mcg/h patch q 72 h	For opiate tolerant pts. Start 25 mcg
Fentanyl oral transmucosal (Actiq)	Mod-severe	1 unit po prn	For opiate toleratnt pts. Start 200 mcg, titrate up to 1600 mcg. Dissolve in mouth, do not chew or swallow
Cyclobenzaprine (Flexeril)	Muscle spasm	5–10 mg po tid	Therapy should be limited to 3 wks maximum
Pamidronate (Aredia)	Bone mets	90 mg IV q 3–4 wks	Monitor renal function. Dental exam prior to treatment
Zolendronic acid (Zometa)	Bone mets	4 mg IV q 3–4 wks	Monitor renal function. Dental exam prior to treatment

Note: Drug selection, method and duration of administration, and dosage should be verified by the reader with the most current product information provided by the manufacturer.

MISCELLANEOUS

Name	Use	Dose	Comments
Epinephrine	Anaphylaxis	0.1–0.5 mg SC (1 : 1000) q 10–15 min or 0.1–0.25 mg IV (1 : 10,000) over 5–10 min	For urticaria, give benadryl 25–50 mg. For hypotension, add IV fluids, elevate legs, and add O2. May need atropine 0.6 mg IV push (repeat up to 3 mg total)
Diphenhydramine (Benadryl)	Anaphylaxis	25–50 mg po/IV q 6–8 h	Max 100 mg/dose, 400 mg/d

Note: Drug selection, method and duration of administration, and dosage should be verified by the reader with the most current product information provided by the manufacturer.

Index